F. H. Stefani   G. Hasenfratz

Macroscopic Ocular Pathology

An Atlas Including Correlations with Standardized Echography

With 320 Figures, Mostly in Color

Springer-Verlag
Berlin Heidelberg New York
London Paris Tokyo

Professor Dr. med. FRITZ H. STEFANI

Dr. GERHARD HASENFRATZ

Augenklinik der Universität,
Mathildenstr. 6,
D-8000 München 2

Gedruckt mit Unterstützung des Förderungs- und Beihilfefonds Wissenschaft der VG Wort

ISBN-13: 978-3-642-71798-7 e-ISBN-13: 978-3-642-71796-3
DOI: 10.1007/978-3-642-71796-3

Library of Congress Cataloging-in-Publication Data
Stefani, F.H. (Fritz H.), 1941– Macroscopic ocular pathology.
Bibliography: p. Includes index.
1. Eye – Diseases and defects – Atlases. I. Hasenfratz, G. (Gerhard) II. Title. [DNLM: 1. Eye Disease – pathology – atlases. 2. Ultrasonic Diagnosis – atlases. WW 17 S816m]
RE71.S68 1987 617.7′1 87-9505

Softcover reprint of the hardcover 1st edition 1987

2122/3130-543210

Preface I

Today, ophthalmic pathology deals more and more with pathogenesis using highly sophisticated techniques. In recent decades, it has expanded to such an extent that it now fills several volumes of a modern comprehensive atlas or textbook. Black and white prints of the macroscopic appearance of dissected eyes are standard in modern textbooks. Color photographs, although providing more visual information and a better insight into the sometimes complex disease processes of the eye, are however costly. Nevertheless, many ophthalmologic colleagues expressed their desire to have me prepare such an atlas. It is not intended to replace one of the textbooks in this field but rather to supplement existing texts and to stimulate clinical and diagnostic thinking. Hence it should be used in conjunction with textbooks on anatomy and ocular pathology. The reader will find references on the different subjects in the excellent modern textbooks listed below.

Diagnosis and treatment in ophthalmology is to a great extent based on morphologic examination. Clinical ophthalmologists have available such excellent tools as the slit-lamp, the gonioscope, and the ophthalmoscope to study and document ocular disease in vivo under high magnification. Both external eye structures and transparent ocular structures can be observed better in vivo than in the pathology laboratory. Therefore the pathology of these is only presented in conditions in which direct visualization is normally difficult. There are also regions within the eye itself which cannot easily be observed either directly or with a wide angle lens or the view of which is obscured by a range of opacities. My objective was not to cover every known pathologic condition but to include illustrations which may contribute to the understanding of clinical findings. Moreover, students, registrars, clinicians, and practitioners may need the macroscopic image of a diseased organ to correlate the technical findings of ultrasonography, CT scanning, or scintigraphy with clinical conditions. Anatomy, pathophysiology, clinical signs and symptoms, as well as the macroscopic pathology of the lids, skin, conjunctiva, and orbit are not included. For these subjects the reader should refer to the special textbooks of ophthalmology and/or dermatology.

The first chapter aims to familiarize the observer with artifacts, so that he or she is easily able to differentiate these from the relevant information. The subsequent chapters deal with the various ocular structures in sequence and address mainly malformations, inflammatory reactions, degenerative lesions and secondary tissue reactions, glaucoma, ocular trauma (both accidental and surgical), tumors, and so-called pseudotumors. Since intraocular microsurgery has become routine over the past decade, vitreoretinal reactions have attracted more interest and are hence documented in greater detail. Where there was difficulty in determining the appropriate heading for changes involving multiple ocular structures, that of the most affected region is used. Because complex changes are expected in posttraumatic and tumorous conditions, a separate chapter on each of these subjects was introduced. The number of illustrations in each chapter varies according to availability and importance. A given lesion may be illustrated by several photographs to demonstrate either dynamics or different stages of intraocular tissue changes. The actual size of a lesion may be estimated from the thickness of adjacent structures such as the cornea, sclera, or retina and the diameter of the cornea, lens, or optic disc.

All the material has been collected and prepared at the Ophthalmic Pathology Laboratory of the Augenklinik der Universität München. Most of the surgical material has been obtained from the Augenklinik der Universität München, while most of the autopsy material stems from the Institut für Rechtsmedizin der Universität München. As film material Agfachrome 50L professional (35 mm color reversal film for artificial light and long exposure) had been used. Unfortunately, this film is no longer produced because of technical reasons.

Since the author's major responsibilities lie outside ophthalmic pathology, the time he could devote to this field was limited to a few hours a day. This atlas represents his experience over a period of 15 year in the field.

It is hoped that this presentation will be a useful contribution to those interested in ophthalmology and pathology.

Acknowledgements

I wish to express my gratitude to the many colleagues who provided this material. In preparing this atlas, I enjoyed the great interest in the progress of the work shown by my many colleagues. To all of them, especially Prof. O.-E. Lund, I am greatly indebted. I am also grateful to Miss Helgard Kuhlman and Miss Helga Treibs who assisted with the preparation, and to Miss J. Whitney M.D., FRACS, FRACO (Australia) and Mr. J. Switzer, M.D. (U.S.A.) who served as English editorial consultants. I especially owe a deep debt to my wife and children who have seen so little of me for such a long time.

Munich, Summer 1987 FRITZ H. STEFANI

Preface II

Echography, one of the modern clinical diagnostic methods, has in the past two decades developed into a major diagnostic tool. Sophisticated echographic techniques are increasingly able to deliver exact and reliable in-vivo findings in numerous intraocular and orbital diseases.

Clinical echography, particularly the method of Standardized Echography, with its specific identification of both normal and pathologic ocular and orbital structures, bears a true in-vivo correlationship with macroscopic and even microscopic pathology. Standardized Echography provides information about topography in pathologic conditions and to an extensive degree about morphologic features. Thus it clearly goes beyond a pure imaging diagnostic method.

We felt that certain macroscopic color pictures would be well complimented by accompanying typical echograms. However, I wish to stress that this supplementary chapter cannot replace a standard text to clinical echography. The reader may be aware that clinical echography, particularly the described method of Standardized Echography, requires a detailed knowledge of technique on basic principles of ultrasound. It is beyond the scope of this atlas to give a complete introduction to echography. Thus only a brief introductory summary of Standardized Echography and a comprehensive legend to the echograms is provided. Further details may be found in the suggested reading list.

Munich, Summer 1987 G. Hasenfratz

Contents

Suggested Reading

Textbooks of Ophthalmic Anatomy and Pathology

D.J. Apple, M.F. Raab
Ocular pathology: Clinical applications and self-assessment. 3rd ed.
Mosby, St. Louis: 1985

C. Beard, M.H. Quickert
Anatomy of the orbit. A dissection manual.
Aesculapius, Birmingham (Alabama): 1977

B. Daicker
Anatomie und Pathologie der menschlichen retino-ziliaren Fundusperipherie.
Ein Atlas und Textbuch.
S. Karger, London, New York, Sydney, München, Paris: 1972

W.C. Frayer
Lancaster course in ophthalmic histopathology. Unit 9.
F.A. Davis, Philadelphia: 1981

A. Garner, G.K. Klintworth
Pathobiology of ocular disease. A dynamic approach.
M. Dekker, New York, Basel: 1982

C.H. Greer
Ocular pathology, 3rd ed.
Blackwell Scientific, Oxford, London, Edinburgh, Melbourne: 1979

J.W. Henderson
Orbital tumors. 2nd ed.
B.C. Decker, New York
G. Thieme, Stuttgart, New York: 1980

M.J. Hogan, L.E. Zimmerman
Ophthalmic pathology. An atlas and textbook. 2nd ed.
W.B. Saunders, Philadelphia, London: 1962

F.A. Jakobiec
Ocular and adnexal tumors. Aesculapius, Birmingham (Alabama): 1978

L.T. Jones, M.J. Reh, J.D. Wirtschafter
Ophthalmic anatomy.
AAO Manual, Rochester: 1982

I. Mann
The development of the human eye. 2nd ed.
Brit Med. Ass. 1950

J. Marshall
(Macroanatomy of the eye. In preparation.)

G.O.H. Naumann
Pathologie des Auges.
In: W. Doerr, G. Seifert, E. Uehlinger (eds.)
Spezielle pathologische Anatomie, Vol. 12
Springer, Berlin, Heidelberg, New York: 1980

Standardized Echography and its Techniques

The Method of Standardized Echography

Since the introduction of diagnostic ophthalmic ultrasound in the 1950s, echography has advanced greatly. Today due to experimental and clinical research and the development of technology and examination techniques, there are basically three main echographic methods in use, namely biometric nondiagnostic echography, B-scan echography, and Standardized Echography.

The term Standardized Echography applies to a specific echographic examination method introduced by Ossoinig (in the 1960s) and developed since by himself and coworkers. This is the method used at the University Eye Hospital, Munich.

The method of Standardized Echography is based on the use of a standardized A-scan instrument developed specifically for tissue differentiation. For intraocular and orbital conditions it is complemented by a real-time contact B-scan and, for orbital and periorbital conditions, additionally by Doppler echography. Standardized A-scan instrumentation is characterized by special signal processing through defined parameters such as a narrowband receiver, a special S-shaped type of amplification with a well-defined dynamic range and high-frequency filtering, etc. ("internal standardization"). Besides this "internal" standardization provided by the manufacturers an "external" standardization has to be performed by the examiner. This includes the ascertainment of the "tissue-sensitivity" setting (a sensitivity optimal for tissue diagnosis) for the instrument probe combination used. The setting of this sensitivity level is achieved by using a durable tissue model.

The instruments used at the University Eye Hospital Munich are the 7200 MA A-scan (main frequency: 8 Mhz; Kretz-Technik), the Ocuscan 400 B-scan (10 Mhz; Sonometrics) and the 1010-A dual frequency bi-directional Doppler (4.1/9.6 Mhz; Parks). Documentation of the A- and B-scan echograms is performed with a Polaroid camera and film type 667.

The term Standardized Echography implies not only the use of specifically designed and standardized equipment, but includes standardized techniques for both the A-scan and the B-scan examination of the globe and orbit. This standardization of both the A-scan instrument and the examination procedure yields consistent and repeatable echographic findings in a wide range.

Examination Techniques in Standardized Echography

Although a detailed description of the standardized examination technique is available from the literature, some aspects will be outlined here in order to facilitate the interpretation of the echograms. Though Standardized Echography is equally, or even more, important in the evaluation of the orbital and periorbital lesions, the atlas emphasis the use of Standardized Echography of intraocular lesions.

The evaluation of the globe, orbit, and periorbit requires:

- the basic examination
  aimed at detecting or ruling out intraocular or orbital lesions
- special examinations
  ("quantitative", "topographic", "kinetic" echography) to differentiate, localize, and measure intraocular or orbital lesions
- special techniques
  to measure the thickness of the optic nerve and extraocular muscles, and to differentiate diseases of these structures
- biometry (using an immersion technique) for axial eye length measurement.

Apart from certain maneuvers, all examination steps are performed dynamically thus providing the benefits of "real-time" ultrasonography. In all cases both standardized A-scan and contact B-scan methods are utilized thus providing the advantages of the two methods in the evaluation of specific echographic criteria.

Basic Examination

To detect or rule out pathologic conditions in the globe or orbit, a "basic examination" is performed (Tables 1 and 2).

After the instillation of local anesthetic drops, the A-scan probe is first placed on the conjunctiva adjacent to the limbus at 6:00 with the patient looking away from the probe. Thus the sound beam is aimed through the center of the globe towards the 12:00 meridian.

By shifting the sound probe towards the conjunctival fornix and angling it simultaneously, the posterior section of the globe and the orbital tissue along the 12:00 meridian is examined (Figs. 1 and 2). The globe

Table 1. Standardized Echography

Basic examination of the globe
Three sensitivity settings of the standardized A-scan instrument are used:
T ("tissue-sensitivity" setting / standardized A-scan)
Examination of at least eight meridians Detection of vitreous conditions and gross fundus lesions
T−24 dB ("measuring-sensitivity" setting)
Examination of at least eight meridians Detection of rather flat fundus lesions
T+6 dB (increased "tissue-sensitivity" setting)
Examination of 2/4 meridians Detection of particularly fine and homogeneous vitreous opacities

Table 2. Standardized Echography

Basic examination of the orbit and periorbit
Examination at T ("tissue-sensitivity" setting / standardized A-scan)
Transocular examination (identical to the basic examination of the globe)
Detection of lesions in the central, posterior orbit
Display and detection of lesions of the optic nerve
Display and detection of lesions of the extraocular muscles
Paraocular examination
Detection of lesions in the anterior orbit and periorbit

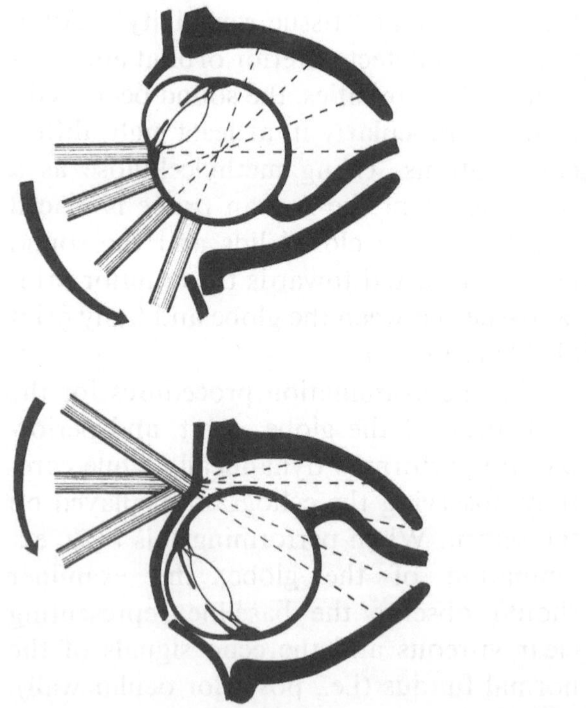

Fig. 1. Schematic illustration of the examination technique. Upper part: Transocular A-scan examination (ocular and orbital evaluation). Lower part: Paraocular A-scan examination (orbital evaluation). (See also Tables 1 and 2.)

and the orbit is likewise examined in at least eight meridians; namely, probe at 6:00 to evaluate the 12:00 meridian, probe at 7:30 to evaluate the 1:30 meridian, etc. To examine the posterior pole including macula, the sound probe is placed adjacent to the nasal limbus and angled sharply towards the posterior pole.

The B-scan probe may be used in a similar fashion to the A-scan examination for topographic evaluation (Fig. 3). However, the large size of the B-scan probe limits its shifting and angling and requires large amounts of methylcellulose as coupling agent. Because of a limited resolution and sensitivity the B-scan is not recommended for performing the basic examination. The B-scan probe may be positioned either for transverse or longitudinal meridional sections.

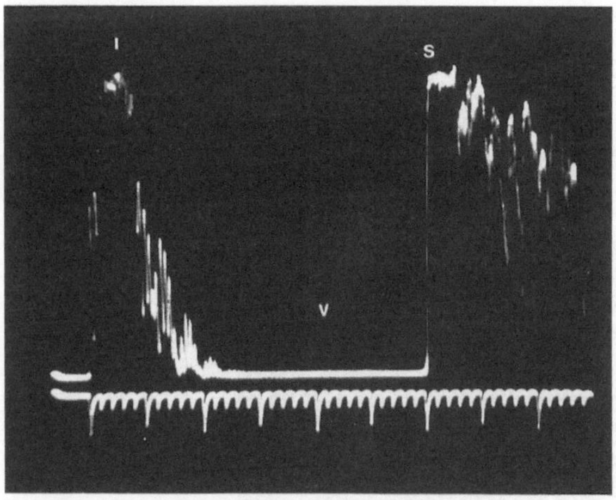

Fig. 2. Standardized A-scan echogram / normal globe. I = initial spike / surface of the globe. V = vitreous. S = sclera.

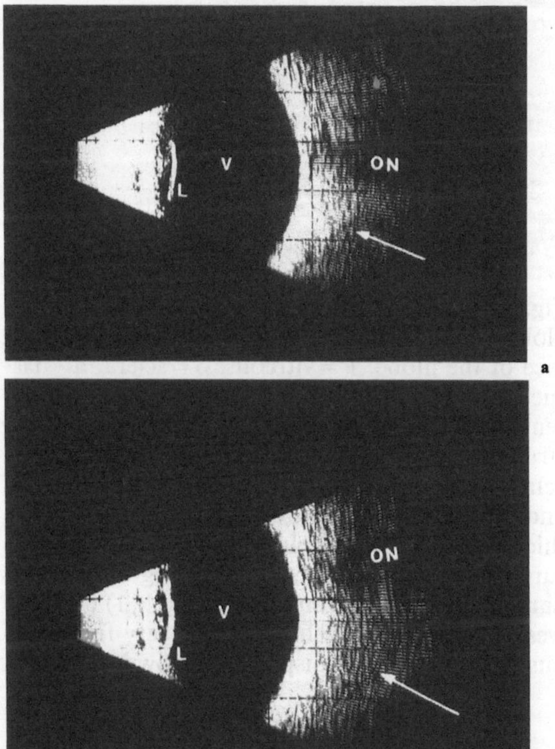

Fig. 3. Contact B-scan echogram / normal globe / normal orbit. Horizontal / vertical axial scans. Horizontal (**a** upper part of the echogram corresponds to the nasal side; lower part of the echogram to the temporal side of the globe) and vertical (**b** top/superior side, bottom/inferior side of the globe) section of a normal globe at the posterior pole. Arrows indicate pattern of normal orbital tissue. (L = posterior surface of the lens; V = vitreous; ON = optic nerve.)

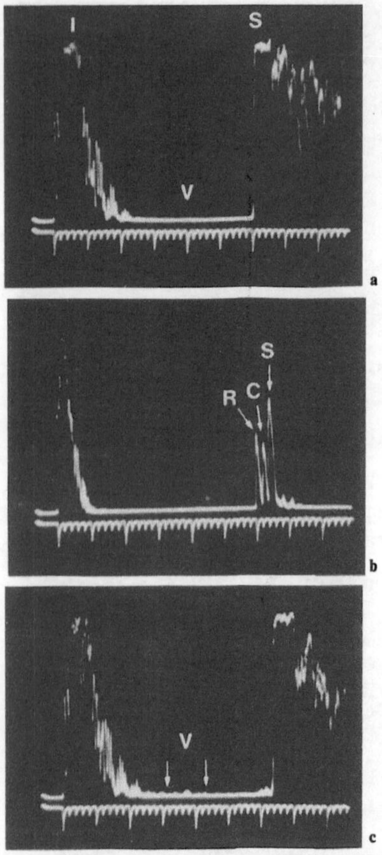

Fig. 4. Standardized A-scan echogram / normal globe / basic examination. *I*=initial spike / surface of the globe. *V*=vitreous. *S*=sclera. **a** "Tissue-sensitivity" setting (see Table 1); **b** Reduced sensitivity setting of the standardized A-scan instrument ("measuring sensitivity"; see Table 1) echo spikes representing retina (*R*), choroid (*C*), and sclera (*S*) can be differentiated. Thus the thickness of the retinochoroid layer can be measured. **c** At a higher sensitivity setting of the standardized A-scan instrument (see Table 1) even the weakest signals (e.g., those due to very fine vitreous opacities) can be displayed (arrows).

During basic examination of the globe, different sensitivity settings of the A-scan instrument are selected, for example, to detect very shallow lesions at the posterior ocular wall or very weak reflecting echo sources in the vitreous (Table 1, Fig. 4). The basic examination of the orbit and periorbit is performed identically but the examination with the standardized A-scan is performed only at "tissue sensitivity". Additionally, to detect anterior orbital and periorbital abnormalities, the sound beam is directed paraocularly in at least eight different positions. Using methylcellulose as a coupling agent the A-scan probe is placed directly on the closed lids and the sound beam is directed towards the anterior orbital tissues between the globe and bony orbit (Table 2, Fig. 1).

All the examination procedures for the evaluation of the globe, orbit, and periorbit, are performed dynamically while carefully observing the echogram displayed on the screen. When performing this basic examination of the globe, the examiner should observe the baseline representing clear vitreous and the echo signals of the normal fundus (i.e., posterior ocular wall). Any change in the normal echo spikes of the posterior ocular wall or the presence of any abnormal spikes or deflections from the baseline indicates pathology. When applying the basic examination to the orbit and periorbit the examiner should look for the appearance of any "defect" in the normally highly reflective orbital pattern. Any such "defect", i.e., a region of more homogeneity or decreased reflectivity, moreover, any increase in the width of the orbital pattern and any echo signal from adjacent sinuses or other periorbital region is indicative of the presence of a lesion.

The basic examination of the orbit is best done with the standardized A-scan at "tissue sensitivity". Adequate evaluation of pathological orbital and periorbital lesions requires a comparison in corresponding sound beam directions in both orbits. For orbital examinations using the A-scan method the horizontal scale on the screen is halved (Fig. 5).

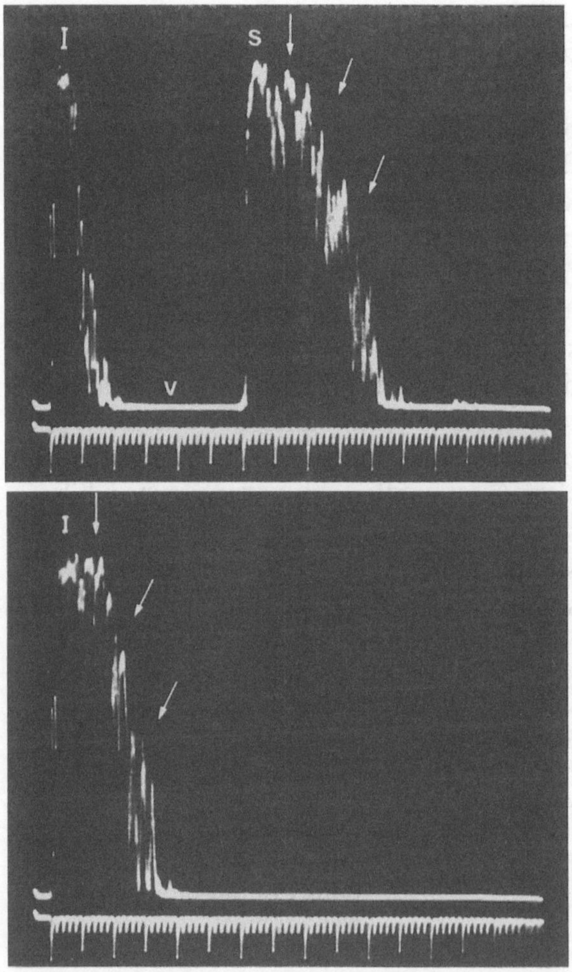

Fig. 5. Standardized A-scan echogram / normal orbit / basic examination. **a** transocular examination: I = initial spike / surface of the globe. V = vitreous. S = sclera. Arrows = orbital pattern. **b** paraocular examination: I = initial echo-signal complex / surface of the lid. Arrows = orbital pattern.

Special Examination Techniques

If the basic examination reveals intraocular or orbital pathology, special examination techniques are used to differentiate, localize, and measure the lesion. A differential diagnosis is reached by a stepwise evaluation of a minimum of nine acoustic criteria using both standardized A- and contact B-scan techniques. These acoustic criteria fall into three categories:

- quantitative echography
- topographic echography
- kinetic echography (Table 3)

Table 3. Standardized Echography

Special examination techniques	Acoustic criteria	Method used
Quantitative Echography	Structure	A-scan
	Reflectivity	A-scan
	Sound attenuation	A-scan / B-scan
Topographic Echography	Borders	A-scan / B-scan
	Shape / Size	B-scan / A-scan
	Location	B-scan / A-scan (globe)
		A-scan / B-scan (orbit, periorbit)
Kinetic Echography	Vascularization	A-scan / Doppler
	Mobility	A-scan / B-scan
	Consistency	A-scan / B-scan

Differential Diagnosis of Intraocular Lesions

A given intraocular lesion is first examined using the technique of topographic echography (Tables 3 and 5), which lies in the domain of the contact B-scan. This technique provides optimal information on both the topographic relationship of pathologic lesions to normal ocular structures (e.g., retinal detachment with insertion of the retina into the optic disc) or to other pathologic lesions (e.g., adhesion of vitreous strands to detached retina) and also on the shape of the lesion (e.g., mushroom-shaped appearance of a malignant melanoma). If the condition is located in the far periphery. i.e., near the ora serrata or the ciliary body, the A-scan method must be applied additionally. For measurements, for example, of an intraocular tumor, the A-scan is always used.

Next, quantitative echography (Tables 3 and 4), which is performed after topographic echography, provides particularly important acoustic criteria for the differential diagnosis. These criteria, internal structure and reflectivity, are determined almost exclusively using the standardized A-scan. Special techniques which compare the reflectivity of abnormal echo signals with known "standard signals", enable differentiation of, for example, vitreous membranes from retina and of intraocular foreign bodies. A- and B-scan techniques determine the sound attenuation within a lesion. In standardized A-scan echograms weak sound attenuation is characterised by a slow pace of decrease of the signals from within a lesion (e.g., malignant melanoma), while in strong sound attenuation a rapid rate of signal decrease is seen. A parameter for sound attenuation is the angle ("angle

Table 4

Standardized Echography Acoustic criteria	Quantitative Echography Classification
Structure	regular – homogeneous – heterogeneous irregular
Reflectivity	extremely high high medium-high medium medium-low low extremely low
Sound attenuation	strong medium weak

Table 5

Standardized Echography Acoustic criteria	Topographic Echography Classification
Borders	diffuse poorly outlined well outlined sharply outlined
Shape	regular irregular description of shape
Size	measurement of elevation (intracular lesion) measurement of width/depth (orbital lesion)
Location	intraocular – meridian – anterior / equatorial / posterior – topographic relation to lens / optic disc / ora ciliary body orbital / periorbital – meridian – anterior / middle / posterior / apex – topographic relation to globe / muscles / muscle-cone / optic nerve / periorbit

kappa") between the baseline and a projected line through the center of a lesion's echo signals. If the sound attenuation is very high due to maximum absorption or to total reflection of the sound beam, the phenomenon of acoustic "shadowing" can be observed, as seen with intraocular foreign bodies, for example.

Kinetic echography (Tables 3 and 6) evaluates the movement of echo signals whether generated spontaneously or after an eye movement on command. Contact B-scan echography will, on requested eye movement, nicely demonstrate an extensive mobility of structures such as freely mobile vitreous membranes or vitreous opacities. But again, standardized A-scan is crucial in determining any more subtle motions of the echo signals. Examples include the fast flickering echo spikes observed in some lesions which occur independent of eye movement and which indicate blood flow (particularly important in the diagnosis of malignant melanomas), or the fine trembling "aftermovements" of vitreous membranes or retina after an eye movement on command (important for differentiating solid from nonsolid intraocular lesions).

Table 6

Standardized Echography Acoustic criteria	Kinetic Echography Classification
Vascularization	distribution intensity artery / vein
Mobility	immobile partly mobile freele mobile
Consistency	solid nonsolid soft firm hard

Differential Diagnosis of Orbital and Periorbital Lesions

Orbital and periorbital abnormalities are evaluated first by means of quantitative echography (Tables 3 and 4). Standardized A-scan is the method of choice in determining the acoustic criteria. Within the normally highly reflective and heterogeneous orbital pattern, the A-scan, at "tissue sensitivity", provides the requisite resolution and sensitivity to determine the reflectivity, the internal structure, and the sound attenuation of an orbital lesion.

Next, using topographic echography (Tables 3 and 5), attention is paid to determining the borders of a given orbital or periorbital lesion. Taking A-scan sections through the lesion trans- and paraocularly, its maximum width and depth is measured. Its relationship to normal orbital structures such as the optic nerve is documented with the contact B-scan.

Kinetic echography (Tables 3 and 6) detects spontaneous motion of the echo signals within a lesion indicating blood flow (A-scan, Doppler sonography) and any pulsation of the whole lesion or the orbital patterns. The mobility of a given lesion is judged during an eye movement on command or for very anterior lesions, during passive movement performed manually by the examiner while the lesion is displayed with the A-scan. By pressing on the globe during transocular examination, the small and easily guidable A-scan sound probe enables determination of the consistency of an orbital lesion. Thus the orbital tissues between globe and bone and a given lesion are compressed taking care to constantly display the lesion. A soft lesion will decrease in size while a hard lesion will remain unchanged.

To display and measure the optic nerve and extraocular muscles, a transocular approach and specific A-scan techniques are used.

Using these examination techniques with optimal instrumentation, the method of Standardized Echography provides abundant information about ocular and orbital pathologic conditions. Thus this method of ophthalmic echography is designed to allow objective judgment of acoustic criteria to yield repeatable and comparable results and, although the examiner's skill and experience plays a role, a wide range of ocular, orbital, and periorbital diseases may be differentiated. This in our opinion is the basis for this very valuable and helpful method of clinical ophthalmic echography.

1. Artifacts

Postmortem autolysis · Preparational tissue changes · Fixational changes

Macroscopical inspection of the globe determines abnormalities in form, size, color, surfaces (elevations or depressions), firmness, texture of cross-sectioned surfaces, and fluids escaping during dissection. Usually the globe with its delicate internal structures is dissected and examined after fixation. The fixative hardens the soft intraocular structures and prevents autolysis as well as tissue drying. Formaldehyde is most commonly used as routine fixative.

Artifacts of enucleated eyes or autopsy eyes may occur as tissue disarrangement, dislocation, shrinkage, discoloration, and mechanical tissue damage. They result from autolysis, fixation, and mechanical forces during dissection. Postmortem changes found in autopsy eyes are retinal folds, distortion of the pigment epithelial layer, liquefaction of the vitreous body, and autolysis of the retina and pigment epithelial layers with pigment dispersal throughout the eye. Mechanical forces at autopsy or enucleation may result in the expression of optic nerve myelin onto the optic disk or retina. Despite the use of a sharp razor blade, dissection of the globe may be another factor causing mechanical tissue deformation. Anterior chamber depth, in particular, cannot be estimated because the thin iris is quite flexible even in the fixed state. Fixatives result in a netting and/or coagulation of tissue protein thus altering tissue consistency. While subretinal fluid in retinal detachment becomes gelatinous and rather soft, for instance, malignant melanomas appear as firm tumors. Formaldehyde fixation also causes a tissue shrinkage averaging 3–4% and usually a whitish-gray opacification of the clear cornea, lens, retina, and other protein-rich structures. Opacification may be reversed by alcohol treatment. In malignant melanomas for instance shrinkage must be considered. Glutaraldehyde fixation preserves clarity but causes a mild yellowish discoloration. Drying of the fixed tissue also leads to changes in color and structure and to tissue shrinkage. Blood vessels collapse in these specimens and are thus not comparable with the in vivo filled state. Decalcification results in marked color change of the tissue. The photographs often show light reflexes and usually no attempt was made to avoid these entirely as they lend a more stereoscopic impression to the illustrations.

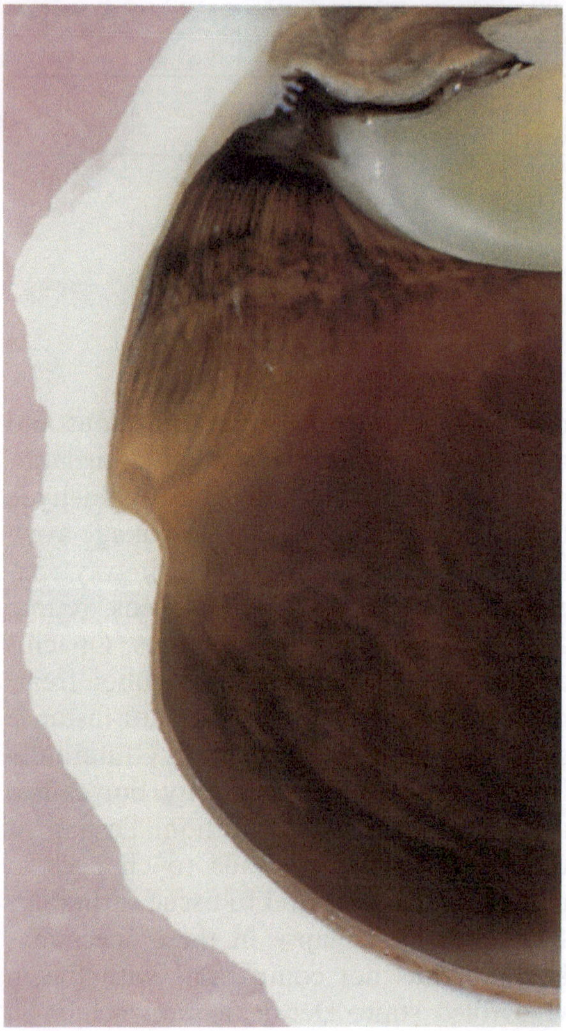

1.1

Postmortem Autolysis

Postmortem autolysis is a progressive self-digestion of cells and tissues of the whole organism. It results from the release of breakdown products (enzymes) of damaged and initially swollen cells into the environment and from bacteria. The first morphological changes begin after a delay of some minutes following the vital defect, as may be shown by electron microscopy. Its rate depends on many factors among which temperature and time are important. Fixatives inactivate cellular enzymes, prevent growth of microorganisms and preserve the structure of cells and tissues.

Scleral Folding

After death the eye loses pressure and becomes increasingly hypotonic. This results in an infolding of the sclera.

Fig. 1.1. The equatorial sclera forms a fold into the soft globe. The pigmented lens nucleus is surrounded by the artifactitious white lens cortex. Formalin-fixed autopsy eye of an adult.

Discoloration

Early postmortem autolysis is accompanied by swelling and opacification of the retina. This opacification is obvious in the unfixed autopsy eye several hours after death and becomes more marked after formalin fixation. All fixatives lead to some discoloration of the intraocular tissues. Formaldehyde results in some loss of color intensity and in a whitish appearance of the transparent ocular structures of the cornea, lens, and retina. The use of nitric acid for decalcification causes a marked opacification and discoloration of the tissues.

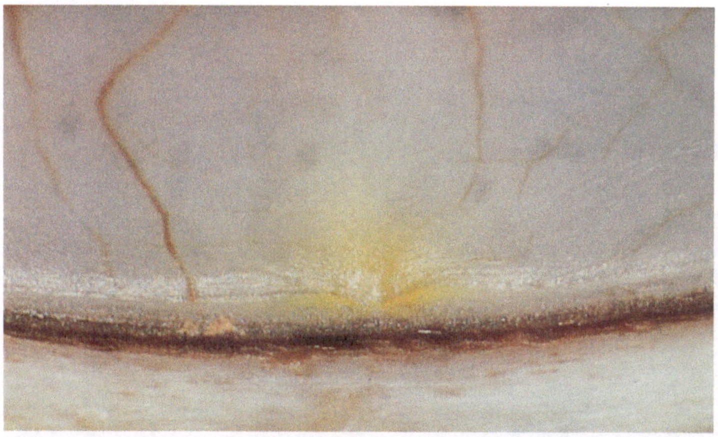
1.2

Fig. 1.2. Bright yellow macula due to retinal xanthophyll deposits contrasted by the formalin-fixed opaque grayish-white adjacent retina. Left of the macula there is some drying of the cut edge of the choroid. M 957/81: 68-year-old female with a malignant melanoma of the ciliary body and iris. Enucleation and formalin-fixed eye.

Retinal Folds

The retinal folds usually seen in autopsy eyes appear fairly early after death.

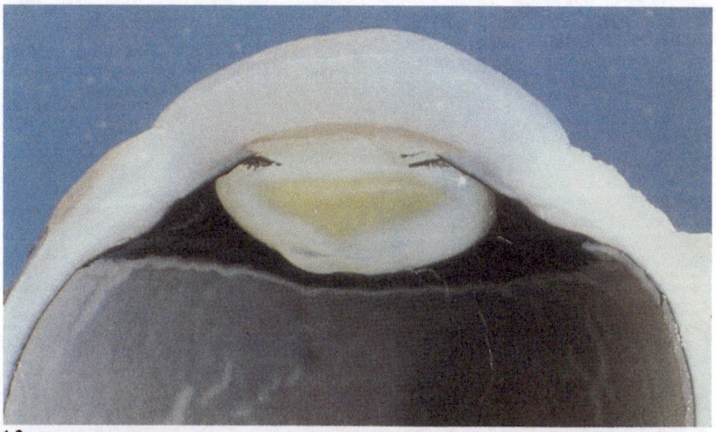
1.3

Fig. 1.3. Postmortem circular retinal fold at the ora serrata (so-called Lange's retinal fold). M 136/80: Formalin-fixed autopsy eye of an infant with congenital corneal opacity.

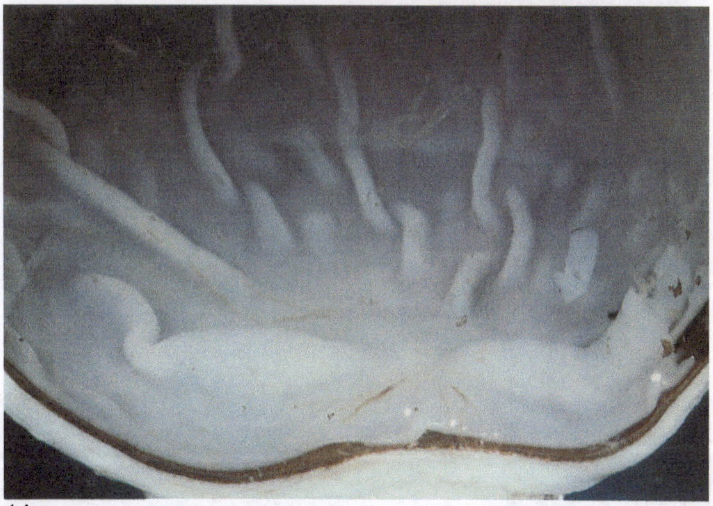
1.4

Fig. 1.4. Postmortem radial retinal folds. At the posterior pole in the macular region, folds appear earlier (see also Fig. 1.5). Formalin-fixed autopsy eye of an elderly person.

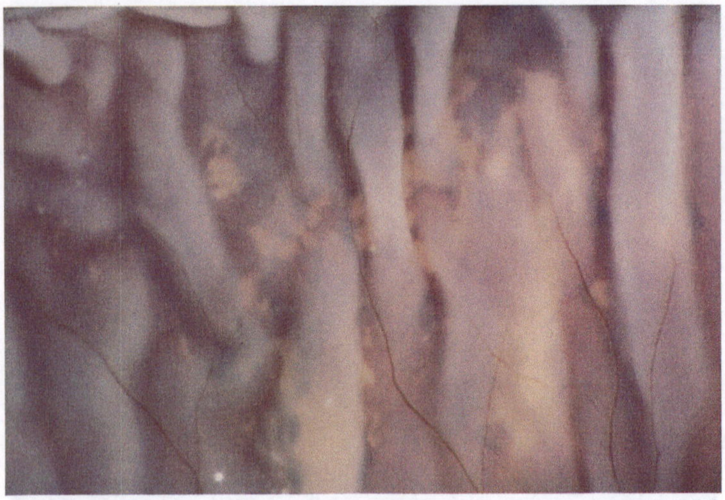
1.5

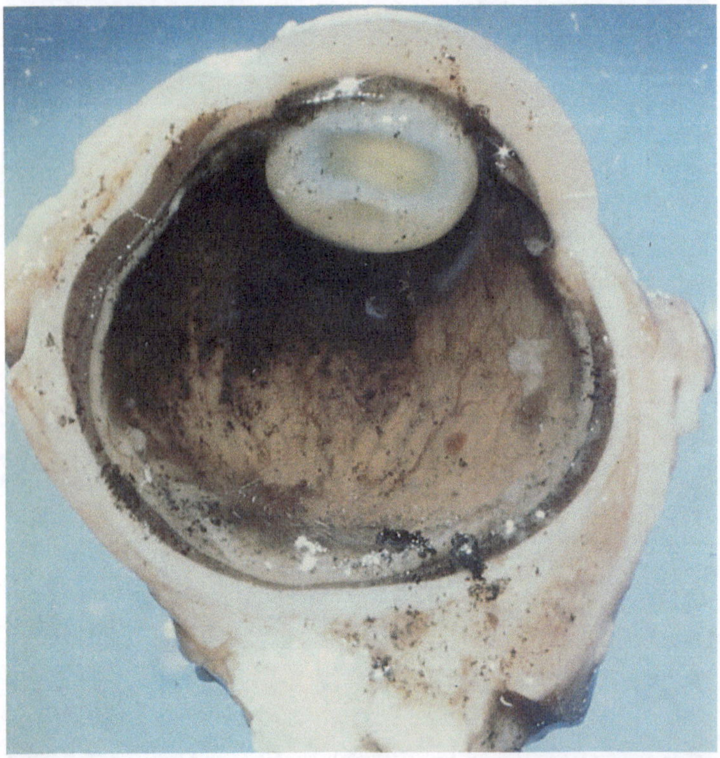
1.6

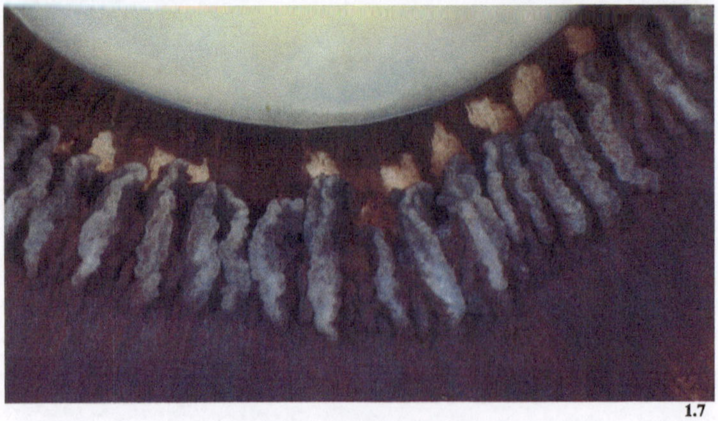
1.7

Changes in the Pigment Epithelium Layer

As time proceeds after death, defects in the pigment epithelium layer develop.

Fig. 1.5. Autolytic defects of the retinal pigment epithelium beneath artifactitious retinal folds. M 54/72: Formalin-fixed autopsy eye of an adult.

Liquefaction

The enzyme liberation in autolysis finally leads to liquefaction of tissues including the zonules, which then leads to subluxation or luxation of the lens.

Fig. 1.6. Marked autolysis with liquefaction of vitreous and a high degree of dispersal of pigment from uveal pigment epithelial cells. M 1149/77: Formalin-fixed autopsy eye of an infant.

Preparational Tissue Changes

Iris Pigment Epithelium Lesions

Fig. 1.7. Circumscribed defects of the iris pigment epithelium opposite to the tips of the ciliary processes caused by pressure during corneal trephining. Artificial opacity of the lens. Formalin-fixed autopsy eye of an adult.

Fig. 1.8. Diffuse defect of the iris pigment epithelium at the zone of lens contact caused by pressure during corneal trephining. Artificial opacity of the lens. Formalin-fixed autopsy eye of an elderly person.

Optic Nerve Pressure

The consistency of unfixed optic nerve tissue is that of tooth-paste. Pressure on the optic nerve during surgical enucleation or at autopsy may force optic nerve tissue (especially myelin) anteriorly.

Fig. 1.9. Accumulation of white material on the disc surface and on adjacent retina. It is optic nerve myelin pressed mechanically through the lamina cribrosa into the eye. Note also the folded white retina and the collapsed blood vessels. Formalin-fixed adult autopsy eye.

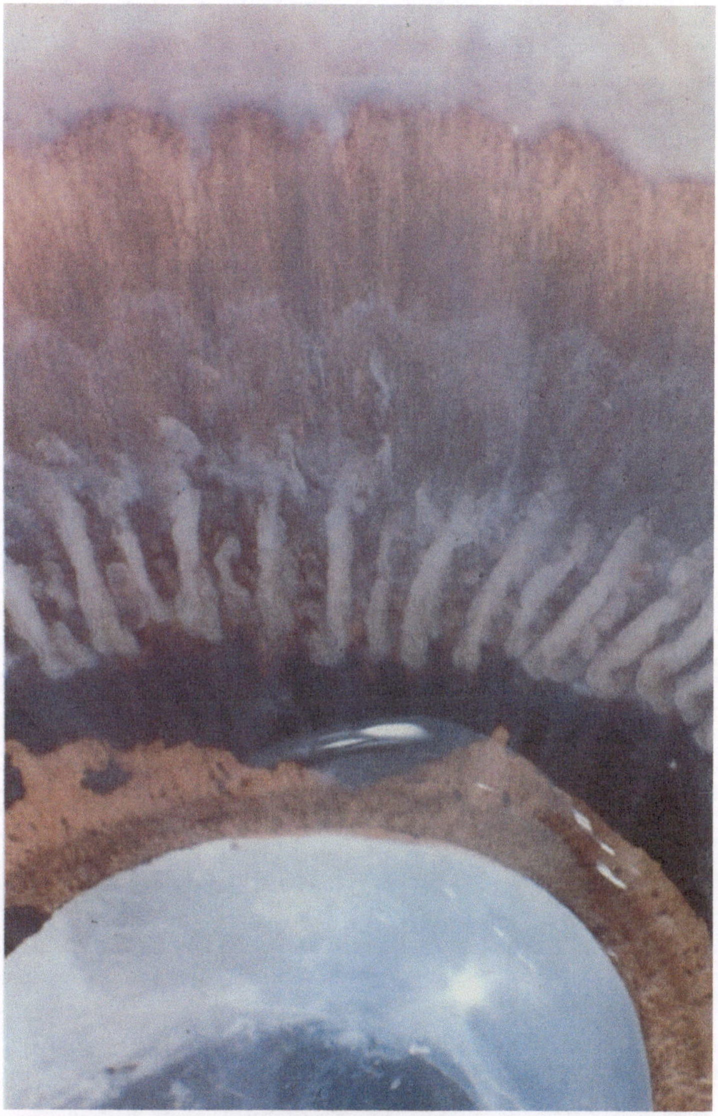

1.8

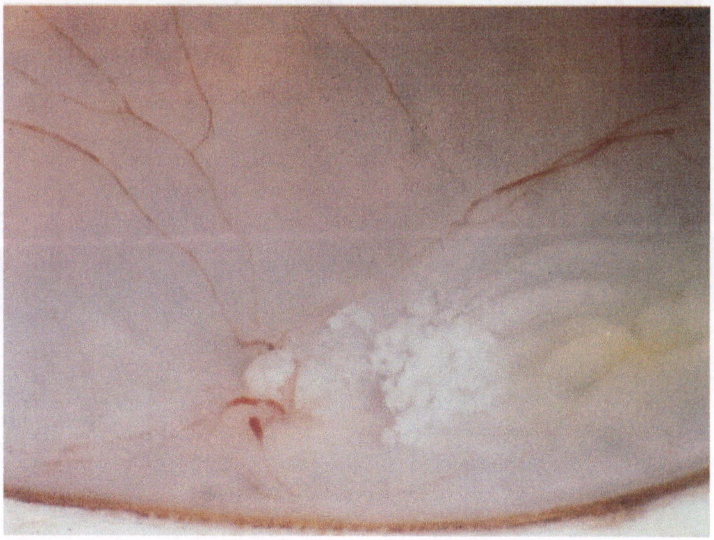

1.9

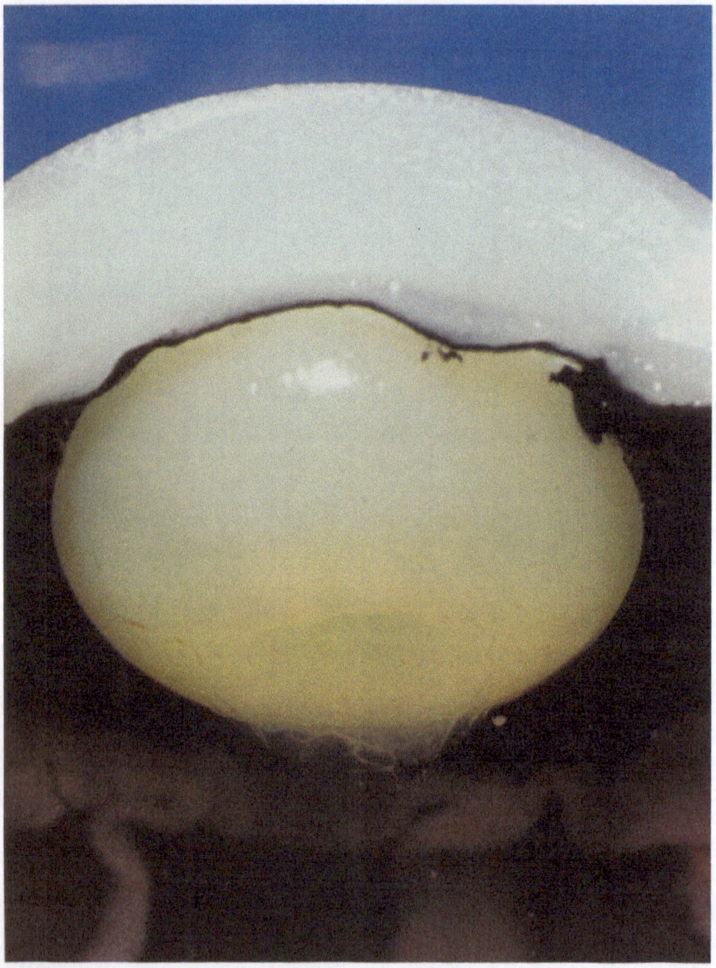

1.10

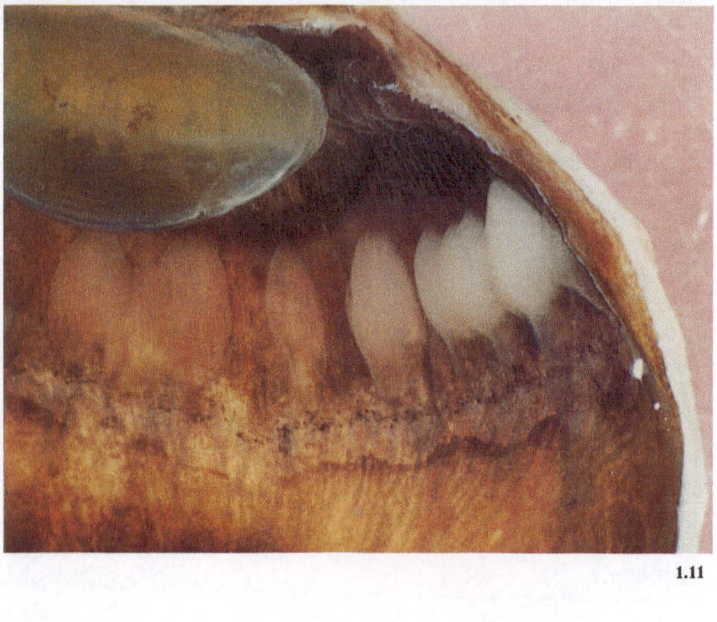

1.11

Changes Due to Fixation

Several fixation fluids are available, most commonly used are formaldehyde (for routine light microscopy) and glutaraldehyde (for electron microscopy). Special examination techniques require special fixation techniques. Fixatives change the protein structure and water content of tissues. This leads to varying degrees of opacification and thus color change, an increase in consistency and shrinkage of tissues. It varies from fixative to fixative. Using formalin or glutaraldehyde proteinaceous fluids such as subretinal exudate in retinal detachment or anterior chamber exudates in anterior uveitis become gelatinous. Clinically fairly soft malignant melanomas of the choroid change into firm tumors. The rather soft lens in children and juveniles changes into a firm structure showing some disconfiguration (umbilication) due to loss of water. The amount of tissue shrinkage in a fixative depends very much on the water content of the tissue.

Fig. 1.10. Umbilication of the posterior aspect of the lens in infancy due to fixation. Note also the white corneal opacity due to formaldehyde fixation, and remnants of the tunica vasculosa lentis. M 1148/77: Formalin-fixed autopsy eye of an infant.

Opacification of Fluids by a Fixative

The degree of opacification of intraocular fluids such as aqueous, vitreous, or cyst contents depends on the amount of protein present.

Fig. 1.11. Transparent and white pars plana cysts. The white discoloration is due to formalin fixation of the proteinaceous contents of the cysts. On the cut edge, some flat ciliochoroidal detachment which may be a preparational artifact. M 449/78: Eye of a 53-year-old female enucleated because of choroidal malignant melanoma.

2. Cornea

Inflammatory disorders · Degenerative lesion · Scarring · Staphyloma

The cornea consists of five layers: the epithelium, Bowman's layer, the stroma, Descemet's membrane and the endothelium. It is transparent and has a lightly oval shape. The central cornea measures about 0.56 mm while the periphery measures about 1 mm. The refractive power of the cornea constitutes almost $^3/_4$ of the total refracting power of the eye. Thus minor changes of the central cornea result in marked visual disturbances.

Primary corneal changes are degenerations (including age-related, senile changes) and epithelial, stromal and endothelial dystrophies. As the cornea develops from surface ectoderm and mesoderm it is associated with many skin and mucous membrane diseases as well as systemic metabolic, collagen, and immune diseases. Tumors arising primarily from the cornea are rare. Malignant or benign tumors usually extend onto the cornea from adjacent structures. The anterior of the eye is constant contact with the precorneal tear film and contaminated skin. Corneal infections by bacteria, fungi and viruses are common and cause keratitis and secondary corneal ulceration. Also common are traumatic lesions of the cornea.

Posttraumatic and postinflammatory corneal scarring are among the common causes of blindness throughout the world. Although rare in general, developmental malformations of the cornea play a role in blindness of infancy. Some of the clinically important traumatic lesions of the cornea are presented in the chapter on trauma. Since corneal transparency is lost by routine fixation in many solutions, postexcisional macroscopic observations under the dissecting microscope are of little value when compared with clinical observations made using the slip-lamp or with histological studies. Therefore only a few examples of inflammatory corneal leukomas are presented.

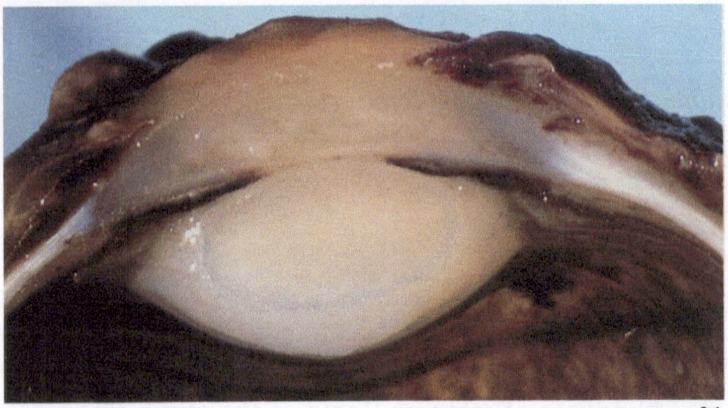

2.1

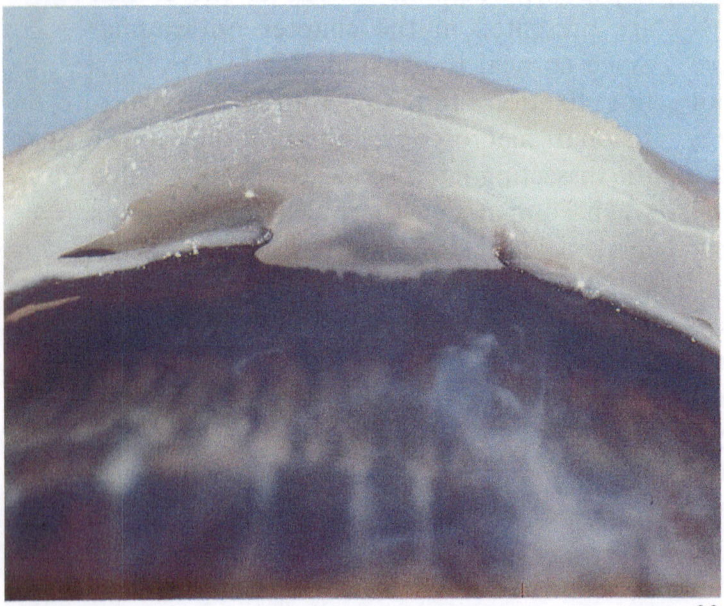

2.2

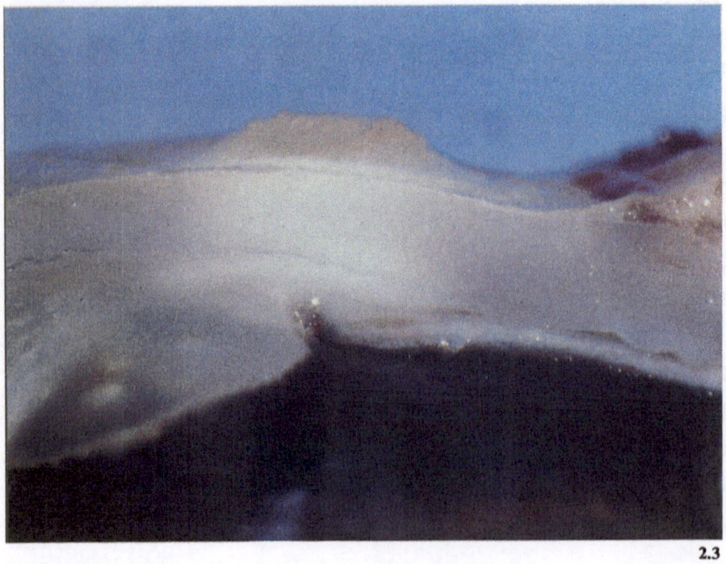

2.3

Inflammatory Disorders

Keratitis

Keratitis with or without corneal ulceration may be caused by bacteria, viruses (especially Herpes simplex virus, and in malnutrition, the measles virus), fungi (especially C. albicans), and amebae, or may result from a hypersensitivity reaction, fifth nerve lesions, exposure, and avitaminosis A. Eventually iritis with hypopyon may develop. A previously diseased cornea with degenerative lesions is more apt to develop keratitis. Keratitis not only impairs vision but carries some risk of corneal perforation and intraocular infection with subsequent loss of the eye.

Bacterial Keratitis

Among the more frequent bacteria causing keratitis are Streptococci species, Pseudomonas aeruginosa, and Staphylococci species. After antibiotic pretreatment, it may be impossible to demonstrate the organism.

Fig. 2.1. Diffuse yellowish cornea due to leukocytic infiltration, massive hypopyon, mature secondary cataract. M 67/81: 46-year-old male with acute bacterial keratitis due to Ps. aeruginosa in a scarred cornea after a severe acid burn (sulfuric acid) and suspected endophthalmitis.

Fig. 2.2. Corneal ulcer with diffuse infiltration of the corneal stroma, peripheral anterior synechias, flattened anterior chamber, corneal wound in the superior corneal periphery, iridectomy, aphakia, and opaque anterior vitreous. M 7/84: 84-year-old male with aphakia, postthrombotic neovascular glaucoma, and ulcer in the inferior third of the cornea. No organism could be cultured after antibiotic pretreatment.

Fig. 2.3. Higher magnification of Fig. 2.2 showing the corneal ulcer, the infiltrated corneal stroma, and flattened anterior chamber.

Degenerative Corneal Conditions

In contrast to bilateral hereditary corneal dystrophies, unilateral corneal degeneration is usually the result of a secondary reaction to an underlying cause such as inflammation, trauma, glaucoma, or a disturbance of the tear film.

Bullous Keratopathy with Degenerative Corneal Pannus

Corneal endothelial insufficiency of various causes (often in glaucoma) leads to chronic edema of the corneal epithelium (bullous keratopathy) and an increasingly developing degenerative subepithelial fibrous pannus.

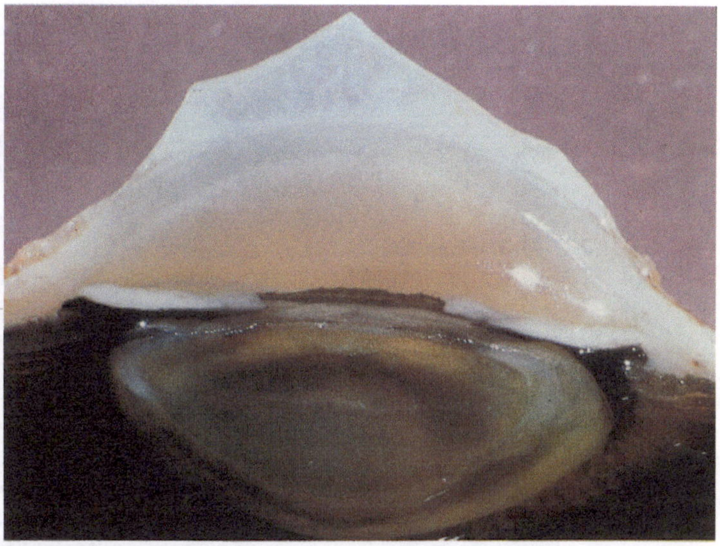

2.4

Fig. 2.4. Unusually large bullous keratopathy. The epithelial layer of the cornea together with a fibrous subepithelial pannus is lifted off Bowman's membrane, forming a large superficial corneal bulla. White inflammatory infiltration of the iris (iritis). M 582/75: 68-year-old myopic female suffering from chronic iridocyclitis, secondary glaucoma, blindness, and pain.

Postinflammatory Corneal Scarring

Healing of keratitis and corneal ulcers is often accompanied by superficial neovascularization (inflammatory corneal pannus) and stromal neovascularization. Early and appropriate treatment may obviate neovascularization but usually leaves an opaque scar. In cases of corneal perforation, the defect may be sealed by iris prolapse with a subsequent anterior synechia. Although usually growing into the corneal stroma from the limbus, neovascularization may sometimes originate from adherent iris.

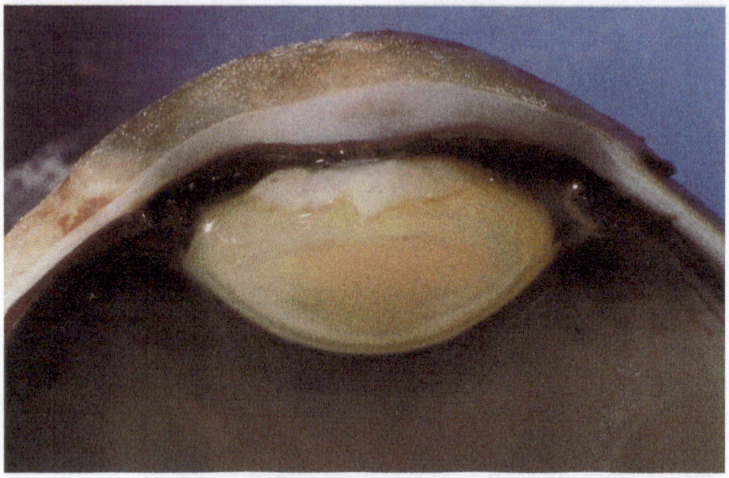

2.5

Leprosy Keratitis

In leprosy an interstitial keratitis may lead to vascularization with scarring of the cornea. Granulomatous iritis is often associated and may lead to posterior synechias and secondary cataract formation.

Fig. 2.5. Corneal scar with thickening and white opacification of the central cornea. Posterior synechias and anterior subcapsular cataract formation as evidence of previous iritis. M 463/79: Lepromatous blind Nepalese patient with corneal scar.

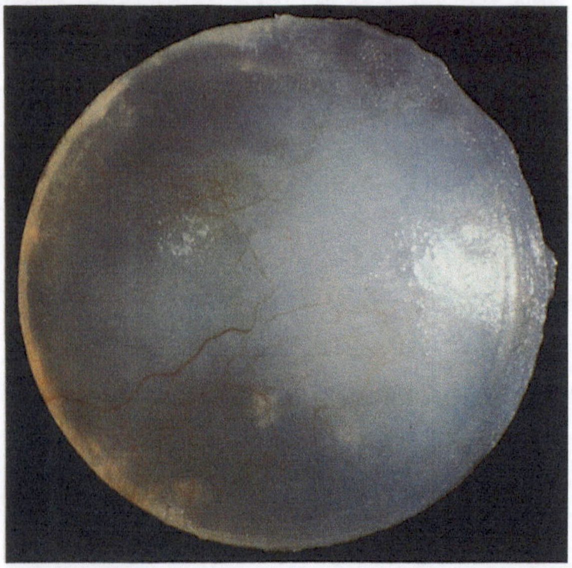

2.6

Measles (Rubeola)

Keratoconjunctivitis with conjunctival Koplik's spots as well as keratitis may develop in measles. Malnutrition is an additional risk factor for secondary bacterial keratitis.

Fig. 2.6. Anterior aspect of a surgically excised cornea. Dense white scar with superficial blood vessels. M 809/81: 17-year-old female who, in childhood, developed measles keratitis resulting in an opaque corneal scar. Perforating keratoplasty was performed.

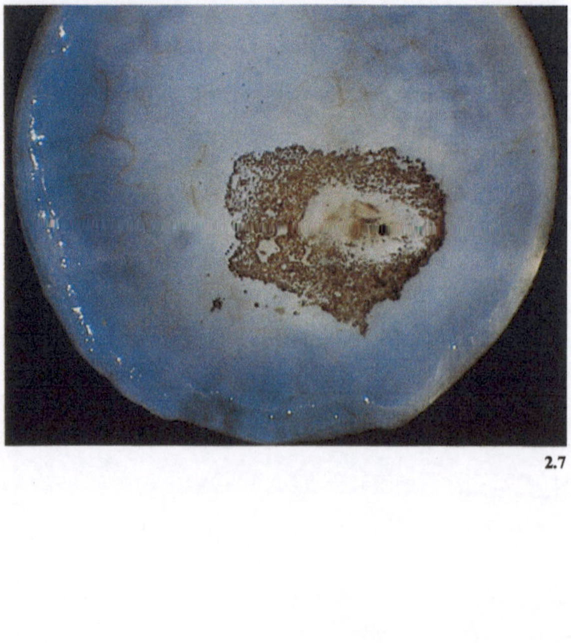

2.7

Fig. 2.7. Posterior aspect of a surgically excised cornea with pigmentation due to phagocytosed pigment, iris pigment epithelial cells, and iris melanocytes surrounding a site of corneal perforation.

Corneal Staphyloma

A staphyloma is an ectasia of the outer coats of the eye (cornea or sclera) internally covered by uveal tissue (iris, ciliary body, or choroid) and thus showing a blue discoloration. Corneal perforation (traumatic or inflammatory) if accompanied by a loss of the anterior chamber and total anterior synechia may lead to corneal staphyloma.

Fig. 2.8. Corneal staphyloma with total anterior synechia due to postkeratitic corneal perforation. Dislocation of the cataractous lens, some vitreous opacities and a white, postinflammatory uveal scar at the ora serrata. Postinflammatory pigment epithelial reaction at the posterior pole. M 740/84: 72-year-old shepherd noticed visual disturbances of 2 years, subsequently developing corneal ectasia. Six months prior to enucleation he developed an enlarging staphyloma with pain.

Fig. 2.8A. Corneal staphyloma. **a/b** Contact B-scan echograms and **c** A-scan echogram of corneal staphyloma. Note the wide anterior chamber (AC) causing an increased axial eye-length (**c**). (L = lens; ON = optic nerve.)

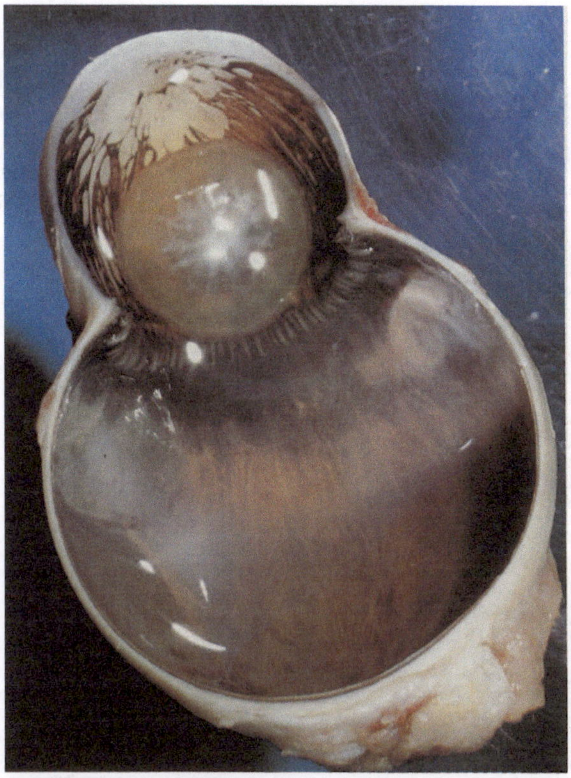

2.8

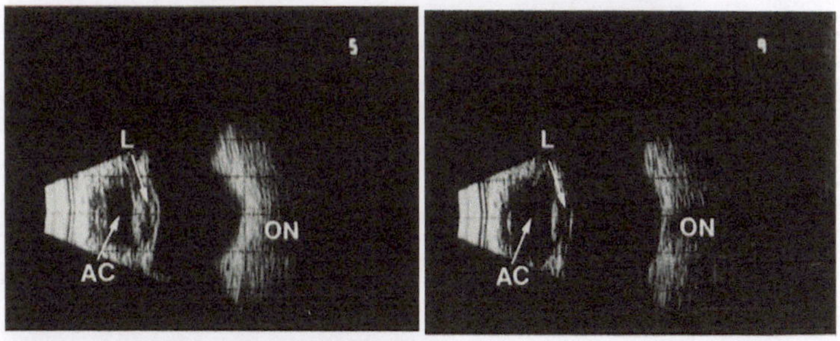

a b

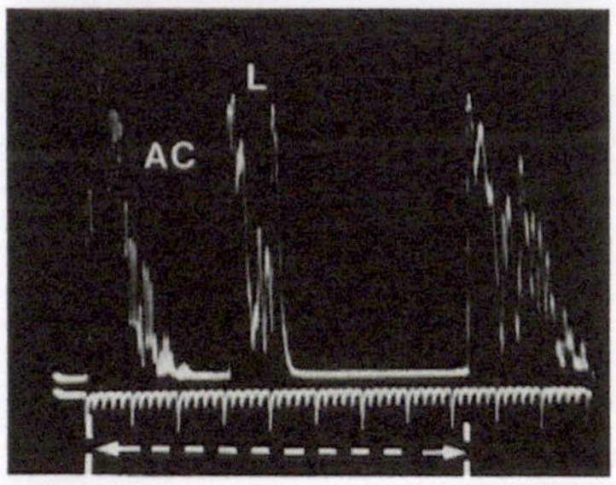

2.8A c

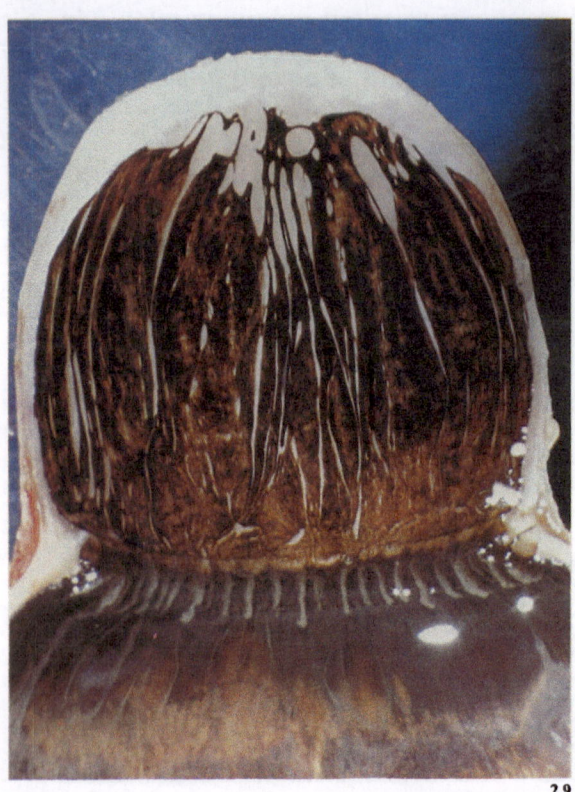

2.9

Fig. 2.9. Close-up view of the callotte of Fig. 2.8 showing the staphyloma with atrophic iris tissue which is pressed into the anterior chamber angle by the elevated intraocular pressure. Additionally, there are larger pars plana cysts (see also chapter 4) and cystoid degeneration of the peripheral retina (see also chapter 5).

3. Sclera

Blue sclera · Scleral thickening · High myopia · Scleral ectasia · Staphyloma · Inflammation · Degeneration

The fibrous sclera is the protective outer layer of the eye and the insertion site of the external eye muscles. Its thickness varies with age and location, the posterior sclera being thickest. It has to withstand normal intraocular pressure unchanged. Glaucoma (especially in children) as well as hypotony results in scleral changes (see chapter on glaucoma and trauma). Congenital disorders are blue sclera, staphylomas, and high axial myopia. Surgical as well as accidental injuries of the sclera are common (see chapters on trauma). A rare but serious disease is scleritis, which is often associated with collagen diseases such as rheumatoid arthritis or Wegener's granulomatosis. A frequently encountered degenerative lesion is the age-related (senile) scleral plaque found anterior to the insertion of the horizontal recti in the elderly. Calcification and ossification of degenerative scleral collagen may occur.

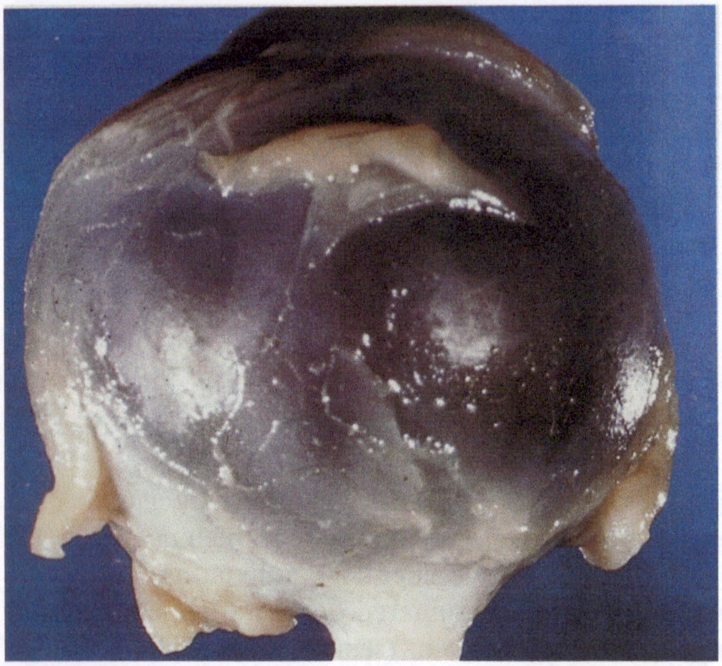

3.1

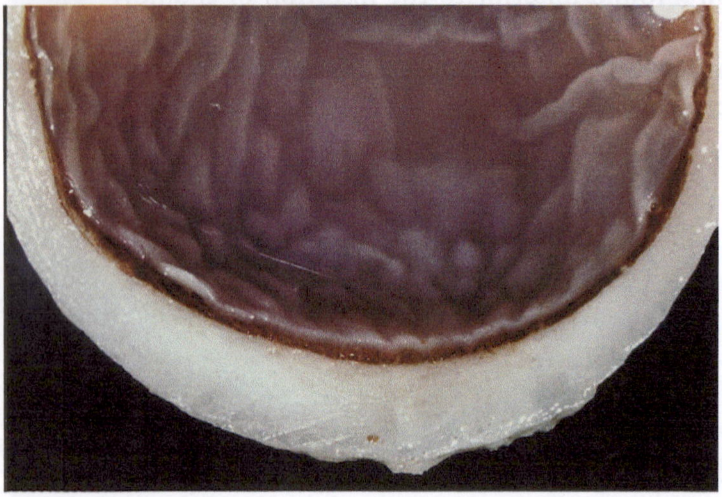

3.2

Blue Sclera

In inherited osteogenesis imperfecta, blue sclera associated with bone fragility, deafness, and other abnormalities may be present at birth. The scleral discoloration is due to the underlying uveal tissues shining through a thinned sclera with abnormal collagen fibres.

Fig. 3.1. Outer aspect of the eye showing an extensive bluish discoloration of the sclera. M 177/81: Newborn female with osteogenesis imperfecta and markedly blue sclera.

Scleral Thickening

Scleral thickening appears either spongy, firm, or inflammatory. Spongy thickening of the sclera is common in hypotonic eyes with ciliochoroidal detachment or in phthisis bulbi (see Fig. 11.51). Diffuse firm scleral thickening is rare. It has been described in mucopolysaccharidosis type VI. Nonnecrotizing scleritis is accompanied by marked scleral thickening.

Fig. 3.2. Markedly thickened sclera with hyalinoid homogeneous appearance. M 641/84: Autopsy eye of a 35-year-old male, who had died of pulmonary embolus.

Scleral Thinning

A thin sclera is present in blue scleras of osteogenesis imperfecta, scleral staphylomas including posterior scleral staphyloma with high axial myopia, scleral ectasis, and necrotizing scleritis.

High Axial Myopia

High axial myopia develops by progressive posterior staphylomatous elongation of the eye close to or around the optic disc. The sclera thins and adjacent structures within the staphyloma develop reactive changes such as chorioretinal atrophy, lacquer cracks, and Fuchs' spot. In addition the vitreous structure degenerates resulting in liquefaction.

Fig. 3.3. High myopia with thinning and staphylomatous ectasia of the sclera at the posterior pole. The choroid shows atrophic white patches just below the macula as well as pigment epithelial changes. Additionally there is cobblestone chorioretinal degeneration (see also chapter 5) between the equator of the eye and the lower temporal ora serrata. M 478/74: 46-year-old male with high myopia, amaurosis and unexplained ocular pain.

Fig. 3.3A. High myopia / Posterior staphyloma. **a** A-scan echogram/section nasally to the disc: the diameter of this myopic globe at this section is 33 microsec / 25.2 mm (*arrow* = sclera; *VO* = vitreous opacities). **b** Axial section at the posterior pole / macula area: the axial length of the globe is increased to 42 microsec / 32.5 mm (*arrow* = sclera, note the difficulty in displaying a steeply rising surface signal in this staphylomatous area of the globe; *L* = lens). **c, d** Contact B-scan echograms: vertical section (**c**) and horizontal section (**d**). *ON* = optic nerve; *VO* = vitreous opacities; *VD* = vitreous detachment; *arrows* = posterior staphyloma.

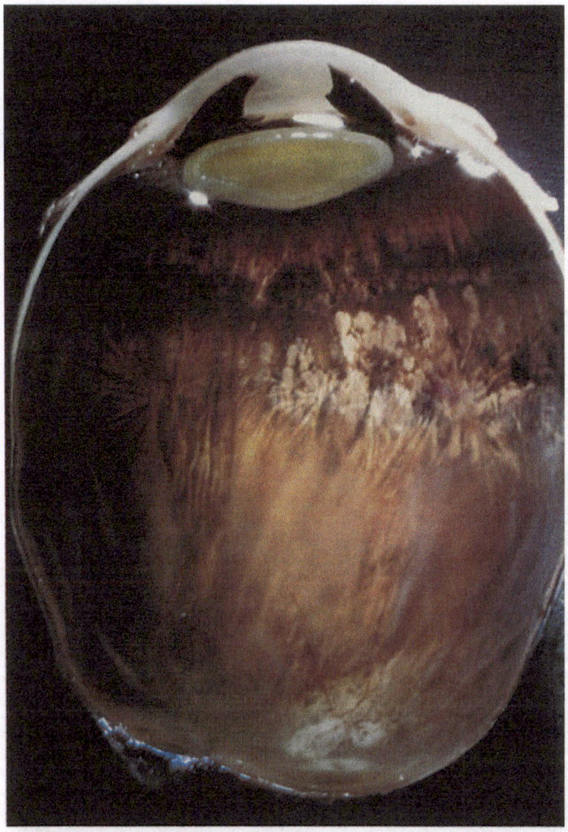

3.3

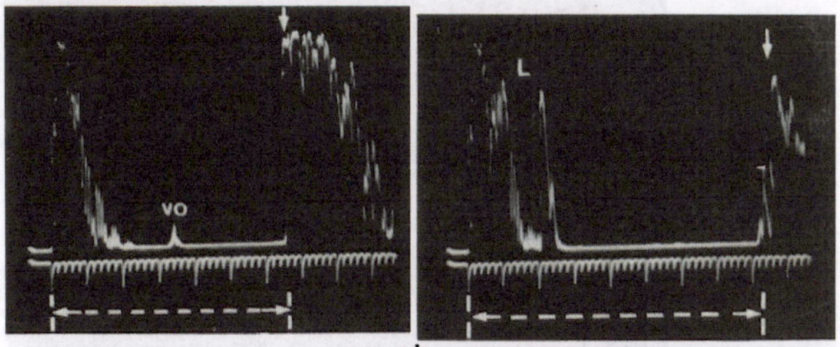

a b

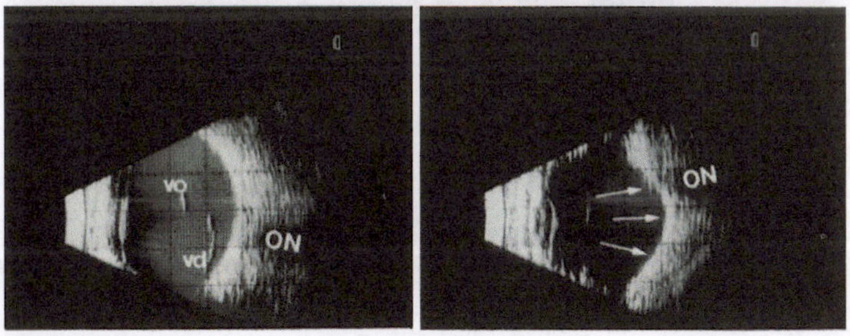

3.3A c d

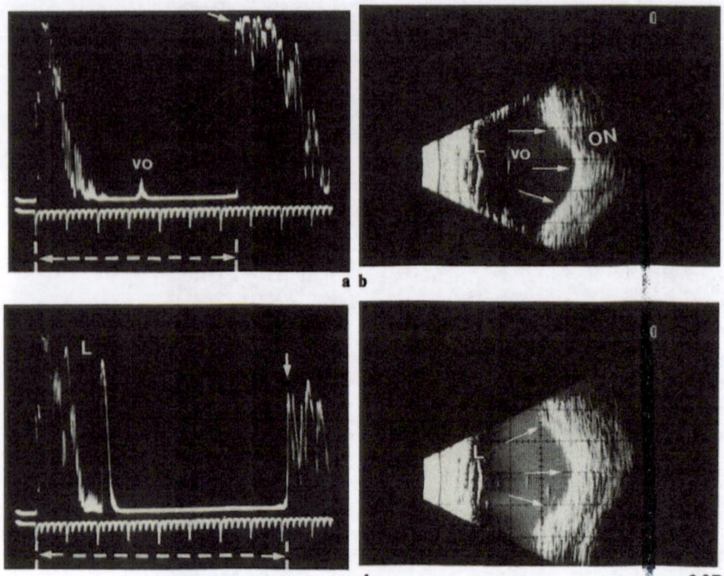

a b c d 3.3B

Fig. 3.3B. High myopia / Posterior staphyloma. **a, c** A-scan echograms: section nasally from the disc (**a**) and from the posterior pole (**c**). Note the difference in diameter and the difficulty in displaying a steeply rising echo signal from the ocular wall in the staphylomatous region at the posterior pole (**c**). *VO* = vitreous opacities; *L* = lens; *arrows* = sclera. **b, d** Contact B-scan echograms: horizontal section (**b**) and vertical section (**d**) at the posterior pole. Note the posterior staphyloma (*arrows*). *VO* = vitreous opacities; *ON* = optic nerve.

Scleral Ectasia

Decreased scleral resistance to intraocular pressure seen in congenital glaucoma, in postinflammatory or in posttraumatic scleral scarring may lead to scleral ectasia. An internal covering with uveal tissue will result in a scleral staphyloma.

Scleral Staphyloma

A scleral staphyloma is a localized area of scleral thinning and ectasia. The usually atrophic uveal tissue shines through the thinned sclera giving it clinically a characteristic blue discoloration. Anterior (ciliary and intercalary), equatorial, and posterior staphylomas are differentiated.

Anterior Intercalary Staphyloma

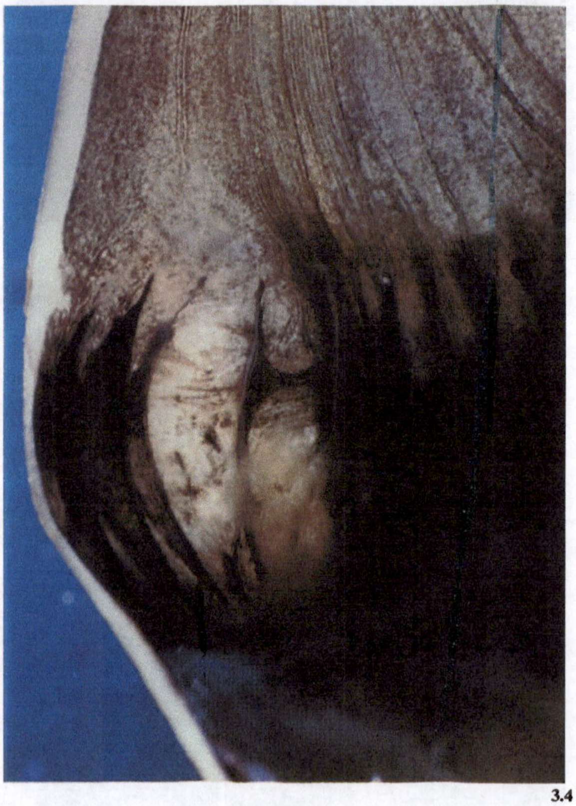

3.4

Fig. 3.4. Thinning and ectasia of the sclera overlying the pars plicata of the ciliary body with atrophy of the lining ciliary body. Total anterior synechia and atrophy of the iris. M 302/84: 17-year-old girl born prematurely. Hydrophthalmos secondary to total anterior synechia. Retinopathia proliferans. Diathermy of the ciliary body had been performed.

Equatorial Staphyloma

Fig. 3.5. Equatorial staphyloma underneath a rectus muscle (insertion of the rectus just anterior to the staphyloma) with choroidal detachment. Note also the goniosynechias (peripheral anterior synechias) and vitreous hemorrhage. M 639/82: 71-year-old diabetic male with diabetic retinopathy, central retinal vein occlusion, vitreous hemorrhage, and rubeosis iridis.

Fig. 3.5 A. Scleral staphyloma / scleral ectasia. Contact B-scan echograms of a scleral staphyloma / ectasia displayed in two sections (**a, b**) in more anterior (equatorial) part of the globe.

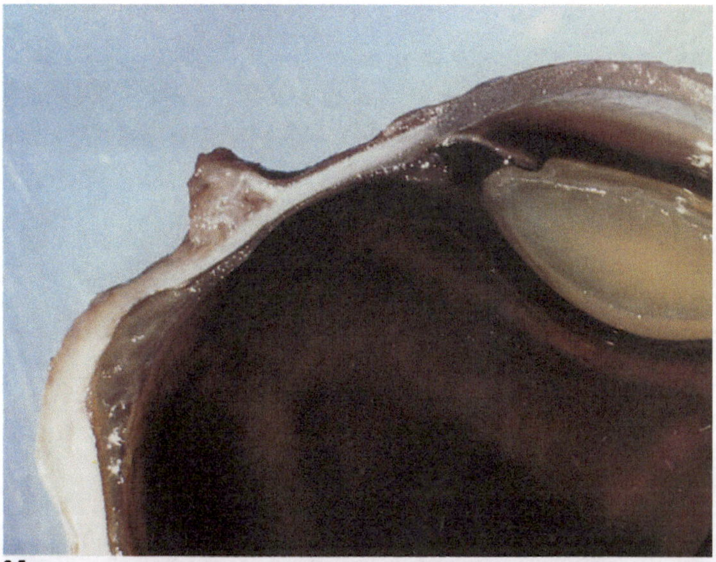

3.5

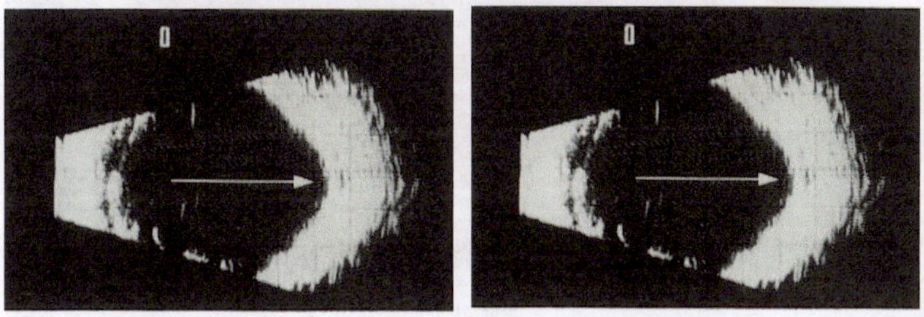

3.5 A a b

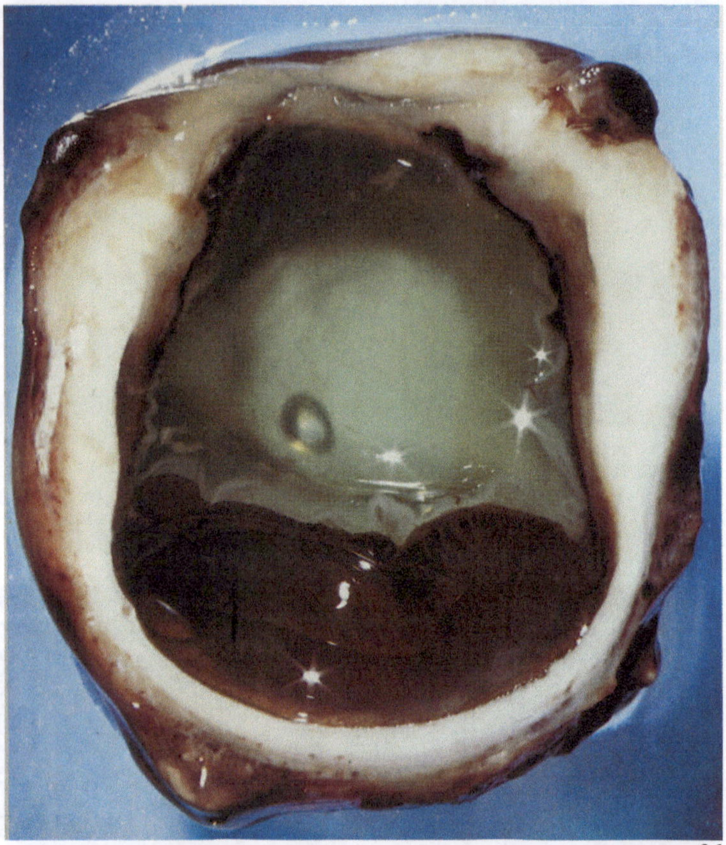

3.6

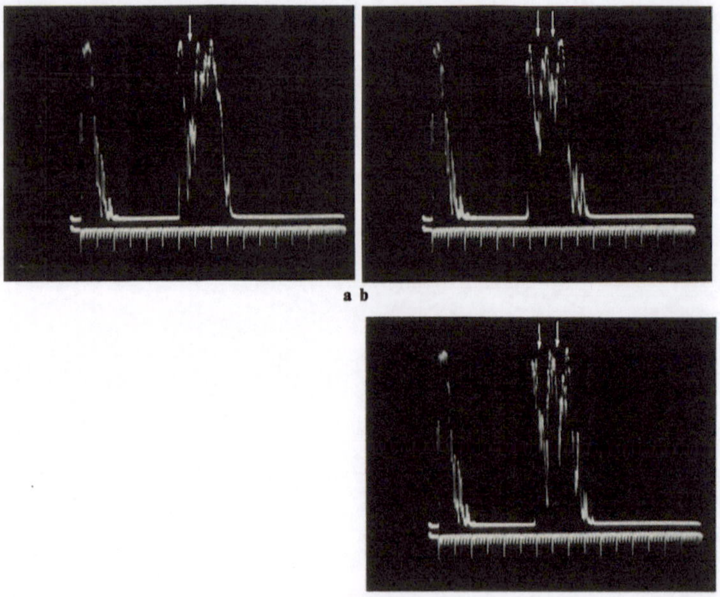

a b

c 3.6A

Scleritis

Unilateral or bilateral scleritis is an uncommon but severe inflammatory ocular disease often associated with systemic disease such as rheumatoid arthritis. Women more frequently are affected. It may lead to keratitis, uveitis, cataract, or retinal detachment. Clinically, anterior and posterior scleritis are differentiated. Initial thickening characterizes the more common anterior scleritis. Histologically, a nodular and diffuse type may be differentiated. Melting of collagen is rare, but results in necrotizing scleromalacia which may lead to scleral perforation with uveal prolapse. Healing leaves a thin sclera which may result in scleral ectasia.

Acute Necrotizing Scleritis

Fig. 3.6. Massive almost diffuse thickening of the sclera and the cornea. Posterior reactive detachment of the cellular infiltrated opaque vitreous. M 1161/80: 51-year-old male with history of rheumatoid arthritis.

Fig. 3.6A. Thickening of the sclera. **a–c** A-scan echograms of thickened sclera (scleritis / episcleritis posterior) with thickened insertion of the medial rectus muscle (arrows).

Fig. 3.7. Sclera thickened at the site of insertion of the rectus muscle but less so than in the previous case. Inflammatory infiltration of adjacent tissues such as the choroid, ciliary body, pars plana epithelium, and peripheral retina. Additionally, there is lattice degeneration of the equatorial retina (see also chapter 5). M 245/84: 82-year-old female with history of rheumatoid arthritis.

Fig. 3.7 A. Thickening of the sclera. **a–c** Contact B-scan echograms of thickened sclera (scleritis / episcleritis posterior) with thickening of the insertion of the medial rectus muscle (arrows).

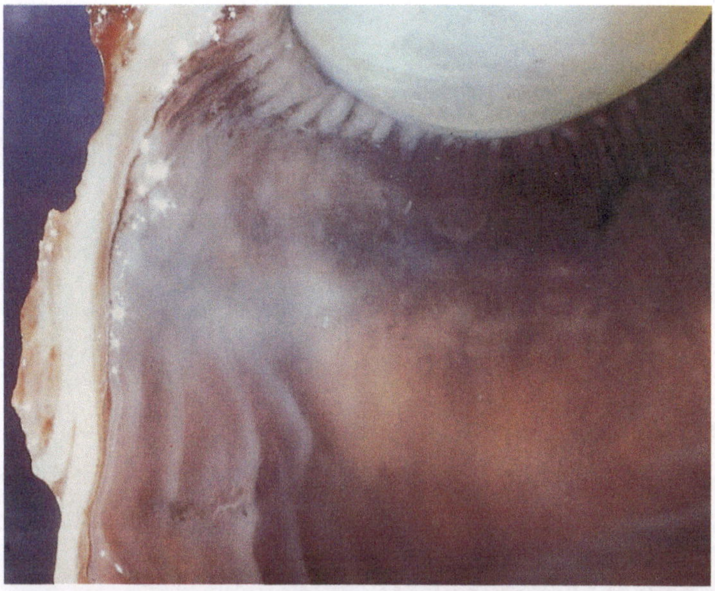

3.7

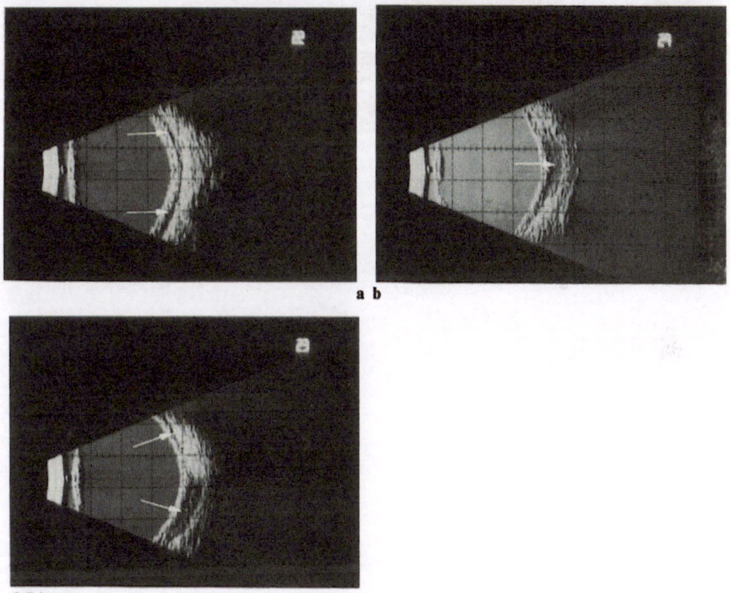

a b

3.7 A c

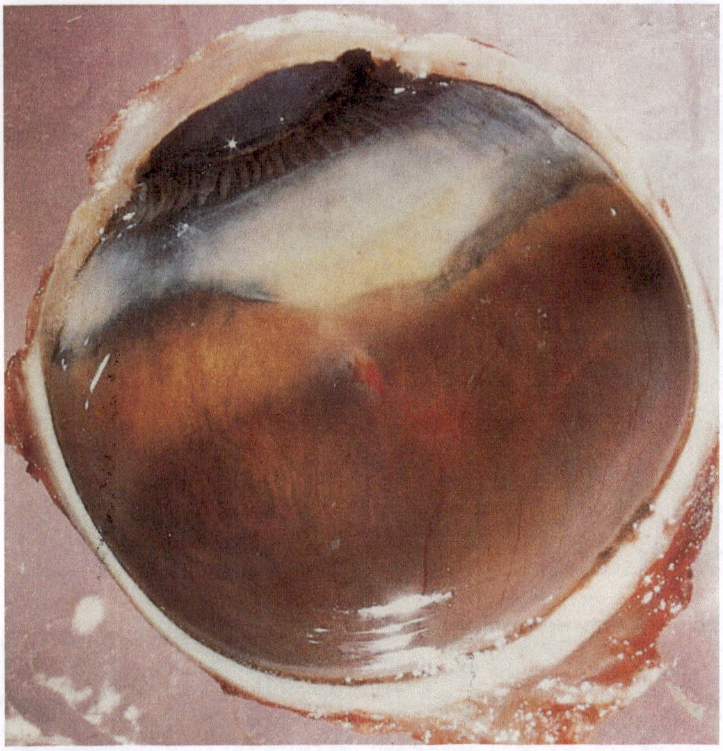

3.8

Chronic Anterior Scleritis

Fig. 3.8. Chronic brownish, partially granulomatous scleritis with loss of scleral collagen. Reactive proliferation of connective tissue within the ciliary body and at the pars plana. Proliferation of retinal pigment epithelium demarcates the zone of inflammation. The cornea is thickened due to pannus formation from additional keratitis. M 755/75: 51-year-old female with polyarteritis nodosa.

Degenerations

Usually, degenerative changes appear as localized collagen disturbances which may finally calcify. Superficial degenerations are clinically visible as gray areas.

Age-Related, Senile Scleral Plaque

A gray "hyaline" scleral degeneration anterior to the insertion of the horizontal rectus muscles is common in patients over the age of 70. In rare instances, a calcified age-related senile scleral plaque may extrude as a sequester.

Fig. 3.9. Oval grayish calcified plaque within superficial sclera anterior to the rectus muscle insertion. M 1185/80: Autopsy material. No clinical data available.

Atypical Scleral Plaque

Sometimes by chance, a calcified plaque is found histologically in the posterior inner sclera. It may cause a localized scleral thickening. The pathogenesis of this atypical sclera is unknown.

Fig. 3.10. Localized thickening of the posterior inner sclera due to an atypical calcified scleral plaque. M 835/81: Autopsy material. No clinical data available.

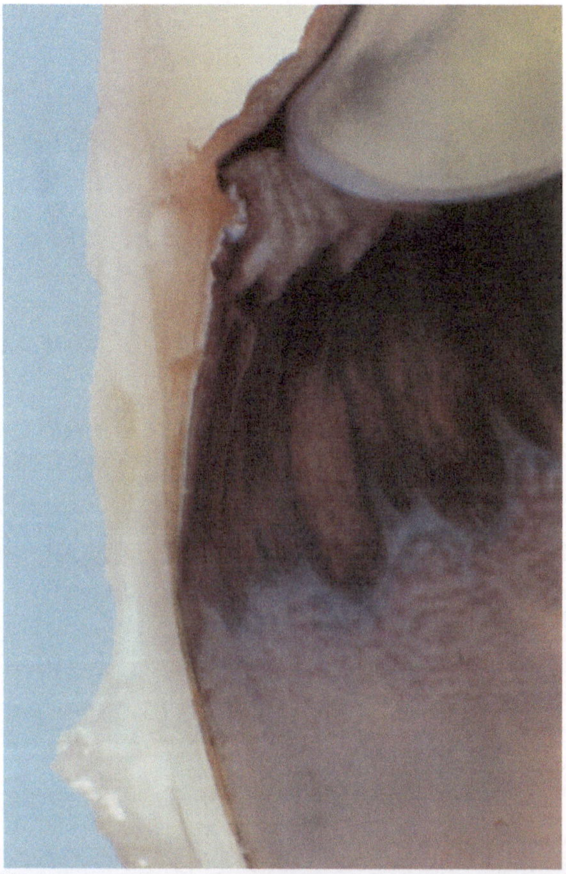

3.9

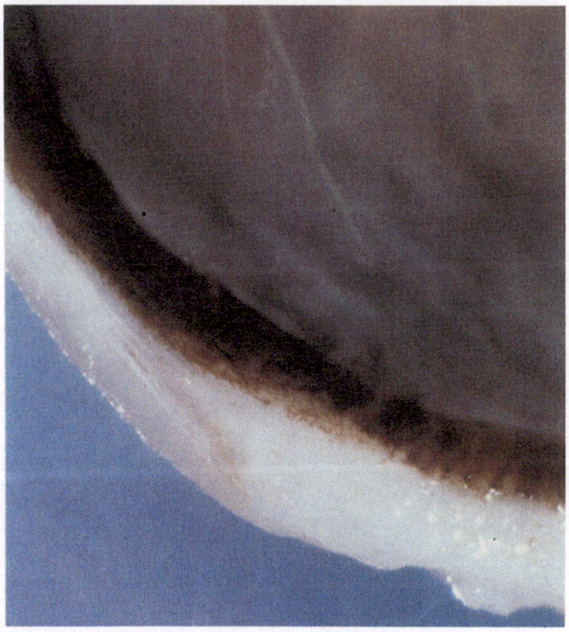

3.10

4. Uveal Tract

Coloboma · Melanosis oculi · Inflammation · Postinflammatory complications · Hyphema · Pars plana cysts

The uvea consists of the iris, the ciliary body, and the choroid. The latter contributes to the oxygen supply of the outer retina. Iris blood vessels have a thick collagenous adventitia. This adventitia prevents a direct view of the blood column. Thus iris blood vessels may be easily seen without magnification in a blue iris as radiating gray strands. In the ciliary body, two zones are differentiated: the anterior pars plicata (corona ciliaris) with the ciliary processes and the posterior pars plana. Although the epithelium lining the internal aspect of the iris and ciliary body develops embryologically from the wall of the primary ocular vesicle and is thus an anterior extension of the sensory retina and retinal pigment epithelium, it is in fact an integral part of iris and ciliary body. Therefore degenerative epithelial changes of the ciliary body are presented in this section rather than under retina. Inflammation is commonly found in any of the uveal structures and may lead to secondary inflammation or degeneration in adjacent structures such as retina or lens. In untreated iritis, inflammatory adhesions to the anterior lens surface (posterior synechias) or to the back of the cornea (anterior peripheral synechias) may develop. Hemorrhages within or from uveal structures result either from trauma (see chapter 11), endogenous systemic diseases, or from local vascular diseases. Serous or hemorrhagic ciliochoroidal detachment may result from trauma, tumors, or inflammation (see chapters 10 and 11). Neovascularization of the iris (rubeosis iridis) is an important complication in extraocular and ocular vascular or systemic diseases such as diabetic retinopathy and central retinal vein occlusion, ocular tumors, or in postinflammatory ocular conditions because it may lead to peripheral anterior synechias and glaucoma.

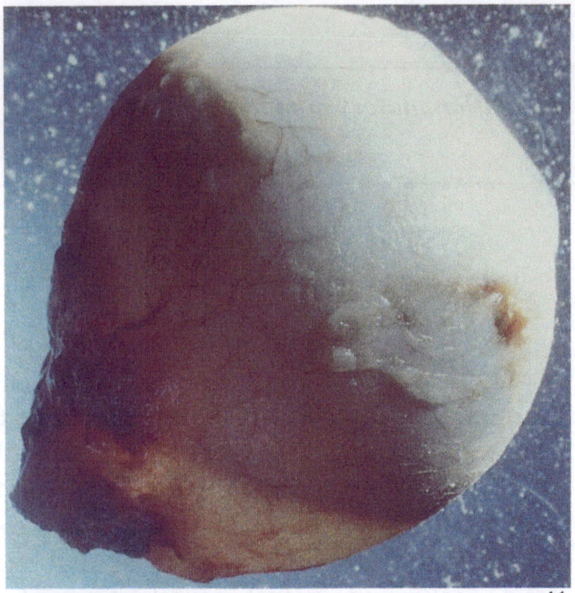

4.1

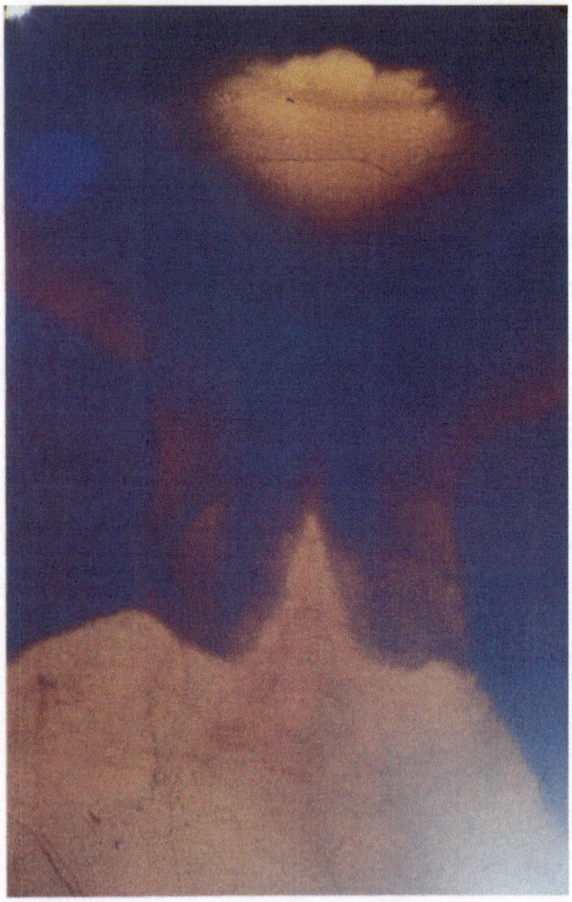

4.2

Colobomas

Colobomas are a result of defective closure of the embryonic cleft of the eye and/or the ocular adnexae. They occur in any part of the uvea and may be genetically transmitted. Clinically, an iris coloboma appears as a keyhole pupil. A ciliary body coloboma may result in a misshapen lens due to the absence of zonules within the coloboma. In postequatorial colobomas the retina and choroid are absent. Colobomas of the optic nerve head may result in cystic changes.

Fig. 4.1. Transillumination of the posterior segment with a large choroidal coloboma. M 911/83: 5-month-old female infant with trisomy 13-q and multiple systemic defects. The eye showed a large uveal coloboma which involved the iris, ciliary body, and choroid. The eye was enucleated because it contained retinoblastoma (see also chapter 10).

Colobomas in Trisomy 13 (Patau's Syndrome)

Uveal colobomas are usually present in trisomy 13, which consists of other multiple ocular and extraocular defects which include amongst others microphthalmos, retinal dysplasia, optic atrophy, cataract, cerebral defects, cleft palate, and heart defects. Life expectancy is poor.

Fig. 4.2. Transillumination of the eye showing a keyhole pupil, a malformation of the ciliary body, and a large choroidal coloboma.

Fig. 4.3. The iris coloboma is shining through the artifactitious opaque lens which is misshapen and forms an edge directed towards the ciliary coloboma. The incompletely closed embryonic cleft in the ciliary body widens into the large choroidal staphyloma.

Fig. 4.4. Neural retina reaching forward onto the ciliary body towards the ciliary body coloboma. The misshapen lens is cataractous showing a small notch at the site of the ciliary coloboma. There are three small additional choroidal defects at the equator. The postequatorial retina shows an oval degeneration with a whitishgray border, which consists of retinal dysplasia. M 23/85: Autopsy eye of a $2^1/_2$-month-old infant with trisomy 13, iris coloboma, cataract, and multiple systemic defects.

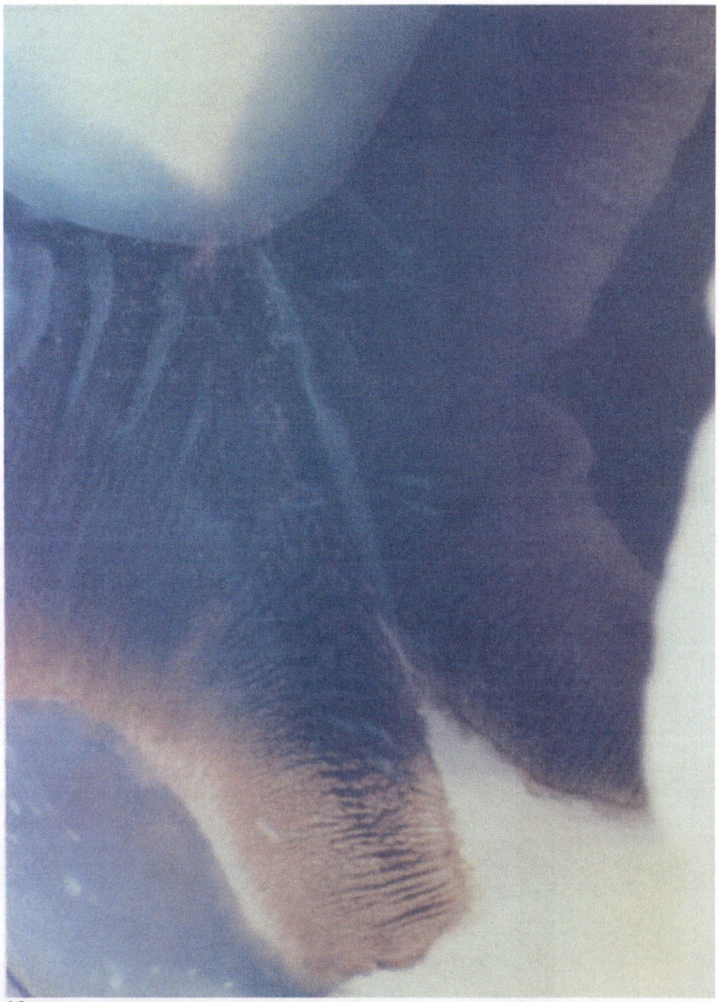

4.3

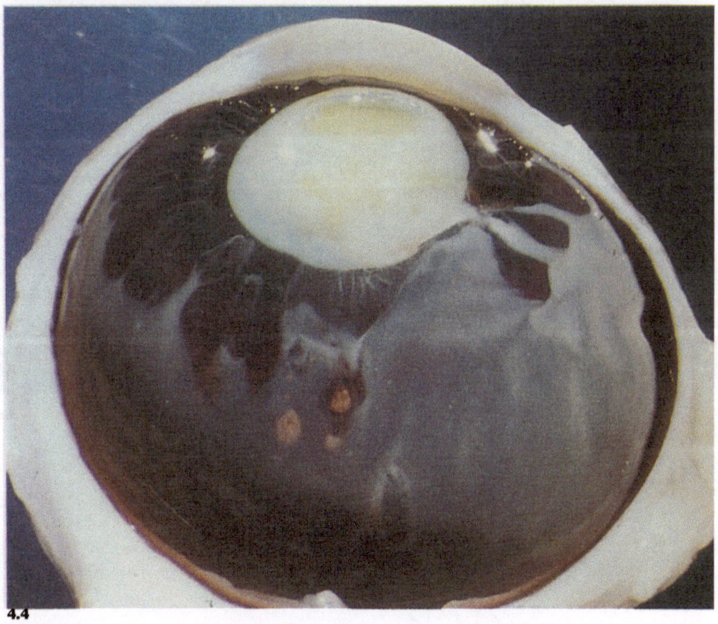

4.4

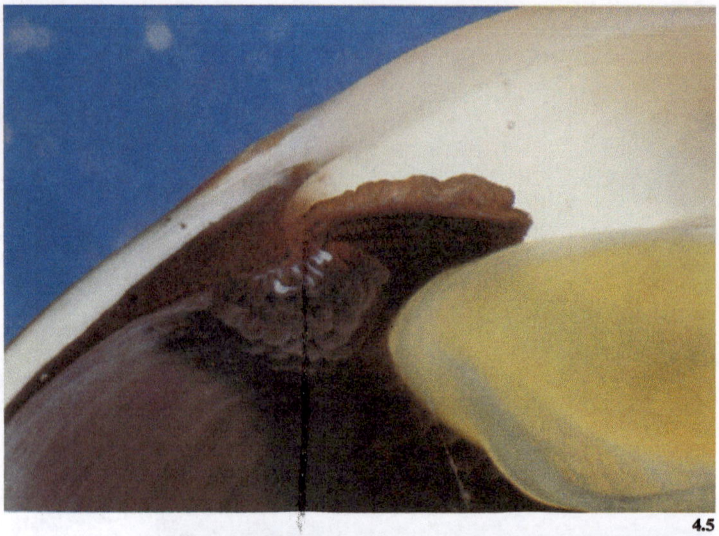

4.5

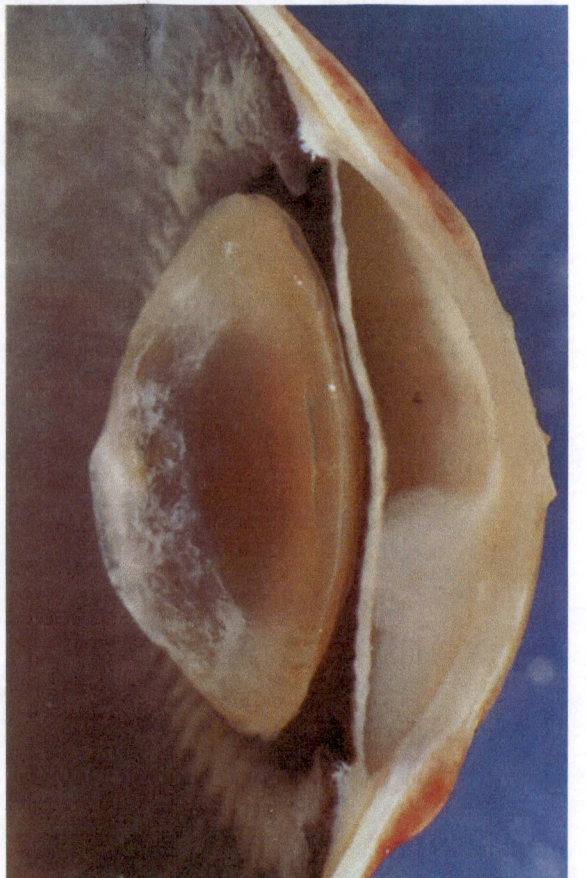

4.6

Melanosis Oculi

The normal content of melanocytes within the uveal structures varies with individuals. In congenital melanosis oculi (which may be part of the rather rare non-inherited usually unilateral nevus of Ota), there is a marked pigmentation of all uveal structures including the ciliary muscle and of the trabecular meshwork. Normally there is little pigmentation of the trabecular meshwork and the ciliary muscle. Melanosis oculi may be complicated by glaucoma and malignant melanoma in rare instances.

Fig. 4.5. Deep brown pigmentation of the iris, ciliary body (including the ciliary muscle), and trabecular meshwork. Additionally there is a yellowish nuclear sclerosis of the lens. M 427/79: 57-year-old male with malignant melanoma of the choroid in congenital melanosis oculi.

Uveal Inflammation

Uveal inflammation is not uncommon and is an an important cause of blindness. Recurrent attacks are common. Anterior and posterior uveitis may be differentiated. Although there are many causes of uveitis, it is usually nonspecific. Specific endogenous uveitis syndromes are those associated

Fig. 4.6. Proteinaceous whitish exudate in the lower anterior chamber. Minimal inflammatory reaction over the ciliary body. Secondary posterior subcapsular cataract formation. M 819/84: Recurrent metaherpetic keratitis and iridocyclitis in a 64-year-old man

with joint diseases, sarcoid, tuberculosis, following ocular trauma (lens-induced uveitis and sympathetic uveitis), and Fuchs' heterochromic cyclitis. Uveitis often accompanies keratitis (iritis, iridocyclitis), scleritis (cyclitis), trauma such as surgery, or infections of the eye (panuveitis in endophthalmitis). Severe iritis may be accompanied by hypopyon. Posterior uveitis affecting the retina is termed chorioretinitis. Complications of uveitis can lead to secondary glaucoma due to synechias (posterior synechias, peripheral anterior synechias = goniosynechias), cataract, cyclitic membranes, cystoid macular edema, vitreous strands, and tractional retinal detachment.

Anterior and Intermediate Uveitis

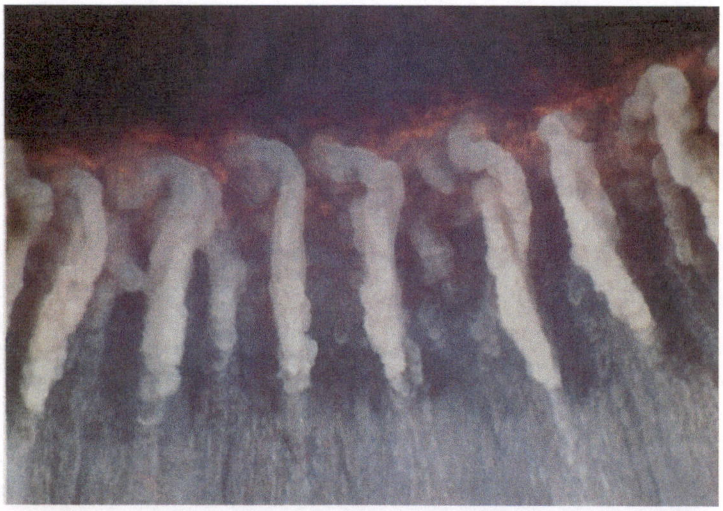
4.7

Fig. 4.7. Loss of pigment epithelium at the base of the upper iris which may be clinically demonstrated by retroillumination.

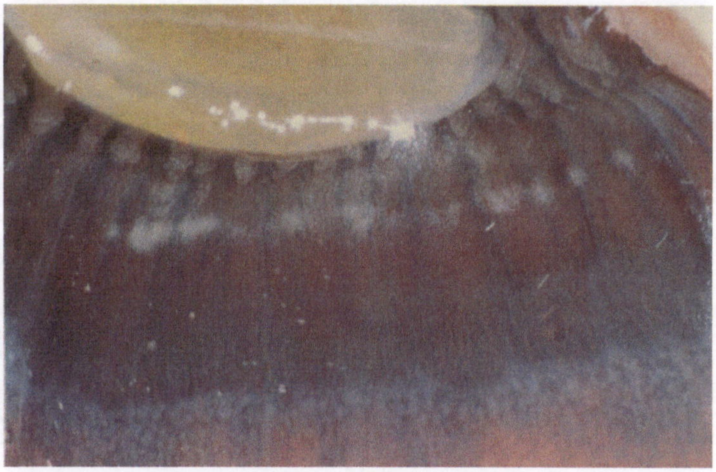
4.8

Fig. 4.8. Cyclitis with small white inflammatory infiltrates in the anterior pars plana epithelium. M 250/74: 68-year-old female with central corneal ulcer and severe hypopyon iritis in an amblyopic eye.

Hypopyon

Pus in the anterior chamber (hypopyon) is seen more commonly in infections than in endogenous uveitis such as Behcet's disease.

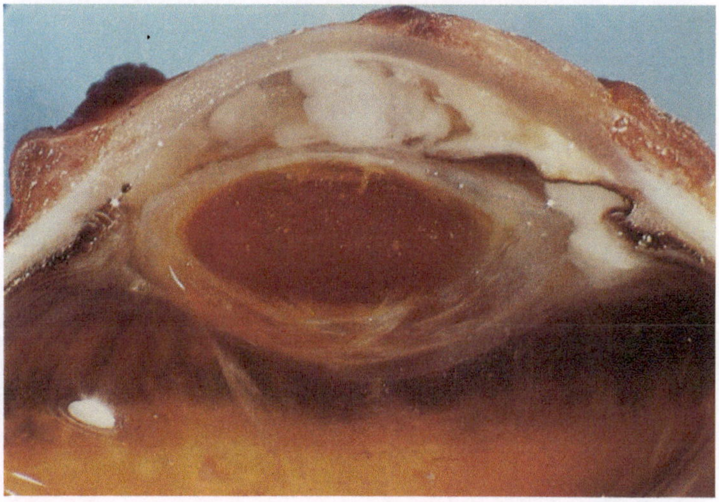
4.9

Fig. 4.9. Pus in the anterior chamber (hypopyon) and lower posterior chamber. Some opacities in the anterior vitreous. Brown nucleus of the cataractous lens. M 1079/78: Acute anterior uveitis with hypopyon in a 66-year-old male with history of glaucoma surgery 6 years previous to this. Cultures and smears from the anterior chamber were negative.

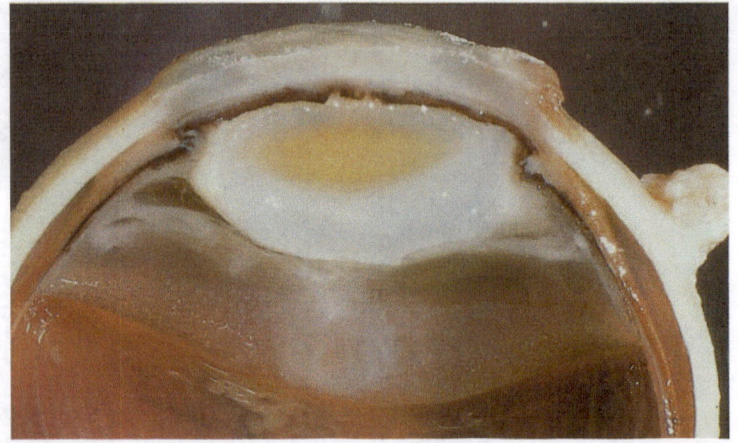

4.10

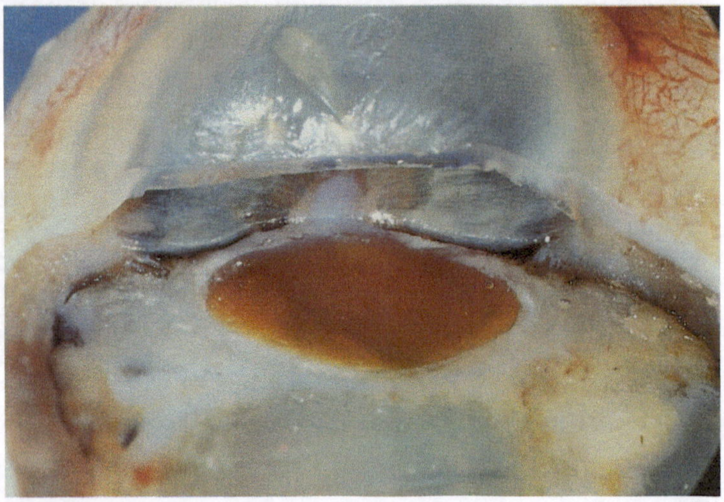

4.11

Lens-Induced (Phacoanaphylactic) Uveitis

After sensitization to lens material following extracapsular cataract extraction or traumatic lens damage, a severe sterile inflammatory hypersensitivity reaction may develop in the fellow eye if the lens is damaged.

Fig. 4.10. Keratitis with thickening and opacification of the cornea. Flat anterior chamber. Mature cataract with yellow lens nucleus and white opaque lens cortex surrounded by whitish infiltrations in the posterior chamber and anterior vitreous. There is an additional posterior vitreous detachment. M 1004/79: 73-year-old male with corneal ulcer, mature age-related cataract, and lens capsule defect.

Synechias and Iridocyclitic Membrane

Healing of anterior uveitis may result in synechias (anterior and/or posterior) and interciliary fibrovascular cyclitic membrane formation which may cause obliteration of the chamber angle, pupil, and posterior chamber. Thus glaucoma or tractional ciliochoroidal detachment with subsequent phthisis bulbi may develop.

Fig. 4.11. Posterior synechia with fibrovascular obliteration of the pupil. The brown cataractous lens is surrounded by fibrovascular tissue (iridocyclitic membrane) which obliterates the posterior chamber angle. Tractional ciliochoroidal detachment with a fibrotic reaction in the suprachoroidal space. The retina is totally detached and adherent to the iridocyclitic membrane. Gelatinous bluish subretinal fluid posterior to the retrolental fibrous membrane. M 423/84: Painful blind eye in a 71-year-old female suffering from recurrent uveitis for many years.

Serous Ciliochoroidal Detachment

In uveitis, an accumulation of serous fluid in the anterior suprachoroidal space may lead to ciliochoroidal detachment and hypotonia bulbi.

Fig. 4.12. Frontal section through the eye and view into the posterior segment showing a large choroidal detachment with folded retina on a smooth choroidal surface. Normal choroidal blood vessels pass through the widened suprachoroidal space to their scleral emissaries. M 1161/80: 51-year-old male with anterior scleritis and keratitis. Same case as in Fig. 3.6.

Fig. 4.12A. Choroidal detachment. Contact B-scan echograms (**a, b**) of serous choroidal detachments. Note the typical dome-shaped appearance and the steep insertion of the "membrane", representing the retinochoroid layer, in the peripheral fundus.

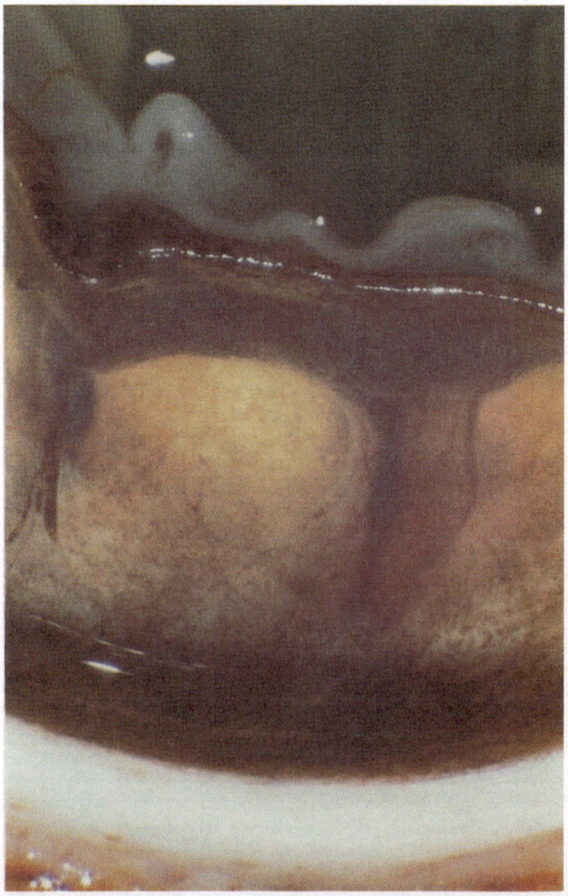

4.12

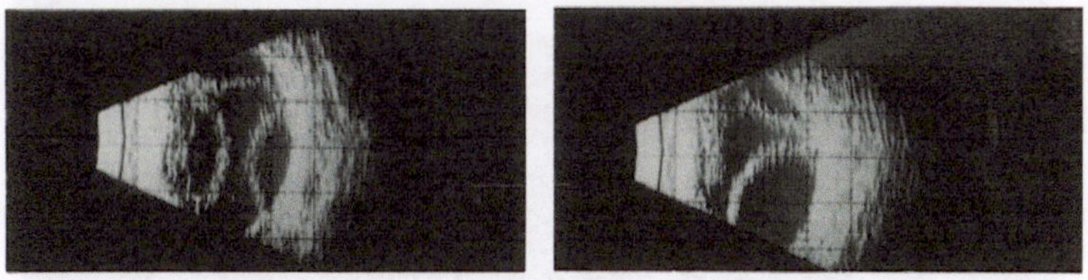

4.12A a b

Chronic Fuchs' Heterochromic Iridocyclitis

Fuchs' heterochromic iridocyclitis is usually a unilateral anterior chronic uveitis (iridocyclitis) without clinical symptoms. An early sign is a unilateral discoloration of the iris which turns grayish-blue. This heterochromia is often present as early as childhood. Slit-lamp examination shows a smooth iris surface with loss of crypts due to inflammatory lymphoplasma-cellular infiltration of the iris stroma and some cellular infiltration of the anterior vitreous body. Complications are unilateral cataract and glaucoma in young adulthood.

Fig. 4.13. Mottled appearance of the iris pigment epithelium and grayish deposits in the ciliary processes. Surgical aphakia. M 802/76: Autopsy eye of a 79-year-old man with Fuchs' heterochromic chronic iridocyclitis. Cataract extraction had been performed 22 years before death.

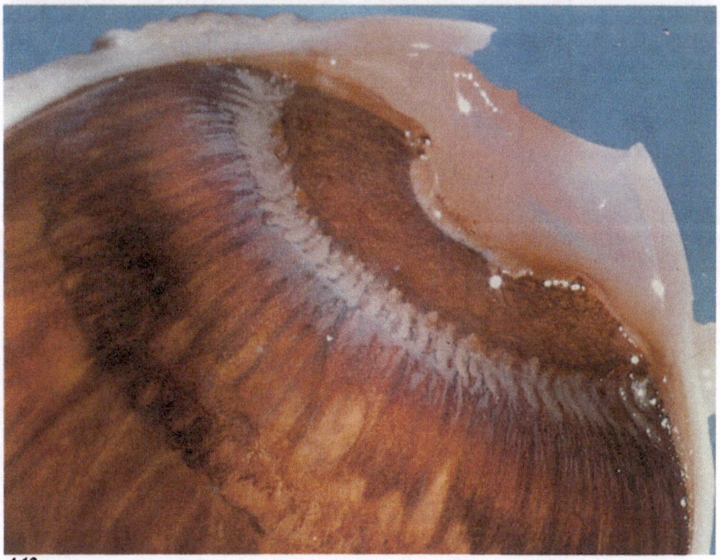

4.13

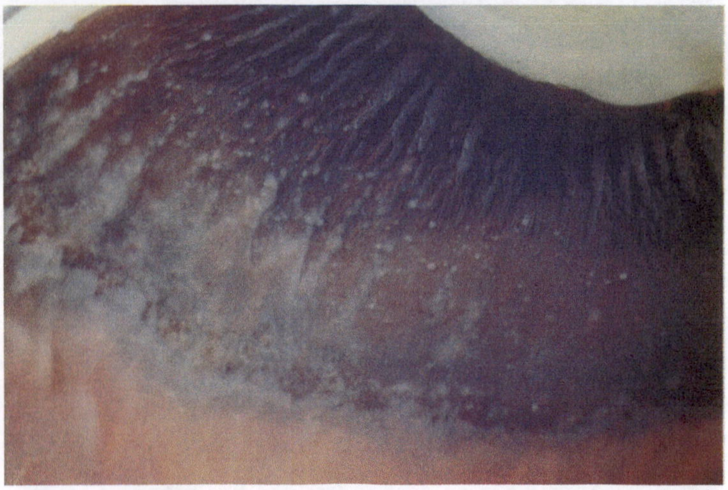

4.14

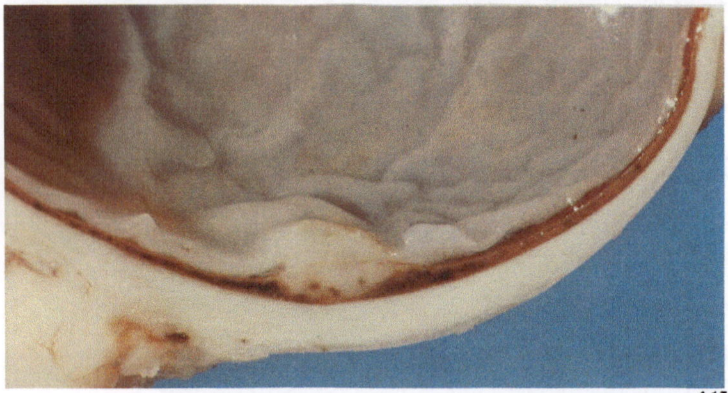

4.15

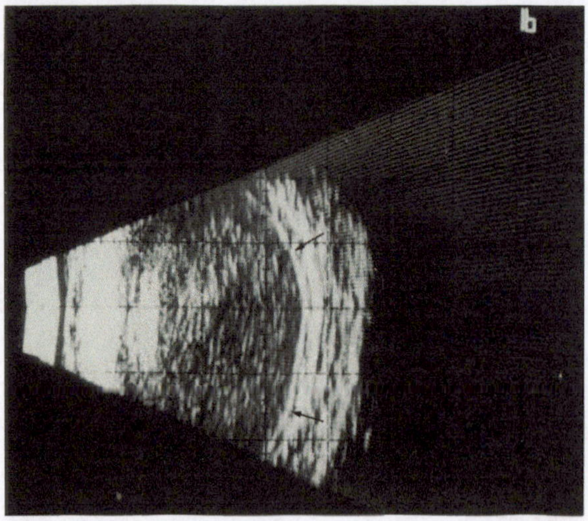

4.15 A

Intermediate Uveitis (Chronic Cyclitis, Pars Planitis)

Pars planitis is an unusual bilateral chronic cyclitis of unknown cause in young adults often without major clinical symptoms. Examination posterior to the lens shows some inflammatory cells in the anterior vitreous and round white agglomerations of cells in the lower vitreous. "Snowbanks" and "snowballs" may be present. Complications are perivasculitis, chronic cystoid macular edema, posterior subcapsular cataract, and scarring over the ciliary body.

Fig. 4.14. Many small whitish-gray nodular agglomerations of cells ("snowballs") overlying the pars plana. M 38/85: Autopsy eye of a 22-year-old male who died during a traffic accident.

Posterior Uveitis

Posterior uveitis has various endogenous causes and in many patients is nonspecific and recurrent. Metastatic posterior uveitis is fairly uncommon. In choroiditis, only the choroid is involved while in chorioretinitis, the inflammation also affects the retina. If the posterior pole including the overyling macula is involved by the inflammatory process, the visual acuity is dramatically and permanently impaired.

Chorioretinitis

Fig. 4.15. Nodular thickening and inflammatory infiltration of the posterior choroid with similar changes in the overlying retina. M 1097/77: Autopsy eye. No medical history available.

Fig. 4.15 A. Uveitis. Contact B-scan of an eye with diffuse dense opacities indicating cellular infiltration of the vitreous and diffuse thickening of the choroid (*arrows*).

Chorioretinitis Scar

Fig. 4.16. Large chorioretinal scar in the periphery of the fundus with hyperpigmentation and depigmentation. From the macroscopic appearance it may be speculated that toxoplasmosis was the cause of this scar. M 1140/77: Autopsy eye with diabetic retinopathy. Details of the medical history are not available.

Fig. 4.17. Total retinal detachment. Marked fibrosis (possible posthemorhagic) at the level of the pigment epithelium. Retrolental membrane and cataract formation. Ciliochoroidal detachment. M 148/81: 71-year-old woman with a long history of recurrent posterior uveitis.

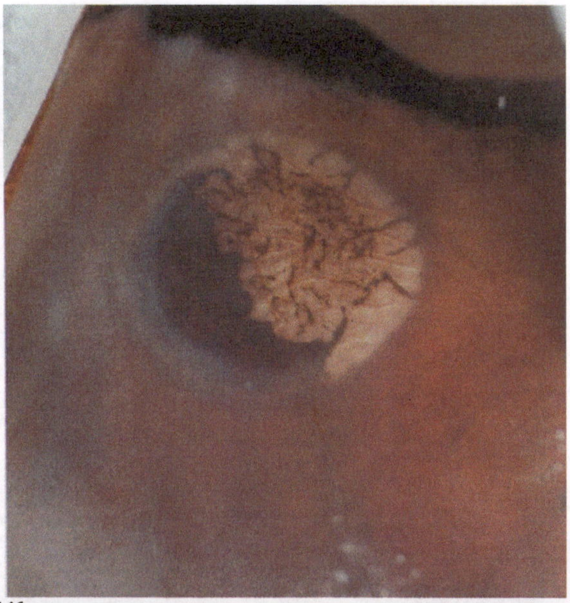

4.16

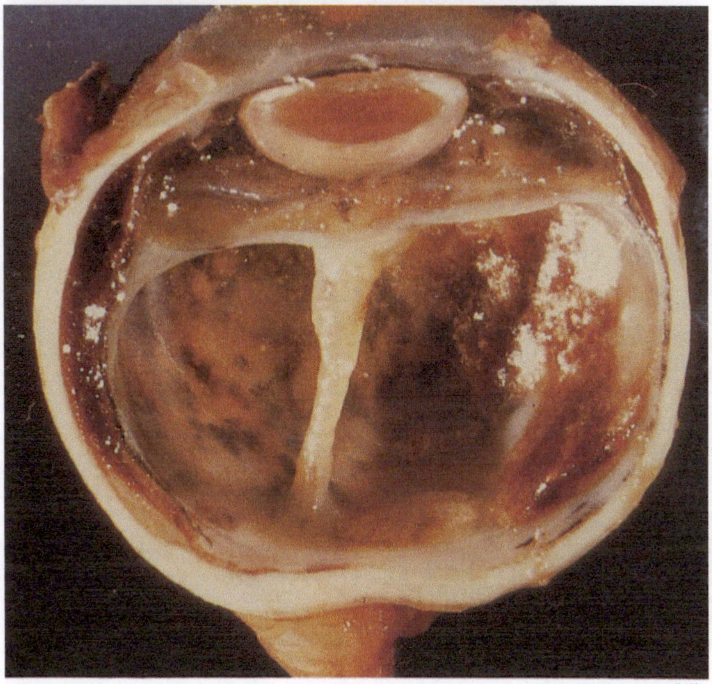

4.17

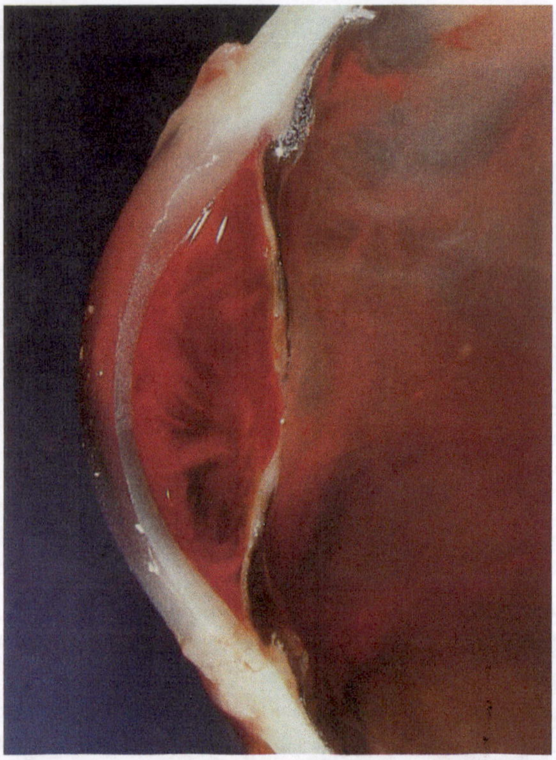

4.18

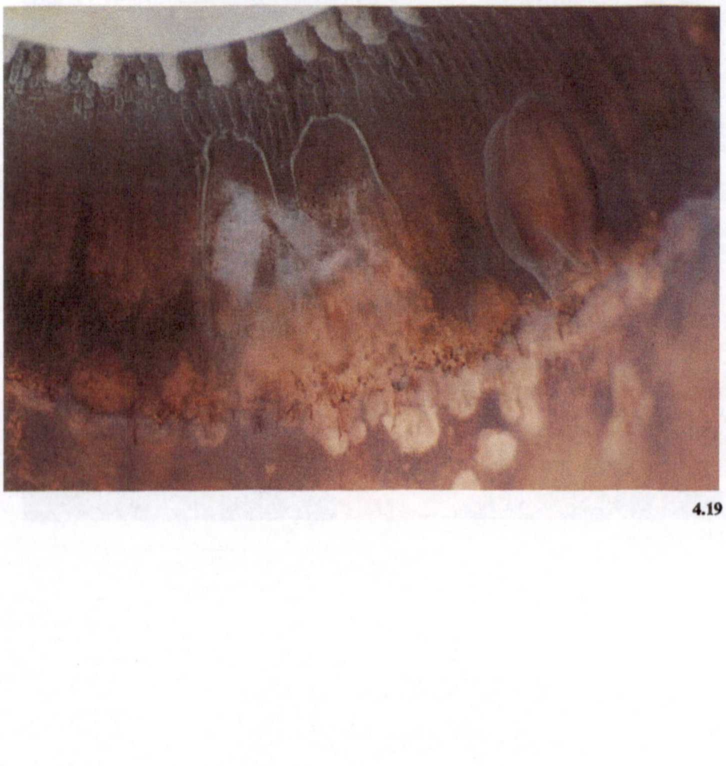

4.19

Hyphema

Anterior chamber hemorrhage (hyphema) from iris or ciliary body blood vessels may result from trauma, inflammation, or develop spontaneously in rubeosis iridis and tumors. Traumatic hyphema, although rapidly adsorbed in most cases, has a tendency to recur. Secondary glaucoma and corneal blood staining are complications of hyphema.

Fig. 4.18. Fresh hemorrhage into the anterior chamber (hyphema) with hemorrhagic imbibition of the cornea and vitreous. M 774/84: 85-year-old man with absolute neovascular glaucoma following central artery occlusion and acute intraocular hemorrhage. Cataract extraction had been performed 8 years prior to enucleation.

Degeneration

Pars Plana Cysts

Pars plana cysts (see also Fig. 1.11) are a localized separation of the nonpigmented from the pigmented ciliary epithelium. With age and in multiple myeloma they are increasingly common. In the latter condition they appear as opaque cysts in the formalin-fixed eye. They are of little clinical importance and are only rarely noticed in indirect routine ophthalmoscopy. Sometimes proliferation of ciliary body blood vessels and connective tissue into the cyst (so-called Snell's plaque) with reactive proliferation of adjacent ciliary epithelium is seen macroscopically at grossing. In rare instances hemorrhage into a cyst may occur and cause diagnostic problems.

Fig. 4.19. Large pars plana cysts with pigment disturbance. Two contain some grayish tissue (Snell's plaque). Additionally there is some cobblestone degeneration at the ora serrata. M 1181/80: Autopsy eye without medical history.

Fig. 4.20. Marked Snell's plaque with reactive proliferation of adjacent pigmented ciliary epithelium.

Fig. 4.21. Cross section of a large pars plana cyst showing the separation of the two ciliary epithelial layers with communication between the cysts. There is artifactitious mechanical impression of the ciliary body tissue. The wide open supraciliary space is regarded as an artifact and not a true ciliochoroidal detachment. M 386/79: Autopsy eye without medical history.

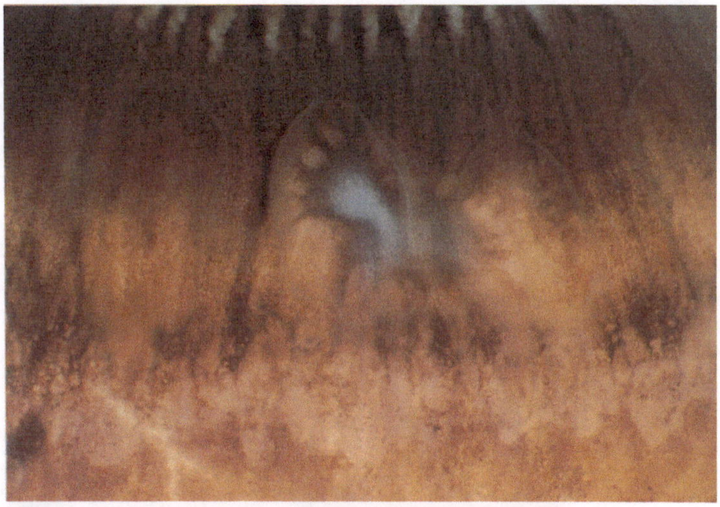

4.20

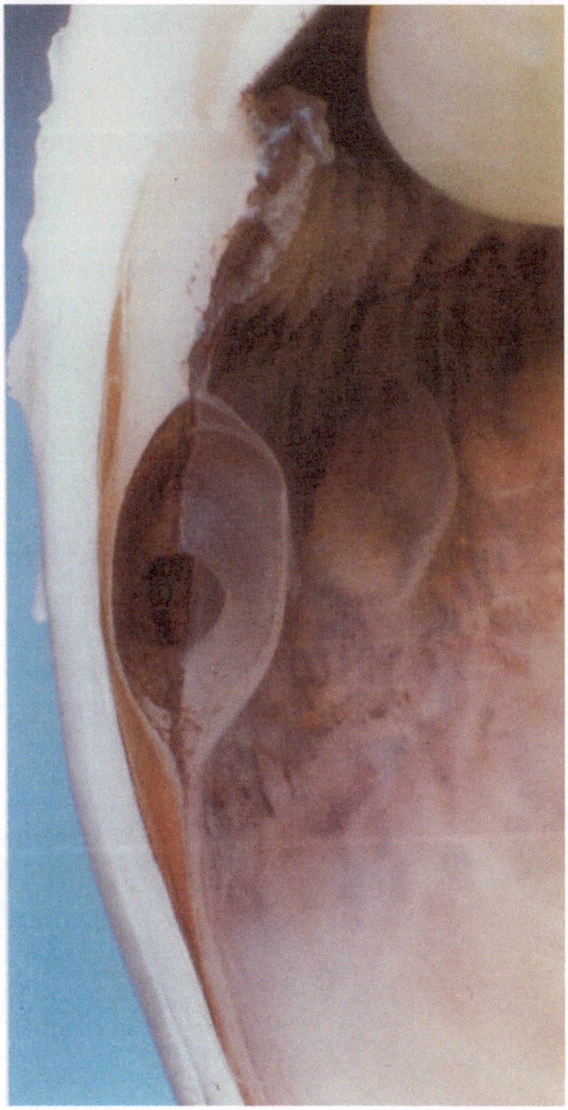

4.21

5. Retina

Congenital anomalies · Inflammation · Vascular disease · Degenerations · Retinal detachment · Macular changes

The thin and transparent sensory retina at the inner aspect of the eye translates visual images into information to the brain. Clinically it is of fundamental importance in the visual functions of color vision, peripheral vision, and visual acuity. It can be well studied functionally and morphologically using various tests provided that the optical media (cornea, aqueous, lens, and vitreous) are clear. With opaque media ultrasonography and electrophysiologic tests may still supply valuable structural and functional information about the retina.

Retinal function is dependent on a normal structure and physiology, which may be affected locally or in association with disease of the adjacent tissues of retinal pigment epithelium, choroid or/and vitreous. Congenital malformations, inflammation, vascular disease (vascular retinopathy including diabetic retinopathy), degenerations, and retinal detachment are major causes of visual impairment. Characteristic features of vascular retinopathy such as vascular sclerosis, narrowing of arteries, increased vessel reflexes, and caliber variations are only seen ophthalmoscopically. Macroscopical changes observed in vascular retinopathy are secondary lesions such as retinal exudates, retinal or vitreous hemorrhages, and proliferative retinopathy. Some retinal diseases preferentially affect the macula. They are dealt with later in this chapter. Proliferative retinopathy causing clinical complications due to intravitreal proliferations are presented in chapter 6. Injuries and tumors of the retinae are presented in later chapters. At grossing various artifacts may be observed (see also chapter 1).

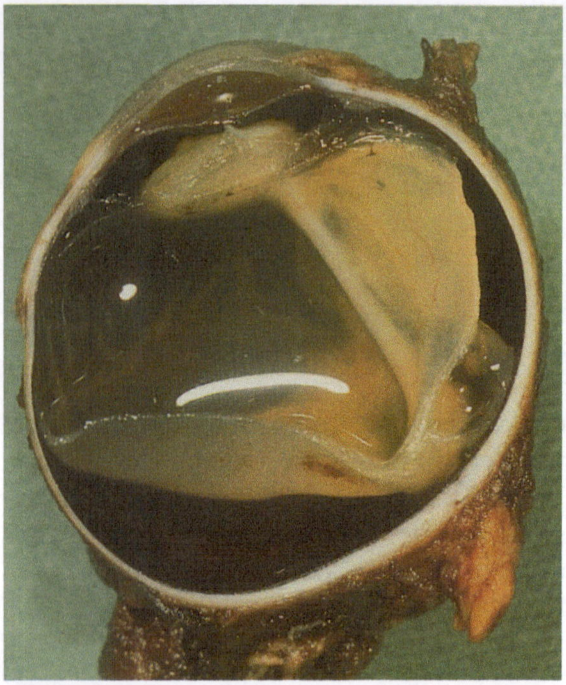

5.1

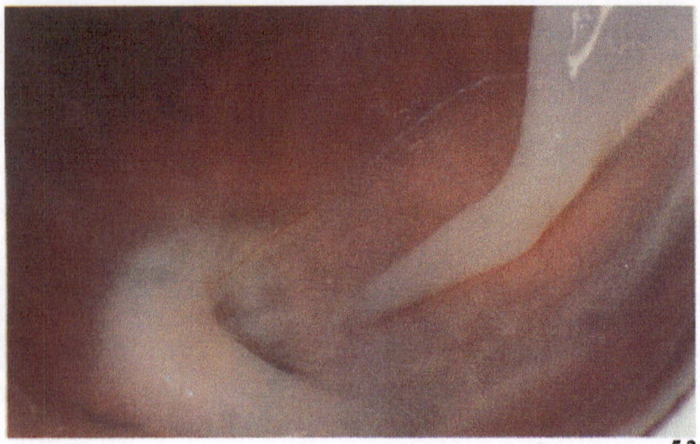

5.2

Congenital Anomalies

Gross anomalies of the retina are rare and if present they are usually associated with marked changes of other intraocular structures. Because of their clinical resemblance to retinoblastoma they are mentioned in the chapter on tumors and pseudotumors. Anomalies associated with uveal colobomas have been shown above in Fig. 4.4. A congenital anomaly associated with the regression of the primary hyaloid system is the congenital (falciform) retinal fold.

Congenital (Falciform) Retinal Fold

This anomaly consists of an inferonasal retinal fold associated with a vascular structure. Typically this fold extends from the optic disc to the nasal back of the lens. But expression is variable and there may only be some distortion of the posterior retina and optic disc.

Fig. 5.1. Thick vascularized strand between the nasal back of the lens and the optic disc. Large retinal fold and retinal detachment (falciform retinal detachment). Partly calcified cataractous lens. M 516/73: 13-year-old boy suffering from absolute glaucoma and cataract since birth.

Fig. 5.2. Congenital (falciform) retinal fold with marked distortion of the optic disc. M 927/82: 3-month-old child with Holtermüller-Wiedemann's syndrome (a congenital dysmorphic craniofacial syndrome that markedly involves the orbit).

Retinal Inflammation

Retinal inflammation may develop at any time of life. It is usually a reaction to organisms (bacteria, viruses, fungi, and parasites) reaching the retina via the blood stream or from adjacent structures. Inflammation without known organisms, such as sarcoidosis, is rare. There is an inflammatory cellular infiltration and edema of the retina and the adjacent structures of retinal pigment epithelium, choroid, and vitreous (see Fig. 4.15). Hemorrhage, retinal detachment, and retinal necrosis may develop. Healing by proliferation of glial tissue and retinal pigment epithelium results in retinal scars.

Prenatal Retinal Inflammation

Important ocular infections in utero are toxoplasmosis (for toxoplasmic chorioretinitis see chapter 4), measles and rubella which causes cataract, glaucoma, and rubella retinopathy.

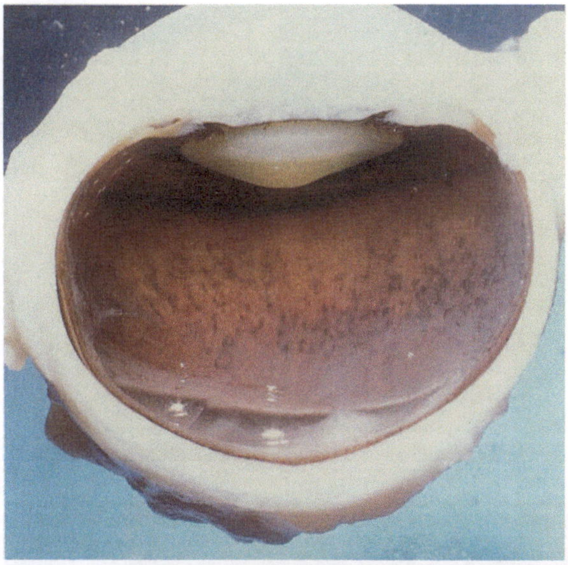
5.3

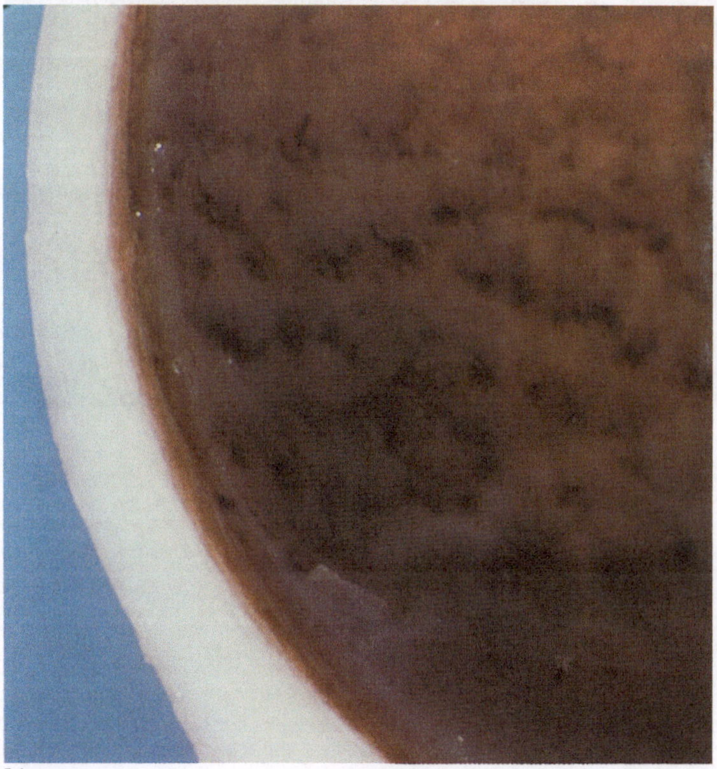
5.4

Fig. 5.3. Rubella retinopathy with hyperpigmented retinal spots and cataract. Additionally there is posterior vitreous detachment and vitreous traction on the retina. M 398/79: 8-year-old boy with history of congenital rubella.

Fig. 5.4. Higher magnification of the hyperpigmented retinal spots in rubella retinopathy.

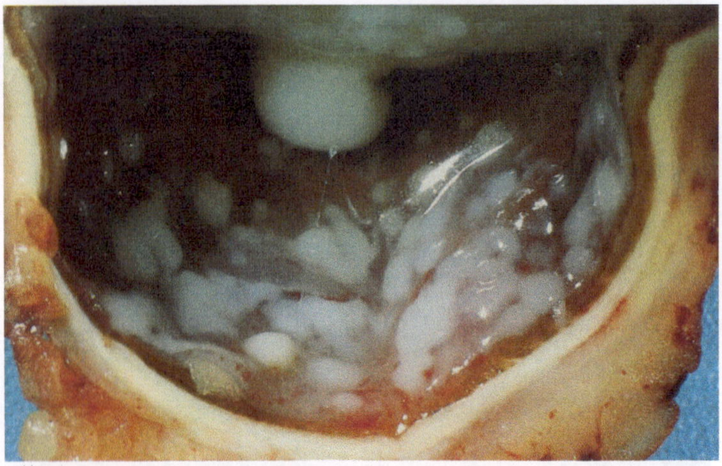

5.5

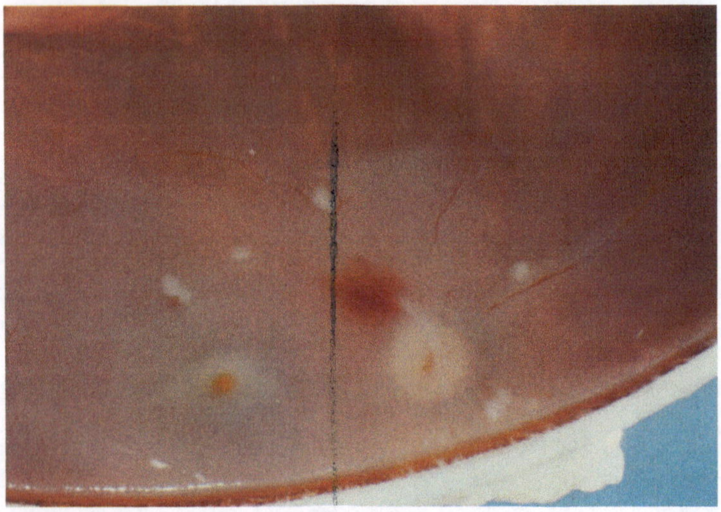

5.6

Metastatic Inflammation

Fig. 5.5. White preretinal inflammatory foci in Candida albicans sepsis. M 636/74: 71-year-old man with diabetes mellitus and leukemia developed Candida albicans sepsis from a venous catheter.

Retinal Vascular Diseases
(Retinal Hemorrhages)

Retinal vascular diseases have various causes. They result in retinal ischemia with edema and venous stasis with intraretinal hemorrhages and may finally lead to secondary vascular reactions such as microaneurysm formation and neovascularization. Except for cotton-wool spots, retinal ischemia is rarely seen macroscopically in pathologic specimens. Retinal and preretinal hemorrhages are a common finding in grossing. They may be seen as a result of venous pressure elevation in autopsy eyes, in neonates, in subarachnoid hemorrhage, and in retinal vein occlusion. They are also a prominent finding in malignant arterial hypertension. In diabetes mellitus, vascular lesions and hemorrhages are especially marked. New vessel proliferation from the retina into the vitreous body may cause tractional retinal detachment, a serious complication of diabetes mellitus, retinal vein occlusion, and retinopathy of prematurity (retrolental fibroplasia). Subretinal hemorrhages usually develop from choroidal blood vessels in disciform degeneration of the macula, choroidal malignant melanoma, or ocular trauma.

Arterial Hypertension

Fig. 5.6. Cotton-wool spots and flame-shaped hemorrhage within the superficial layers of the retina. Autopsy eye without clinical history.

Venous Pressure Elevation

Fig. 5.7. Intra- and preretinal hemorrhages as they are rather commonly seen after birth. M 931/79: Autopsy eye of a newborn with suspected fetal rubella infection.

Fig. 5.8. Large intra- and preretinal hemorrhages around the optic disc as they may develop from final venous stasis at death or following subarachnoid hemorrhage. H 618/80: Autopsy eye without clinical history. Death due to heart failure.

Fig. 5.9. Small hemorrhages into the postequatorial retina. Not the typical finding in subarachnoid hemorrhage (Terson's phenomenon). This type of small hemorrhage into the deeper layers of the peripheral retina is more common in some diabetic patients and Waldenström's macroglobulinemia. M 898/77: Autopsy eye. Death due to massive subarachnoid hemorrhage. Hemorrhage into the optic nerve sheaths was present.

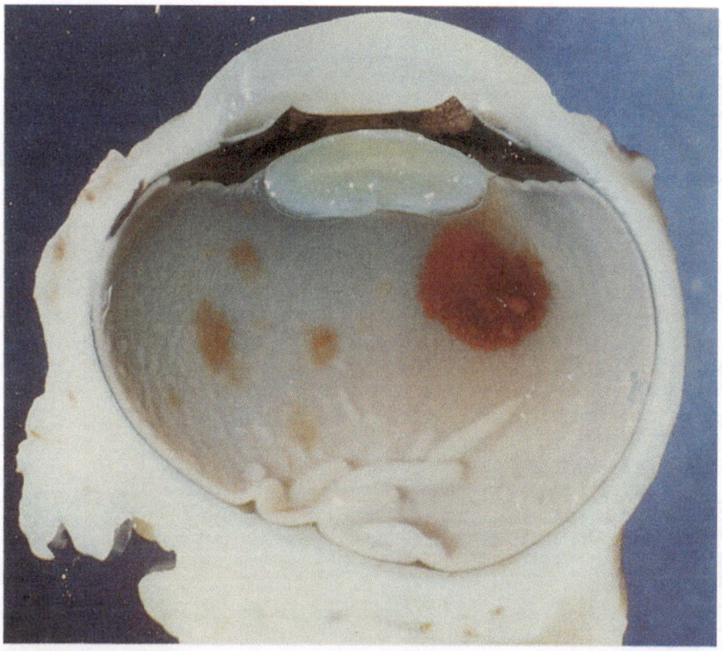

5.7

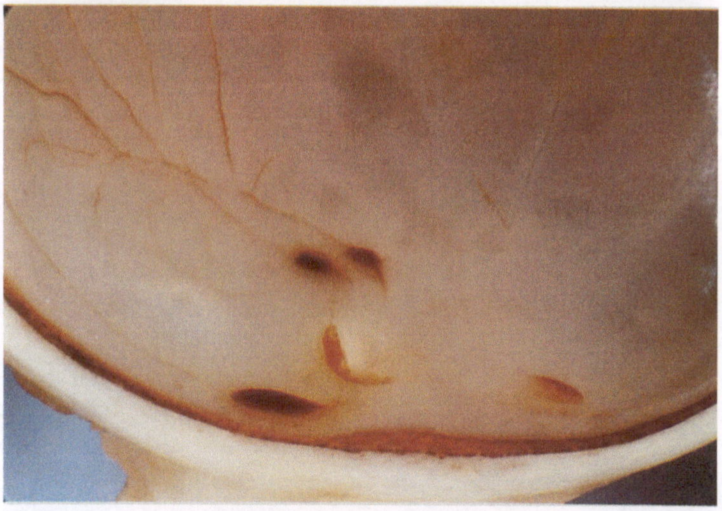

5.8

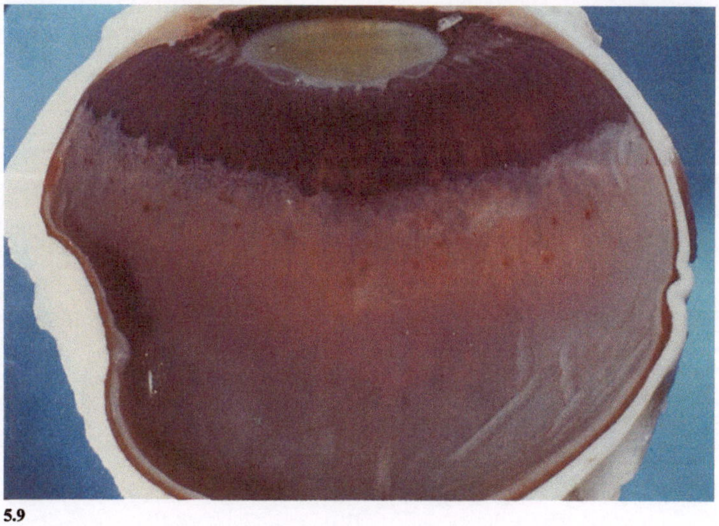

5.9

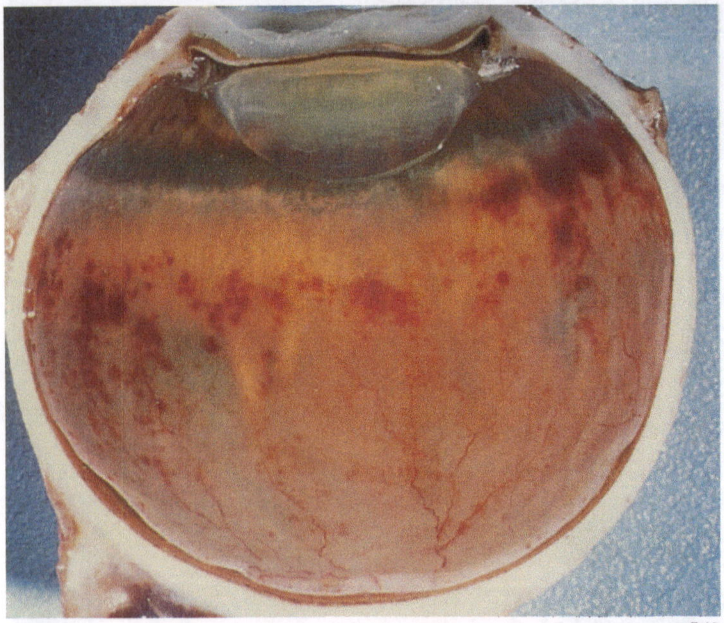

5.10

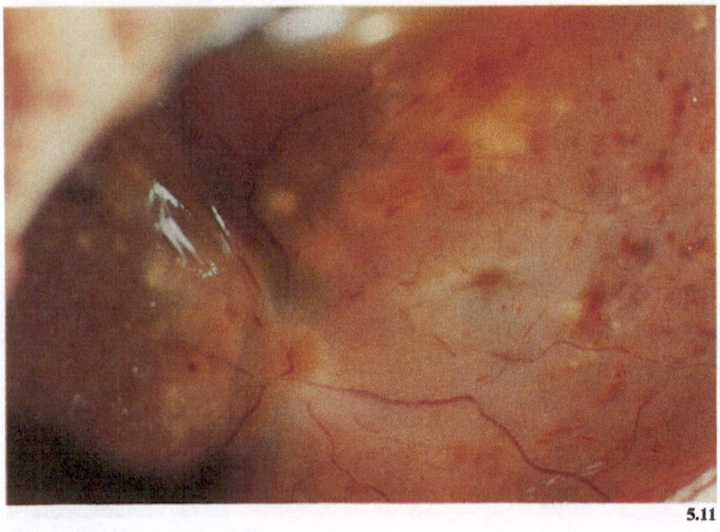

5.11

Retinal Vein Occlusion

Fig. 5.10. Many small deep retinal hemorrhages and microaneurysms. Larger superficial retinal hemorrhages in the periphery of the fundus. M 599/73: 73-year-old male with rubeosis iridis and untreatable glaucoma after central retinal vein occlusion.

Diabetes Mellitus

Diabetic retinopathy is a retinal vasculopathy which leads to permanent blindness when tractional retinal detachment develops. For clinical purposes, a nonproliferative (background) and a proliferative form are differentiated. Background retinopathy consists of intraretinal exudates and hemorrhages from damaged blood vessels, vascular occlusion, and microaneurysms. Treatment today is panretinal photocoagulation to prevent blood vessel proliferation with its attendant complications. In proliferative retinopathy, new vessels grow from the retinal and the optic disc vessels into the preretinal vitreous body. In rare cases, the normally progressive proliferation of new vessels arrests spontaneously. Tissue contraction along with proliferation of vessels into the vitreous leads to retinal detachment. Massive hemorrhage into the vitreous may occur. If rubeosis iridis develops, secondary glaucoma may develop, which does not respond well to pressure-lowering procedures. Intraocular microsurgical vitrectomy is sometimes helpful in these patients.

Fig. 5.11. Marked diabetic background retinopathy with retinal edema of the posterior pole, many small retinal hemorrhages, and yellow intraretinal exudates. M 963/81: 71-year-old woman with nonproliferative diabetic retinopathy. The eye was enucleated for malignant melanoma.

Fig. 5.12. Posterior segment of the eye showing intra- and preretinal hemorrhages as well as hemorrhages into the vitreous. The retina is partially detached due to epiretinal proliferation. The yellow nonpigmented dots represent chorioretinal scars after xenon photocoagulation. M 2/76: Advanced stage of diabetic proliferative retinopathy with neovascular glaucoma due to rubeosis iridis in a 56-year-old male.

Fig. 5.13. Proliferative diabetic retinopathy and early endophthalmitis with some inflammatory infiltration of the vitreous. M 388/79: Autopsy eye of a diabetic patient without detailed clinical history. The patient died from septicemia.

Fig. 5.14. Vitreous strands from proliferating retinal blood vessels and retinal folds from fibrous contraction. Same patient as previous Fig. 5.13.

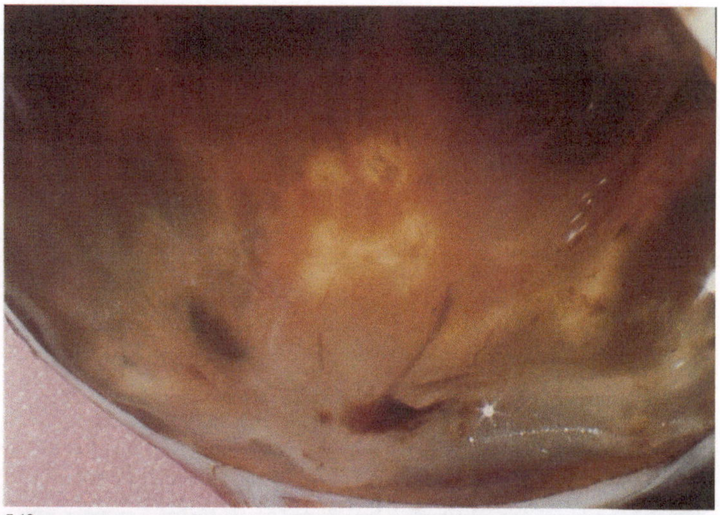

5.12

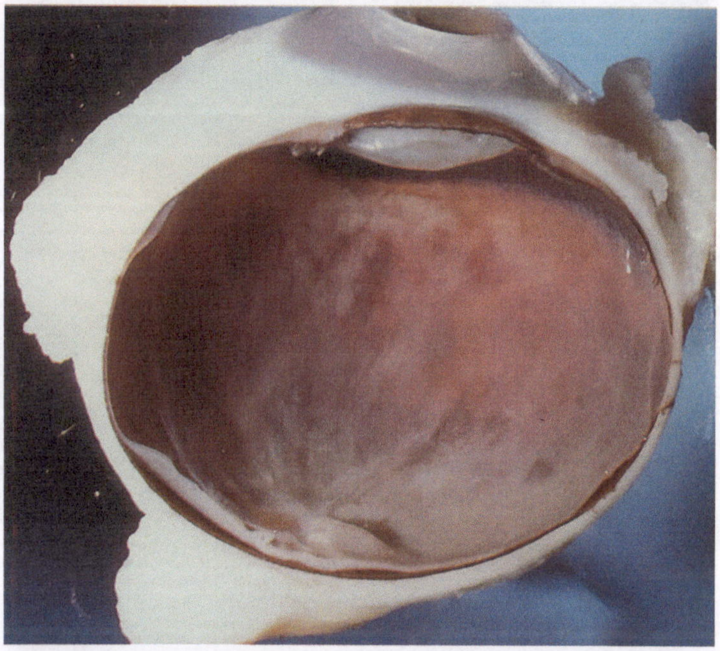

5.13

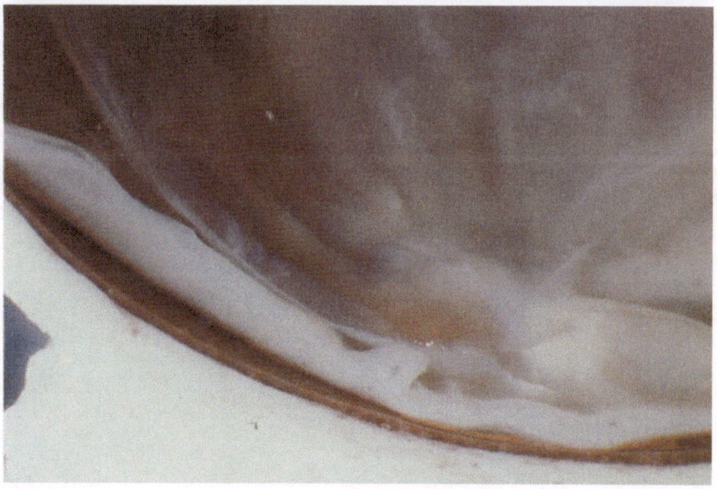

5.14

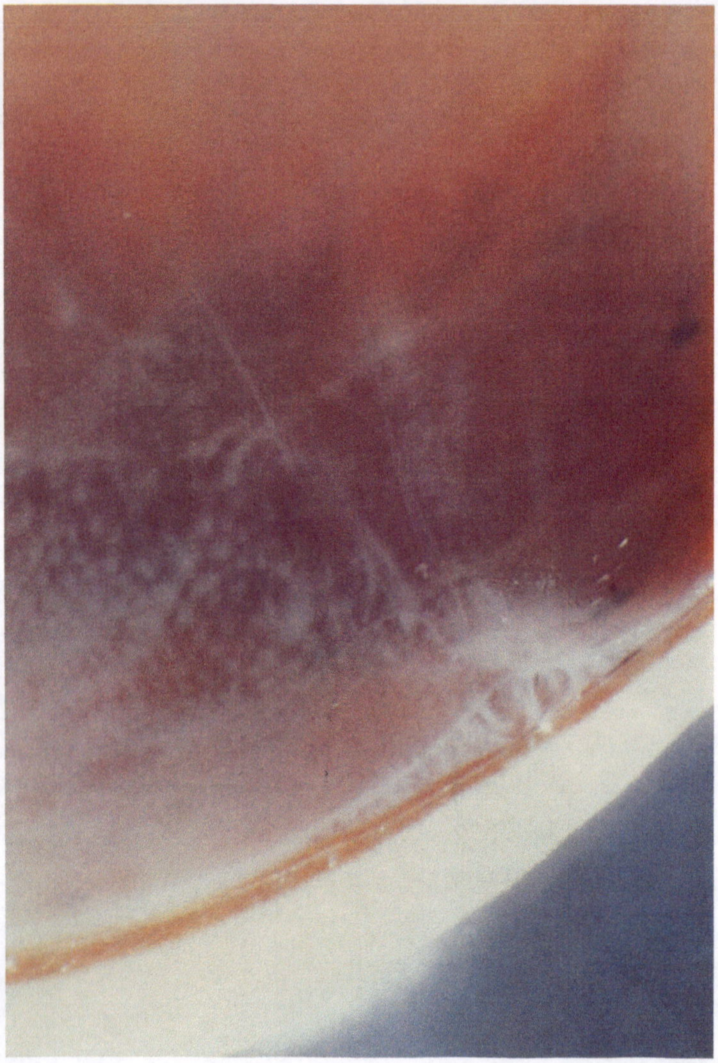

5.15

Fig. 5.15. Secondary cystoid degeneration of the retina at the site of vitreous traction.

Fig. 5.16. Retinal detachment in proliferative diabetic retinopathy with chorioretinal adhesions after photocoagulation. Protein leakage into the vitreous which remains attached. M 734/75: 50-year-old man. Diabetes mellitus recognized for 6 years. Xenon-arc photocoagulation had been performed eight times in this eye. Enucleation for neovascular glaucoma.

Fig. 5.16 A. Proliferative diabetic retinopathy. Contact B-scan echograms (examination with Ophthascan-S B-scan / Biophysic Medical) of traction retinal detachment in proliferative diabetic retinopathy with tent-like or hammock-like appearance. **a** posterior vitreous detachment (*small arrows*). **b, c** Sections at vitreoretinal adhesions (*arrows*). **d** Retinal stalk at the optic disc (*ON* = optic nerve).

Fig. 5.17. Total retinal detachment in proliferative diabetic retinopathy with chorioretinal adhesions after photocoagulation. M 270/81: 54-year-old man. Diabetes mellitus known for 5 years. Xenon-arc photocoagulation had been performed several times. Enucleation for neovascular glaucoma.

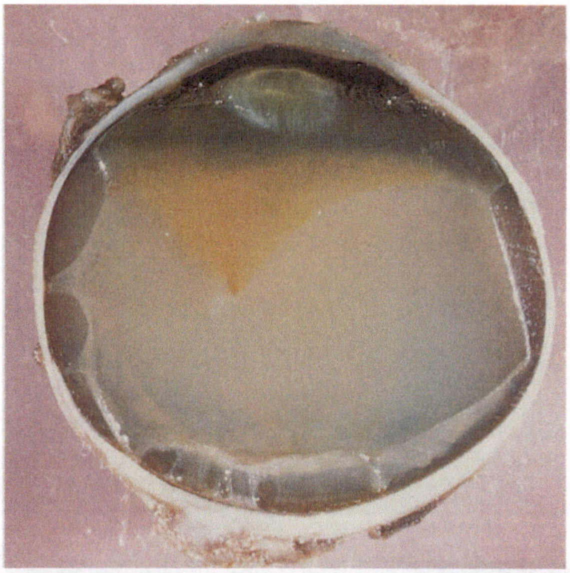

5.16

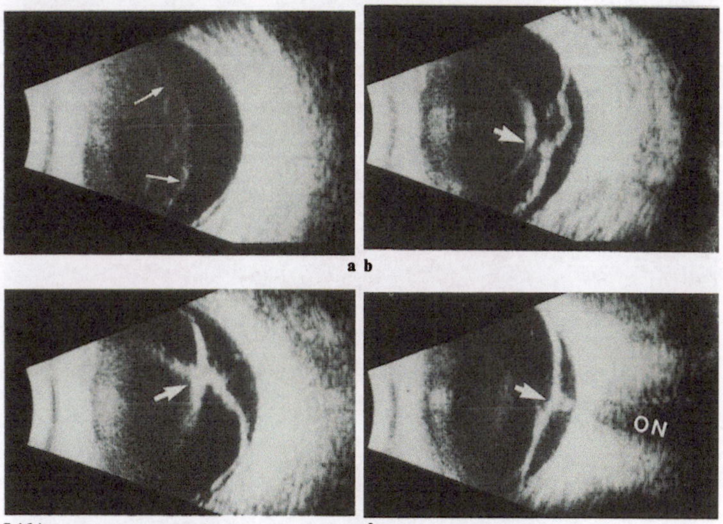

a b

c d

5.16A

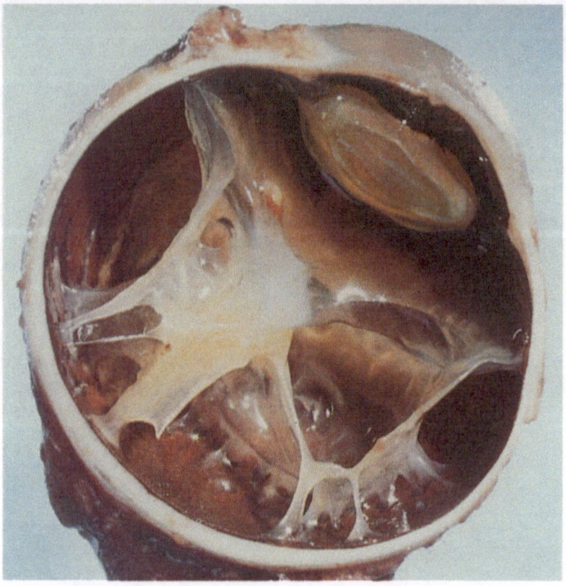

5.17

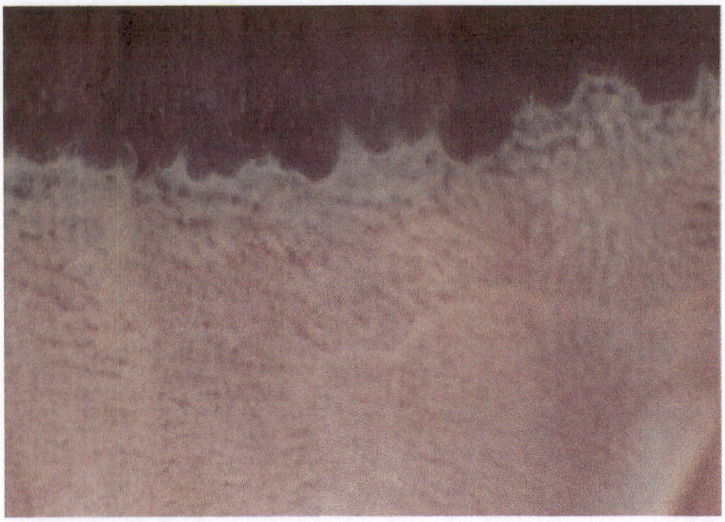

5.18

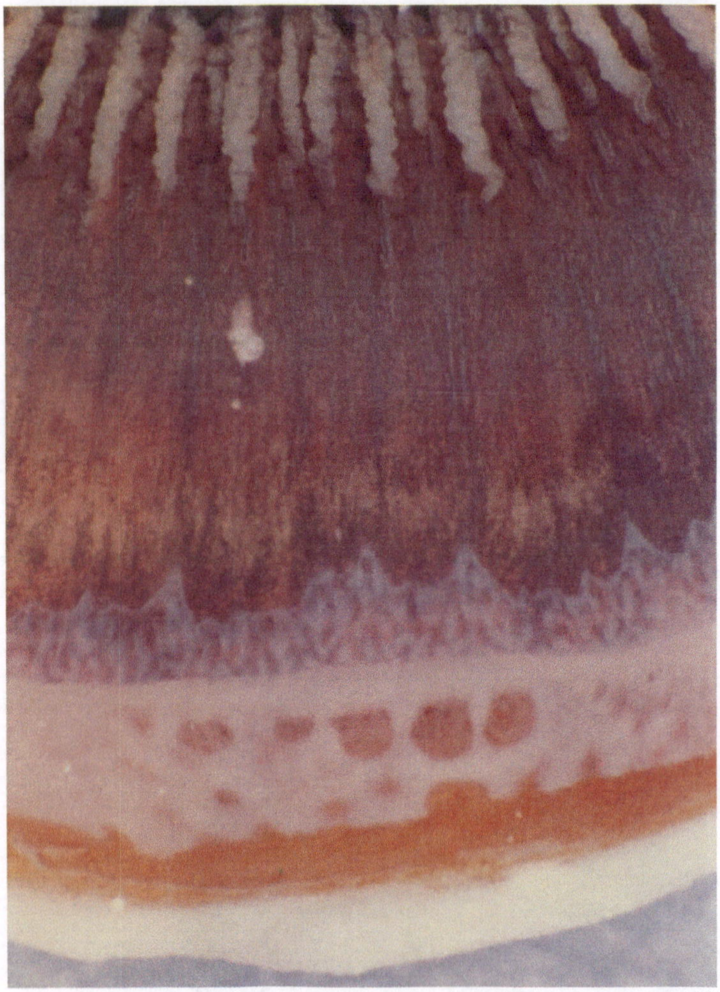

5.19

Retinal Degenerations

Changes of the normal dual oxygen supply of the retina as well as changes in the adjacent choroid and/or vitreous result in structural degenerative retinal lesions such as cystoid retinal degeneration, retinoschisis, lattice degeneration, retinal holes, and tears.

Peripheral Cystoid Degeneration

Two types are differentiated: Typical peripheral cystoid degeneration (Blessig-Iwanoff cysts) and reticular peripheral cystoid degeneration. Blessig-Iwanoff cysts are very common bilateral cystic degenerations of the peripheral retina at the level of the outer plexiform layer which represents the borderline between retinal and choroidal oxygen supply. They may be seen as early as childhood, but increase in frequency with age. In reticular peripheral cystoid degeneration, the cysts are located in the nerve fibre layer mainly of the inferotemporal retinal periphery. Both types may lead to retinoschisis.

Typical Peripheral Cystoid Degeneration (Blessig-Iwanoff)

Fig. 5.18. Typical peripheral cystoid degeneration of the retina (Blessig-Iwanoff cysts). Autopsy eye without medical history.

Fig. 5.19. Section through typical peripheral cystoid degeneration of the retina Blessig-Iwanoff cysts with elevated cut edge of the retina.

Retinoschisis

Splitting of the retina into two layers results from advanced degenerative cystoid change in the retina. Typical (age-related, senile) degenerative retinoschisis, reticular degenerative retinoschisis, and secondary retinoschisis are differentiated.

Typical (Age-related, Senile) Degenerative Retinoschisis

This type is fairly common in adults and usually appears bilaterally especially in the peripheral inferotemporal and superotemporal retinal quadrants as a round transparent cystoid space in the retina with "beaten metal" appearance of the elevated inner layer wall. Rarely the splitting continues as far back as the posterior pole. Degenerative hole formation may appear in the inner and/or outer wall. Holes in both layers may occasionally lead to retinal detachment.

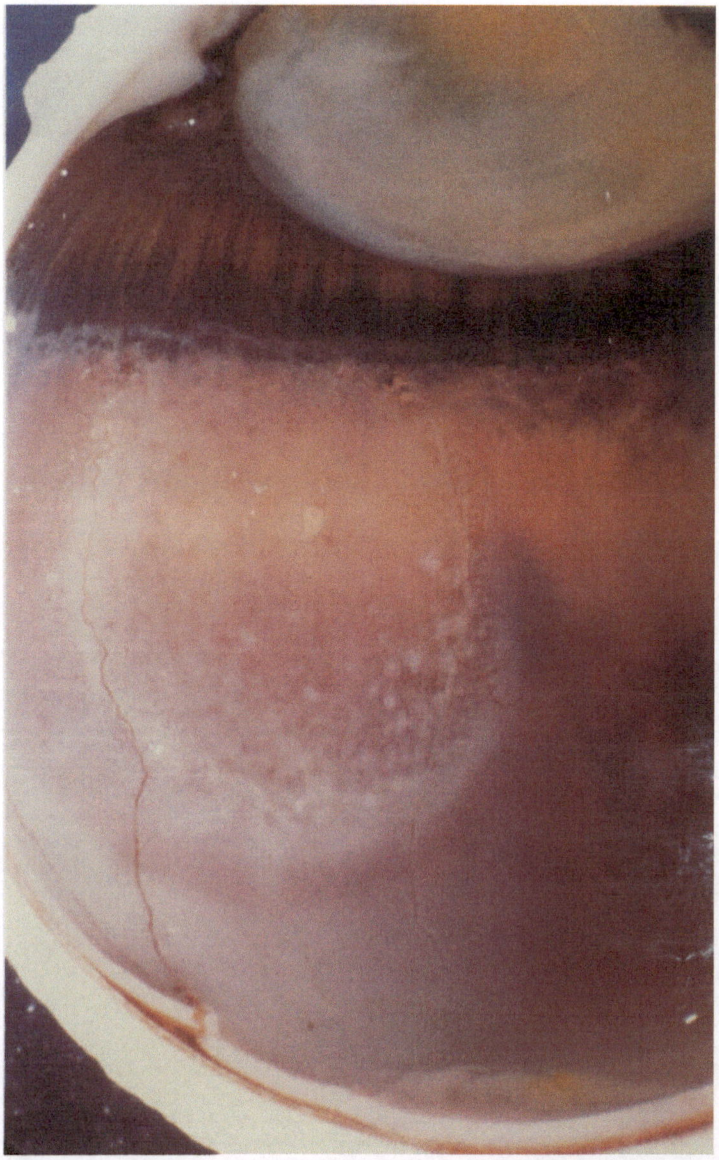

5.20

Fig. 5.20. Typical (age-related, senile) degenerative retinoschisis with whitish dots in the inner wall from the split columnar retinal tissue of peripheral cystoid degeneration. Note that the area of retinoschisis is more transparent than the surrounding artifactitious opaque normal retina. There is yellow nuclear sclerosis of the lens. M 217/77: Autopsy eye without clinical data.

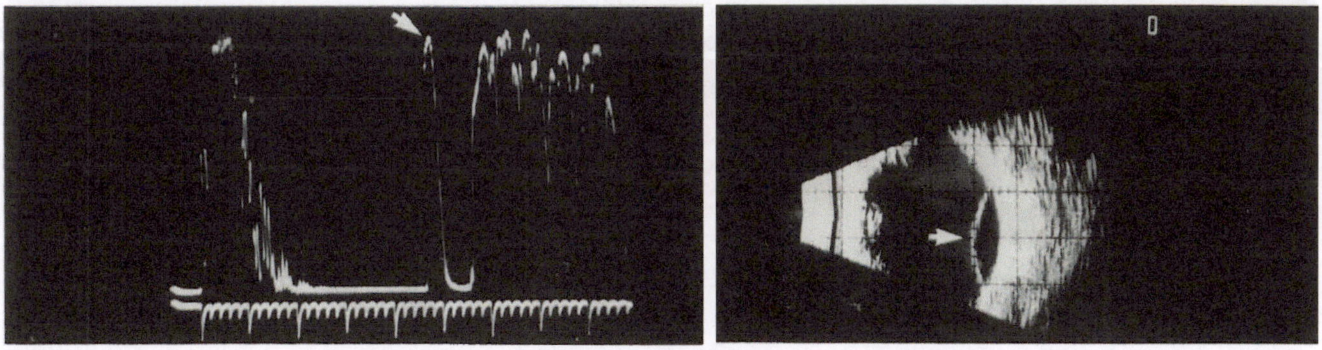

5.20A a b

Fig. 5.20A. Retinoschisis. A-scan echogram (**a**) and contact B-scan echogram (**b**) of typical degenerative retinoschisis (*arrows*).

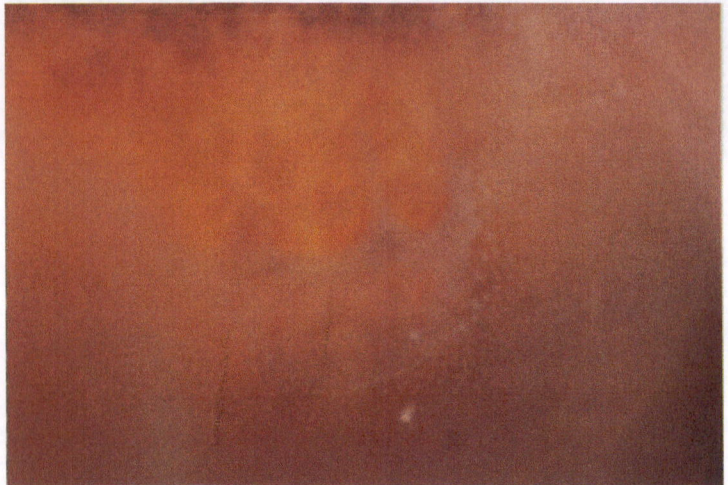

5.21

Fig. 5.21. Degenerative hole formation in the inner wall of typical (age-related, senile) degenerative retinoschisis. M 750/78: Autopsy eye without clinical history.

Reticular Degenerative Retinoschisis

This is an oval or round cystoid space developing from reticular degenerative cystoid retinal degeneration usually posterior to the location of typical degenerative retinoschisis. As retinal splitting occurs in the nerve fibre layer, the elevated inner wall of the retinal cystoid space is so thin that it may be barely visible.

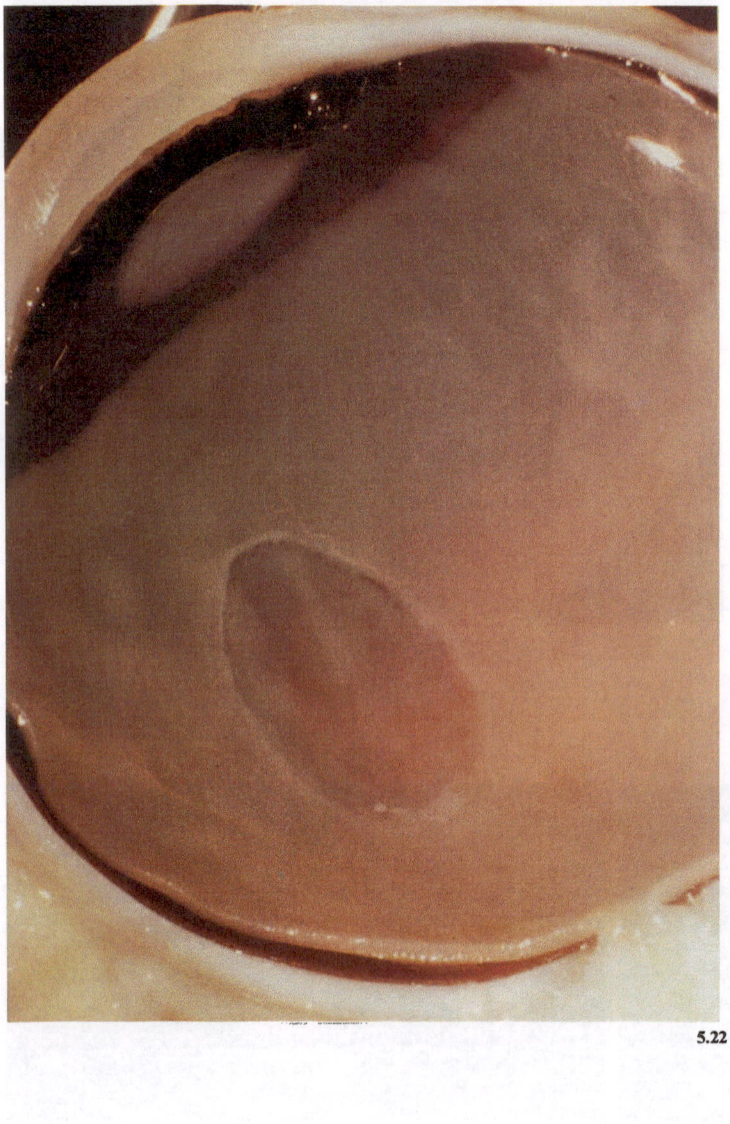

5.22

Fig. 5.22. Large oval-shaped reticular degenerative retinoschisis. The inner wall is not visible macroscopically. Histology showed some retinal dysplasia in the whitish-gray border. M 23/85: Autopsy eye of a $2^1/_2$-month-old infant with trisomy 13–15 (same case as in Fig. 4.4).

Cobblestone (Pavingstone) Chorioretinal Degeneration

Localized choroidal ischemia leads to a sharply outlined loss of outer retinal tissue and associated retinal pigment epithelial changes (degeneration and/or hypertrophy). It is a very common bilateral clinical finding between the equator and the ora serrata especially in the lower quadrants but has very few clinical implications. Extensive cobblestone degeneration has been described in the ischemic eye (e.g., in hypotension).

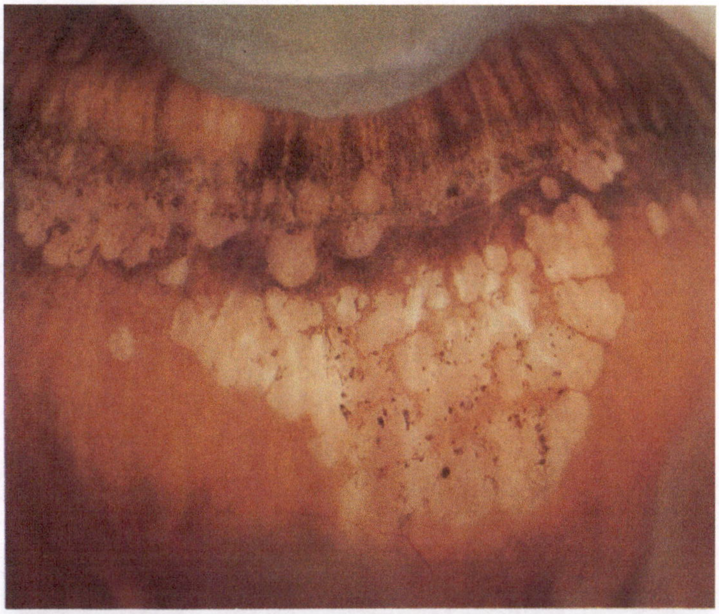

5.23

Fig. 5.23. Confluent cobblestone degeneration in the postequatorial fundus. Autopsy eye without clinical history.

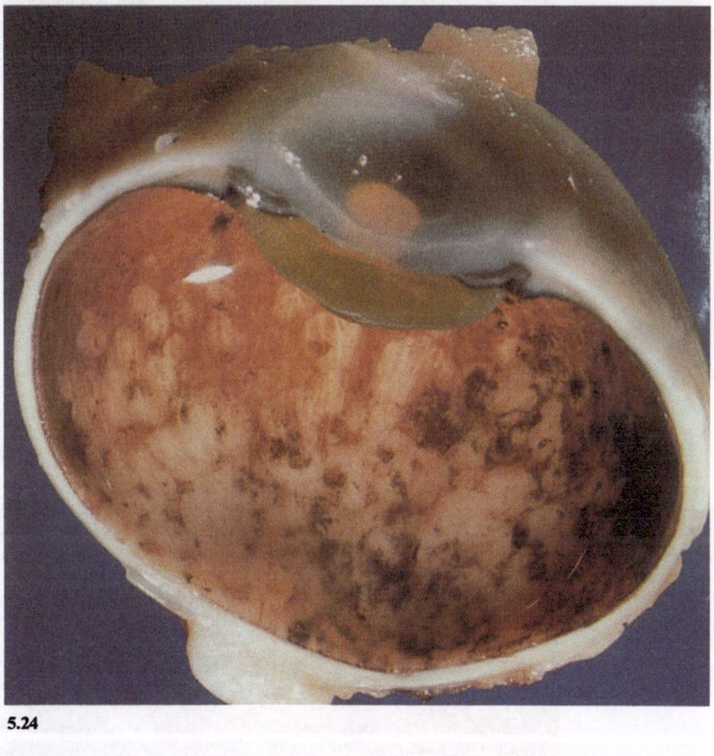

5.24

Fig. 5.24. Extensive confluent chorioretinal degeneration in the posterior segment of the eye. Histology showed signs of arterial hypertension. Small areas of chorioretinal degeneration known as Elschnig spots do occur as a result of hypertensive changes of uveal blood vessels at the posterior pole of the eye. But such extensive lesions are unusual. M 240/78: Autopsy eye of an 85-year-old male without clinical history.

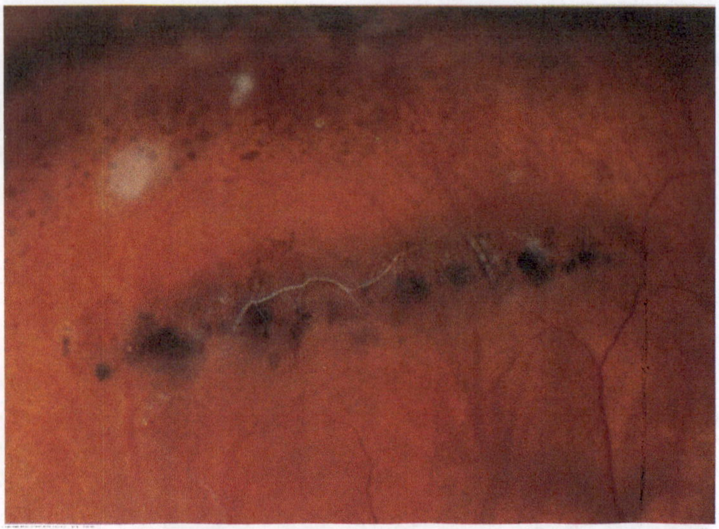

5.25

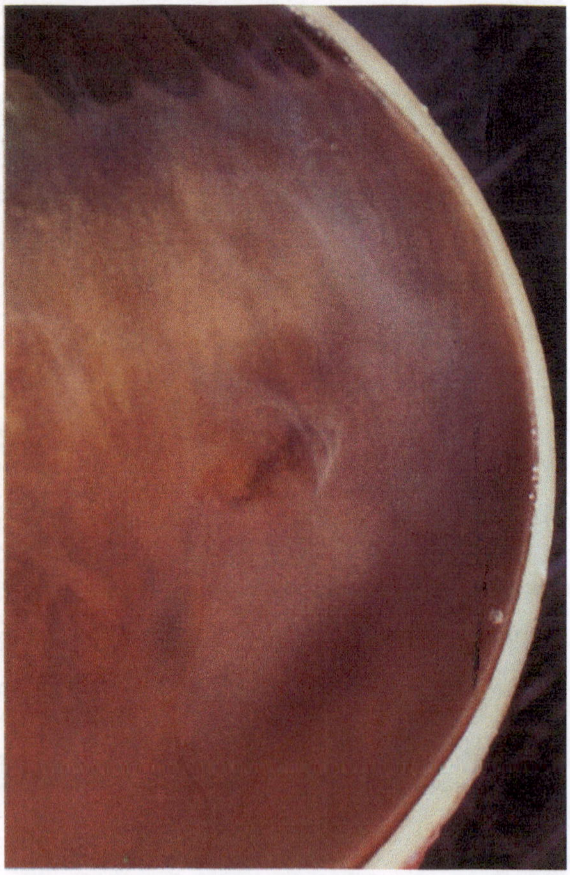

5.26

Lattice Degeneration

The harmless cobblestone degeneration involves the outer layers of postequatorial retina without vitreal changes. By contrast, however, the radially or circularly orientated oval-shaped lattice degeneration involves the inner retinal layers and is accompanied by liquefaction of overlying vitreous and adhesions of vitreous strands at its borders. There may be some hyperplastic reaction of retinal pigment epithelium. Degenerative retinal holes may develop in areas of lattice degeneration. If posterior vitreous detachment occurs, vitreoretinal adhesions at the site of lattice degeneration may produce a retinal pit or tear with subsequent retinal detachment.

Fig. 5.25. Oval-shaped circular lattice degeneration of the equatorial retina with sclerosed retinal blood vessels (white lines) and hypertrophy of retinal pigment epithelium. There is a small round degenerative retinal hole with a small area of local retinal detachment to one side. M 346/75: 71-year-old female enucleated because of malignant choroidal melanoma.

Fig. 5.26. Oval-shaped radial lattice degeneration with overlying vitreous liquefaction and condensations attached to the border of the degenerate retina. M 819/84: 64-year-old male with painful blind eye due to severe herpetic keratitis, iridocyclitis, and glaucoma.

Degenerative Retinal Holes

Degenerative retinal hole formation due to loss of retinal tissue is not infrequently observed within an area of lattice degeneration. The hole is round and sharply outlined as if it were punched out.

Fig. 5.27. Degenerative retinal hole formation in circular equatorial lattice degeneration located posterior to typical cystoid degeneration of the peripheral retina. M 335/80: 43-year-old man with congenitally blind microphthalmic eye and glaucoma.

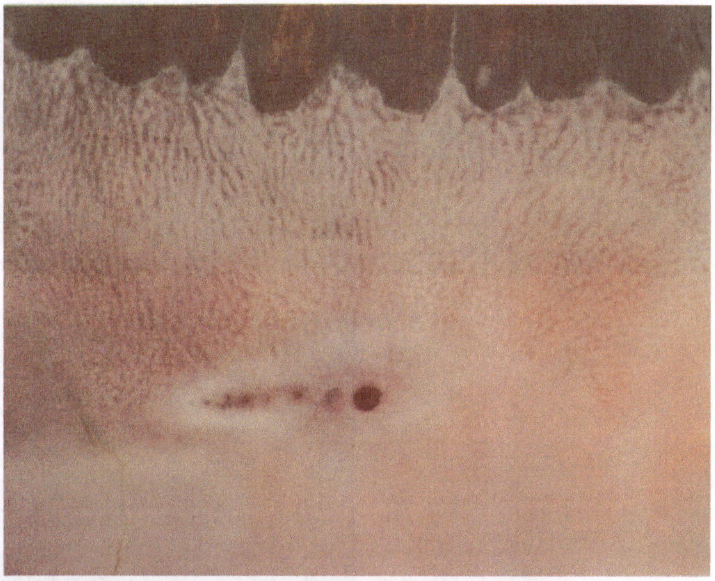

5.27

Retinal Breaks (Pits and Tears)

Retinal pits and tears result from vitreous traction on the retina when involutionary or reactive posterior vitreous detachment develops. If a piece of retinal tissue is completely separated, a retinal pit with a detached operculum results. The operculum floats in the vitreous and undergoes lysis after a time. If retina is incompletely separated, a horseshoe-shaped retinal tear develops. Both types of retinal breaks play an important role in the pathogenesis of retinal detachment.

Fig. 5.28. Horseshoe-shaped retinal tear and surrounding typical peripheral cystoid degeneration of the retina. There is a delicate vitreous strand adherent to the tip of the retinal flap. The retinal tear is the result of traction by this vitreous strand. M 97/77: Autopsy eye without clinical history.

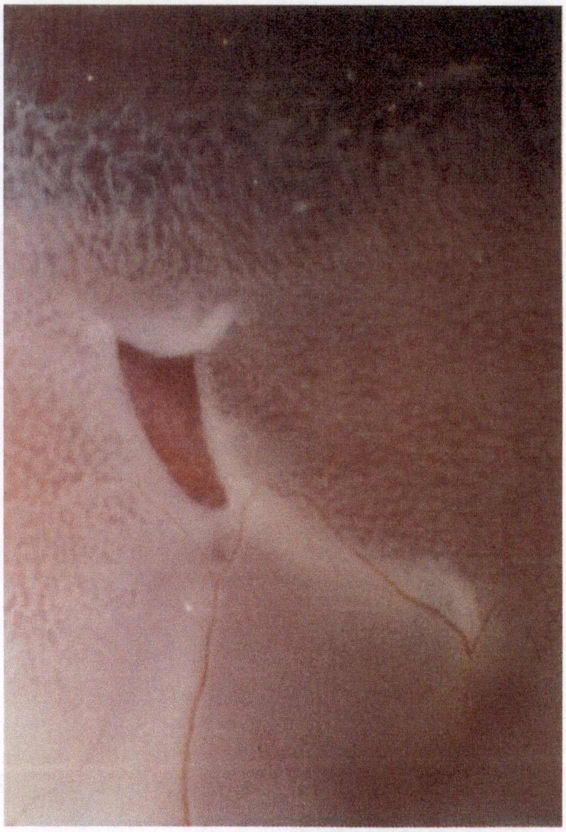

5.28

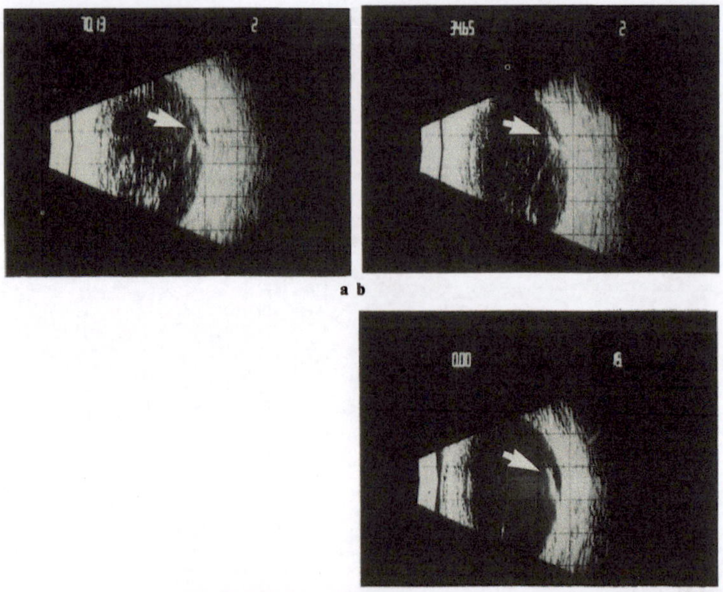

a b

c 5.28A

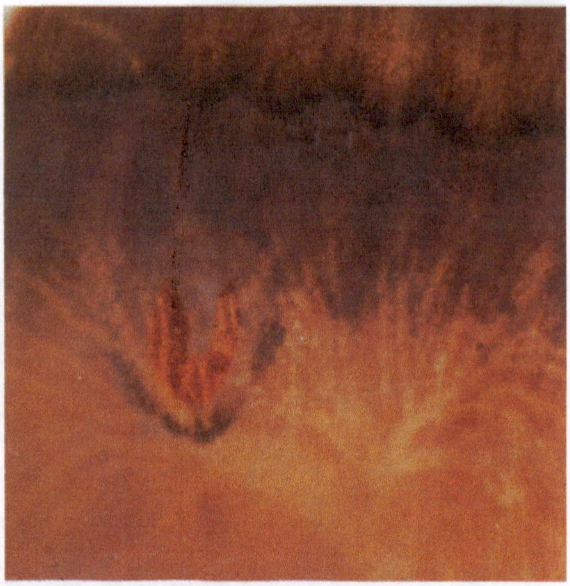

5.29

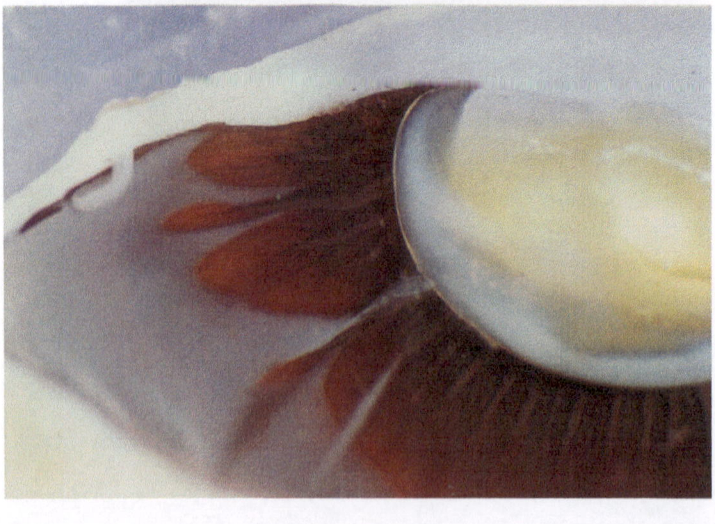

Fig. 5.28A. Retinal tear. Contact B-scan echograms of retinal tear, diffuse vitreous opacities from vitreous hemorrhage, and delicate vitreous adhesion at the retinal flap (**a, b** *arrows*). At reduced sensitivity level (**c**) only the highly reflective retinal tear is displayed (*arrow*).

Fig. 5.29. Horseshoe-shaped retinal tear and surrounding retinal detachment demarcated by hypertrophic reaction of retinal pigment epithelium. M 747/78: Myopic autopsy eye without clinical history.

Meridional Complexes and Retinal Tufts (Tags)

Meridional complexes and retinal tufts (tags) are developmental anomalies often present in otherwise normal eyes. Meridional complexes are anterior extensions of the retina onto the ciliary body. They are a common clinical finding in the superonasal quadrant. The retina posterior to a meridional complex may be somewhat elevated (retinal fold). Retinal tufts (tags) are internal strands of retina which project forward. Traction may lead to cystic retinal degeneration at the retinal insertion site.

Fig. 5.30. Meridional complexes extend forward onto the ciliary body and retinal tufts extend internally forward towards the lens equator. M 642/79: Autopsy eye of a 4-day-old newborn with iris coloboma.

Fig. 5.31. Two retinal tufts with degeneration surrounding the insertion site on the retina. There is also typical peripheral cystoid degeneration of the retina. M 298/81: Autopsy eye without clinical history.

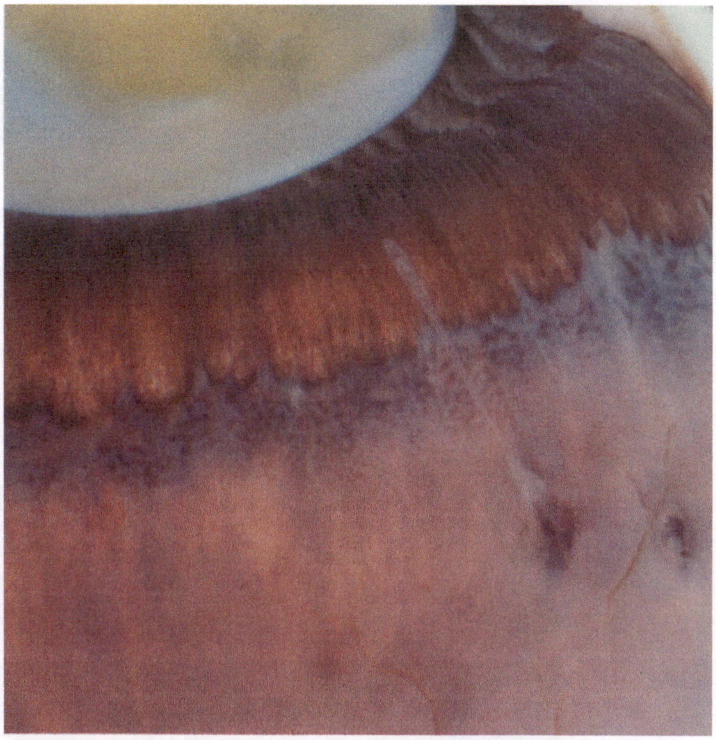
5.31

Ora Pearls

Small yellowish pearl-like structures within dentate processes of the ora serrata may be seen occasionally by ophthalmoscopy and at grossing. They have no clinical implications and are possibly a product of pigment epithelium.

Fig. 5.32. Multiple small yellow ora pearls within dentate processes of the nasal ora serrata. The adjacent retina shows typical peripheral cystoid degeneration. M 464/76: Autopsy eye without clinical history.

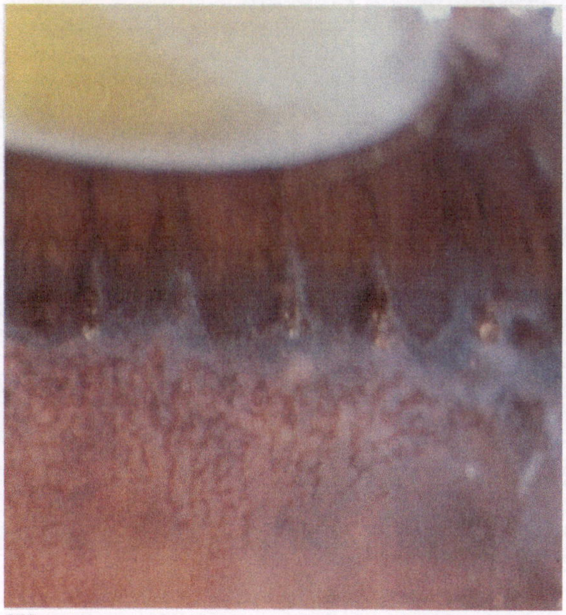
5.32

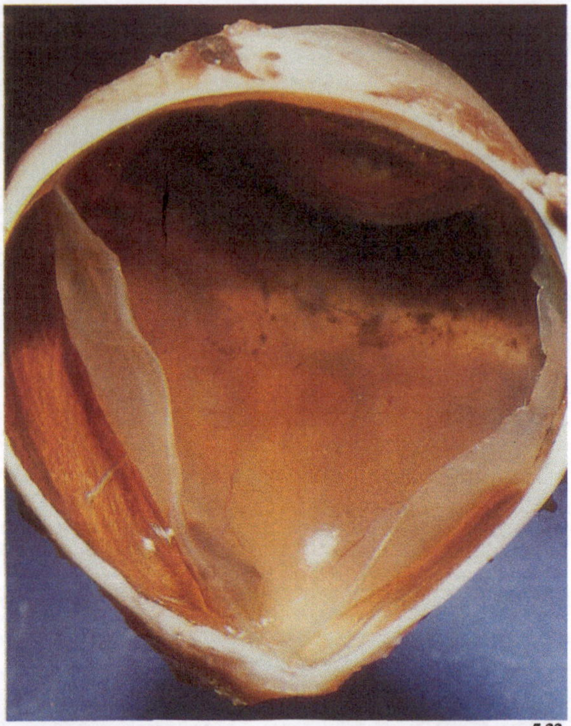

5.33

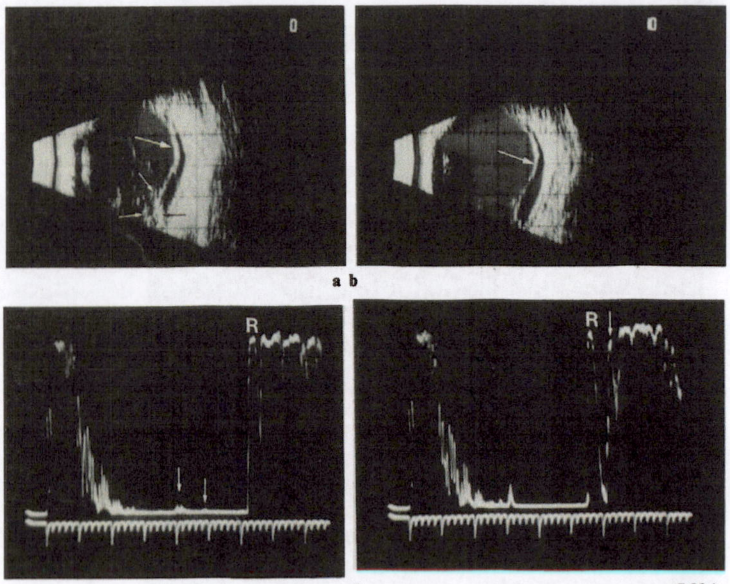

a b

c d

5.33A

Retinal Detachment

The normally weak adhesion of retina to retinal pigment epithelium may fail due to a number of pathologic mechanisms leading to subretinal fluid accumulation, retinal detachment and loss of vision. It may result from a break (degenerative or traumatic), pit or hole in retinal tissue (see above), from barrier dysfunction (inflammation, tumors, retinal and choroidal vascular lesions), from subretinal hemorrhage (retinal or uveal), or vitreous traction (proliferative retinopathy in various diseases). The pathogenesis and secondary tissue reactions in retinal detachment have an impact on the final visual and anatomic prognosis after surgery.

Rhegmatogenous Retinal Detachment

Fig. 5.33. Myopia with posterior staphyloma, total rhegmatogenous detachment and localized peripheral chorioretinal scarring after retinal coagulation. Thin white subretinal strand in the midperiphery and subretinal pigment in the far periphery. M 835/79: 61-year-old myopic female with retinal break and total retinal (rhegmatogenous) detachment.

Fig. 5.33A. Retinal detachment. Contact B-scan echograms (**a, b**) and A-scan echograms (**c, d**) of a shallow, peripheral retinal detachment. **a, b** *long arrows* = retina; *short white arrows* = vitreous opacities; *short black arrow* = subretinal opacities. A-scan echograms show a shallow detachment (*R*), the vitreous opacities (**c** *arrows*) and the subretinal opacities/membranes (**d** *arrow*).

Fig. 5.33B. Retinal detachment. **a** A-scan echogram: Single, very high (100% at "tissue-sensitivity" setting/standardized A-scan; see Table 1/Preface) echo spike of the retina within the vitreous cavity (*arrow*). **b, c** Contact B-scan echograms. **b** Vertical section displaying the insertion of the retina at the disc and moderately high elevation of the retina in the upper part and high elevation of the retina in the lower part of the globe (*arrows* = retina; *ON* = optic nerve; *L* = lens), **c** Horizontal section in a case of a total funnel-shaped retinal detachment (*arrows* = retina; *ON* = optic nerve; *L* = lens).

Fig. 5.33C. Retinal detachment. Contact B-scan (**a, b**) and A-scan (**c**) of a total retinal detachment. Note the attachment of the retina at the disc and the very high reflectivity of the single echo spike that represents the retina (*arrows* = retina; *ON* = optic nerve).

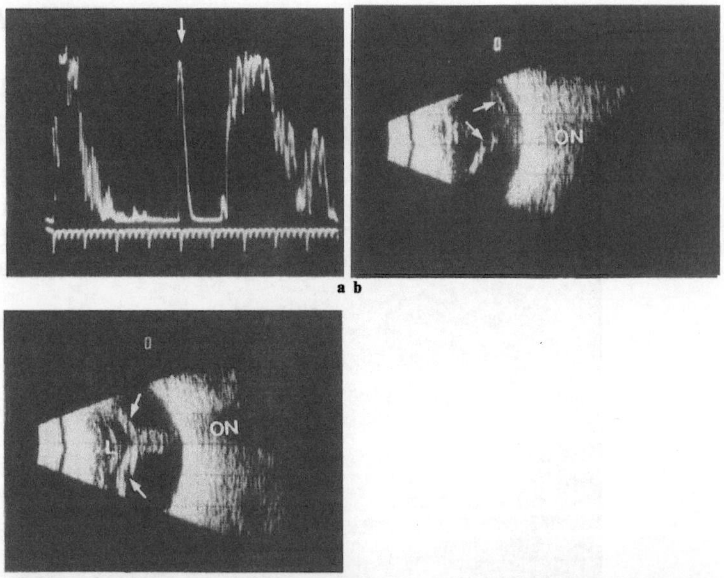

a b

5.33B c

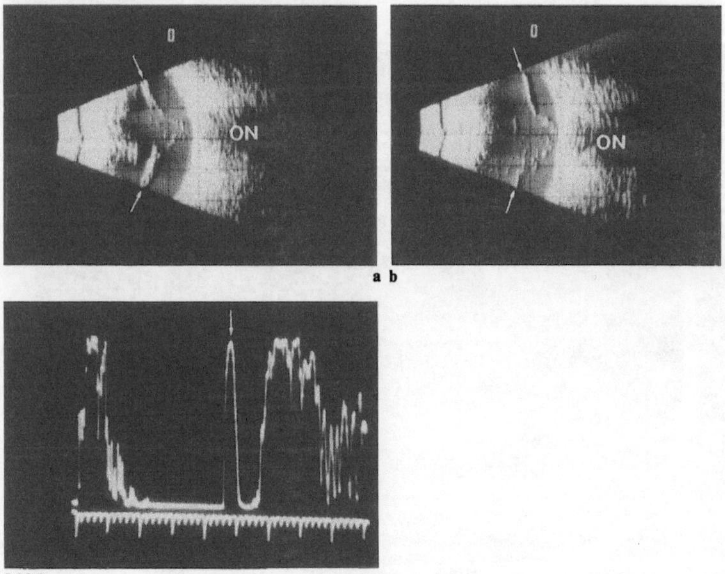

a b

5.33C c

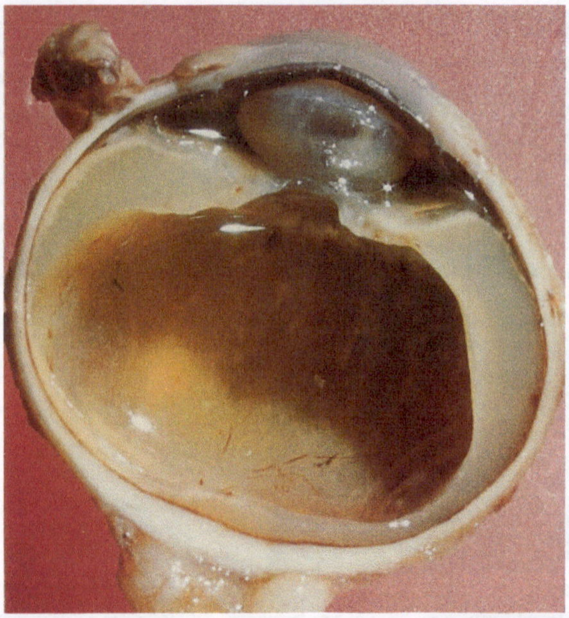

5.34

Exudative Retinal Detachment

Fig. 5.34. Retinal detachment in uveitis. Autopsy eye without clinical history.

Fig. 5.35. Frontal section of the eye showing total funnel-shaped retinal detachment. M 610/74: 63-year-old female with total retinal detachment and history of surgery for breast carcinoma.

Fig. 5.36. Close view into the funnel.

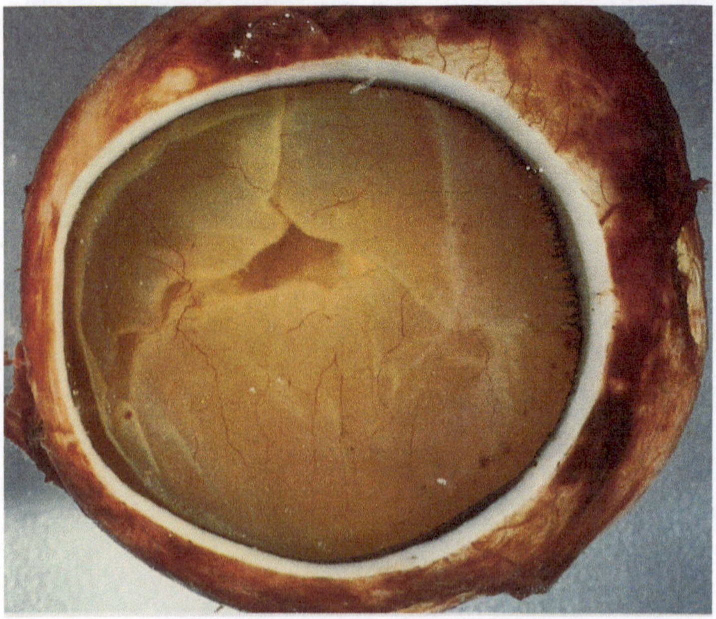

5.35

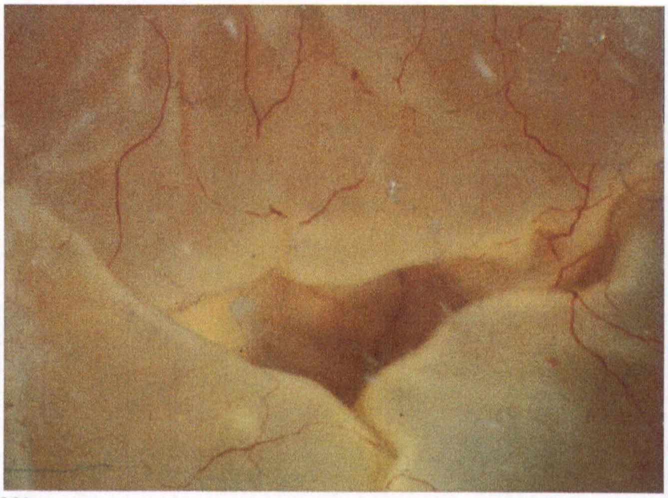

5.36

Tractional Retinal Detachment

Fig. 5.37. Total posterior retinal detachment with vitreous traction on the central retina. M 602/74: 55-year-old male diabetic patient with proliferative diabetic retinopathy and glaucoma.

Fig. 5.37A. Retinal detachment. **a, b** A-scan and contact B-scan echogram of a total retinal detachment. Note the attachment of the retina at the disc (**b**), (*arrows* = retina; *ON* = optic nerve). **c** Contact B-scan echogram of a circumscribed retinal detachment caused by adhesion and traction of vitreous strands (*white arrows* = vitreous strands; *black arrows* = retina).

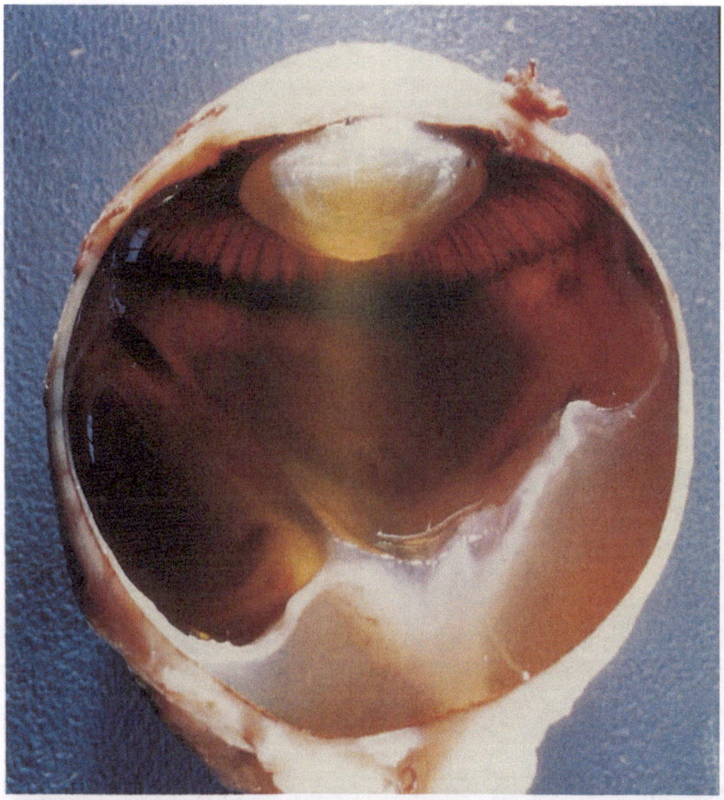

5.37

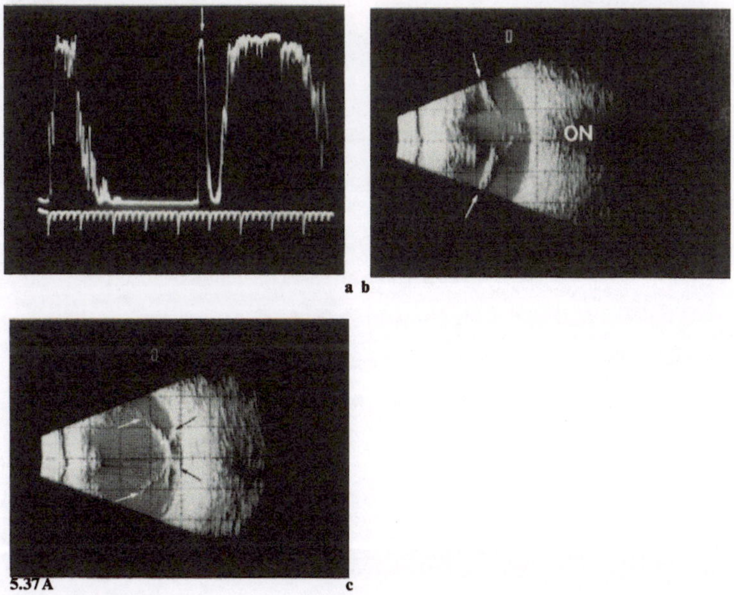

a b

5.37 A c

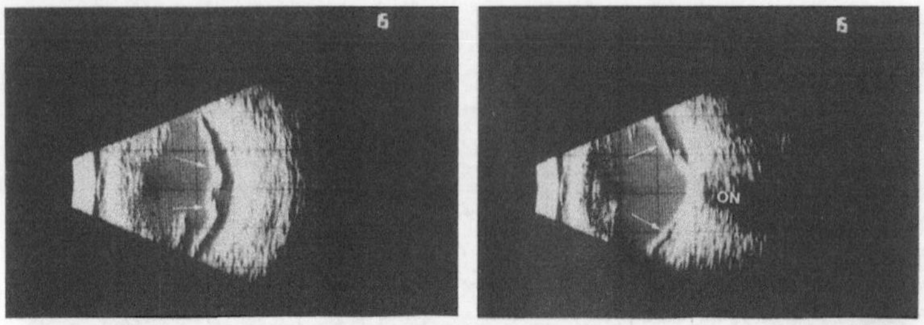

a b 5.37B

Fig. 5.37B. Retinal detachment. Contact B-scan echograms of a total retinal detachment. **a** rather flat elevation of the retina in the temporal periphery with wrinkling of the retina (*arrows*). **b** Vertical section that displays the attachment of the retina at the disc (*ON*=optic nerve) and shows the totally detached retina to be more highly elevated in the upper part and more shallowly detached in the lower part.

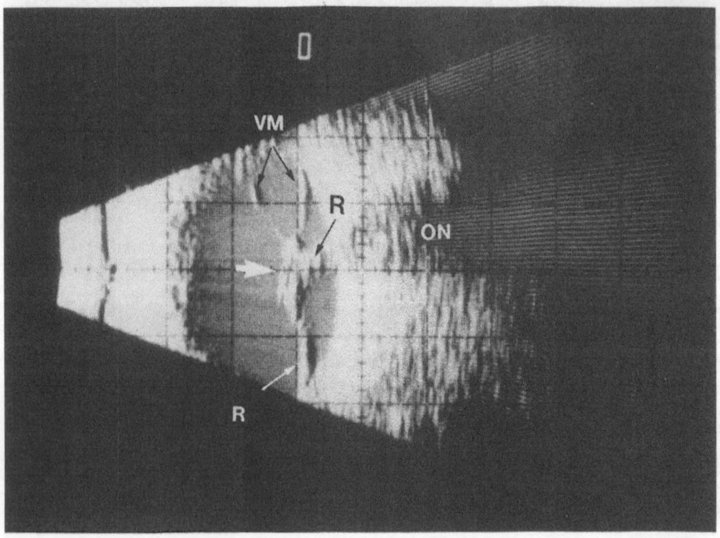

5.37C

Fig. 5.37C. Traction-detachment of the retina. Contact B-scan echogram (horizontal section) of a traction retinal detachment at the posterior pole in proliferative diabetic retinopathy. (*VM*=vitreous membranes; *R*=retina; *thick white arrow*= area of adhesion and traction by multiple epiretinal membranes; *ON*=optic nerve.) Note that the retina is partly dragged over the disc.

Reactive Tissue Changes in Retinal Detachment

In long-standing retinal detachment both the sensory retina and the retinal pigment epithelium show secondary reactive tissue changes. Deposits of crystalline material may occur on the outer aspect of the detached retina (oxalate crystals) in younger patients and at the level of the retinal pigment epithelium (giant drusen).

Macrocystoid Retinal Degeneration

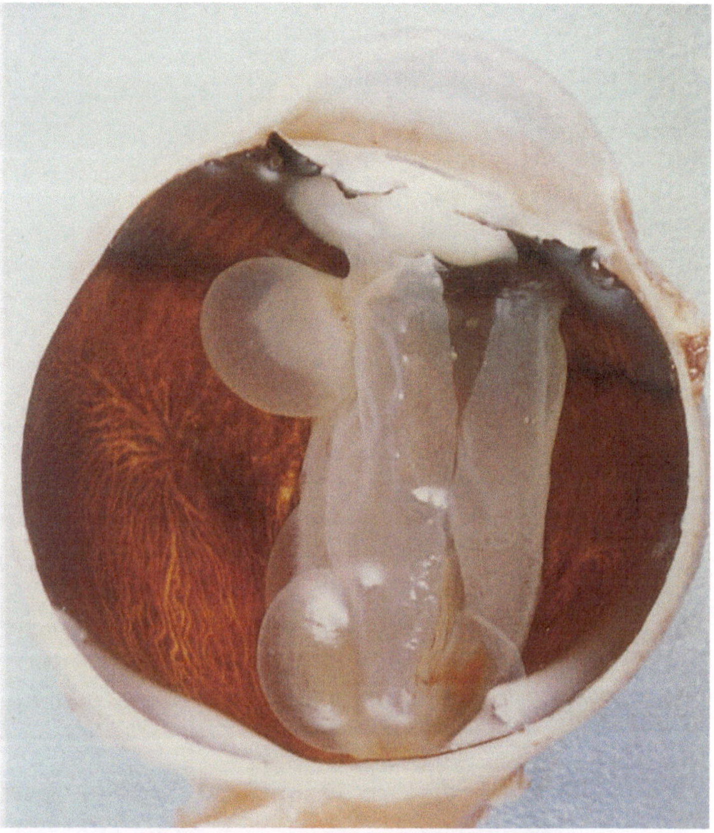

5.38

Fig. 5.38. Macrocystoid degeneration in long-standing total retinal detachment. The retinal detachment also involves the nonpigmented pars plana epithelium. Secondary cataract formation. M 483/72: 26-year-old man with megalocornea, cataract, and scleral staphyloma had been treated with photocoagulation 9 years prior to enucleation which was performed because of a painful blind eye.

Periretinal Fibroglial Proliferation Proliferative Vitreoretinopathy (PVR)

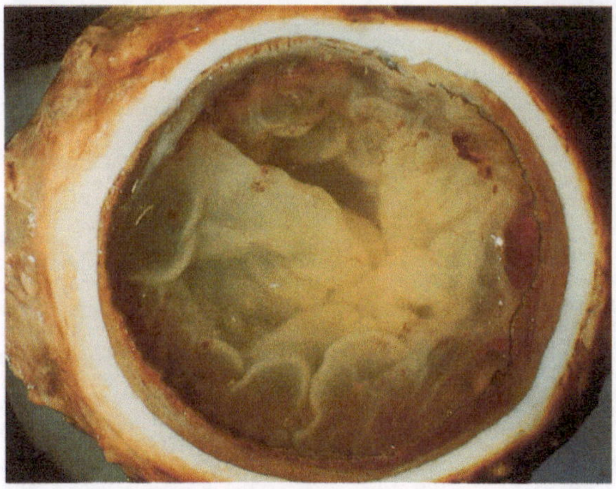

5.39

Fig. 5.39. Frontal section through the eye. Total retinal detachment with wrinkling of the retinal surface (PVR) and an occluded central funnel. M 464/77: 57-year-old man with total retinal detachment and PVR 3 years after a penetrating injury.

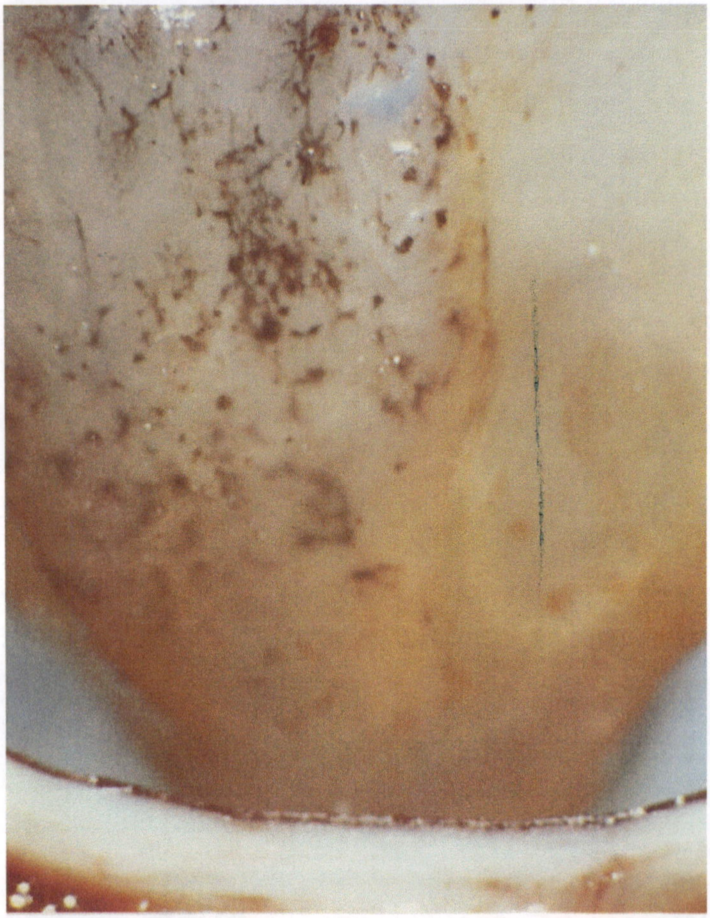

5.40

Subretinal Proliferations

Fig. 5.40. Accumulation of pigmented cells on the outer aspect of the totally detached retina. M 549/82: Posttraumatic total retinal detachment and secondary glaucoma in a 33-year-old man.

Fig. 5.41. Slightly pigmented membrane on the outer aspect of the totally detached retina causing a constriction at the retinal stalk. M 623/76: 58-year-old man with total retinal detachment some years after a perforating injury associated with a metallic foreign body.

Fig. 5.42. Coarse partially pigmented strands fixed to the retinal pigment epithelium within the subretinal space. M 750/84: 24-year-old male with total retinal detachment after several surgical attempts to reposition the retina.

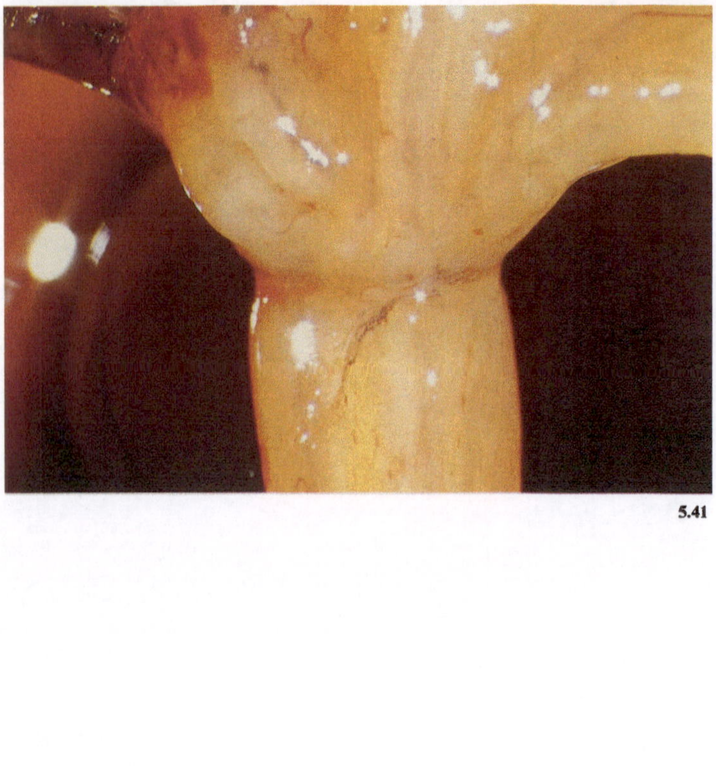

5.41

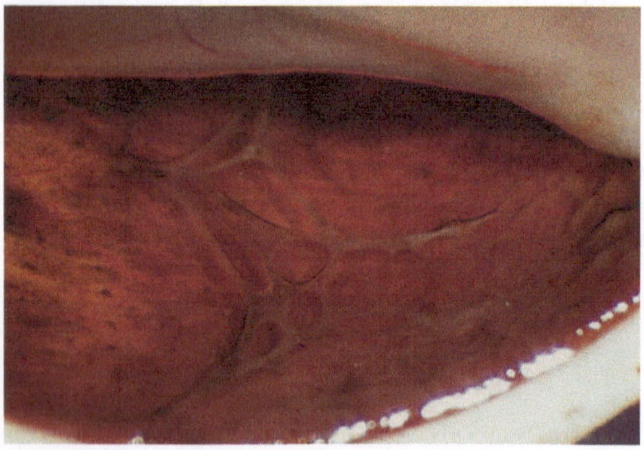

5.42

Fig. 5.43. Subretinal bone formation in long-standing retinal detachment. M 464/77: 57-year-old man who had suffered a penetrating injury 3 years previously. Scleral buckling had been performed unsuccessfully for subsequent retinal detachment.

Deposits in Retinal Detachment

Fig. 5.44. Total retinal detachment with coarse oxalate crystals on the outer temporal retinal surface. The eye is aphakic and shows fine yellowish dots (cholesterol crystals due to previous hemorrhages) in the vitreous space. M 493/76: 37-year-old man who had suffered a penetrating eye injury 16 years prior to enucleation. The aphakic eye showed marked cholesterosis due to recurrent intraocular hemorrhage.

Fig. 5.45. Giant drusen of the retinal pigment epithelium. M 380/85: 24-year-old man with untreated long-standing retinal detachment following penetrating injury from metallic foreign body.

The Macula

All retinal and uveal diseases may involve the macula (central retinal area) and thus reduce visual acuity dramatically. Certain retinal diseases are confined solely to this part of the retina (adult and age-related, senile degenerations, hereditary and metabolic dystrophies), while others preferentially affect the macula (e.g., periretinal proliferation, vascular lesions, inflammation). Since these can be studied well by ophthalmoscopy and fluorescein angiography, only a few of the common conditions are presented here.

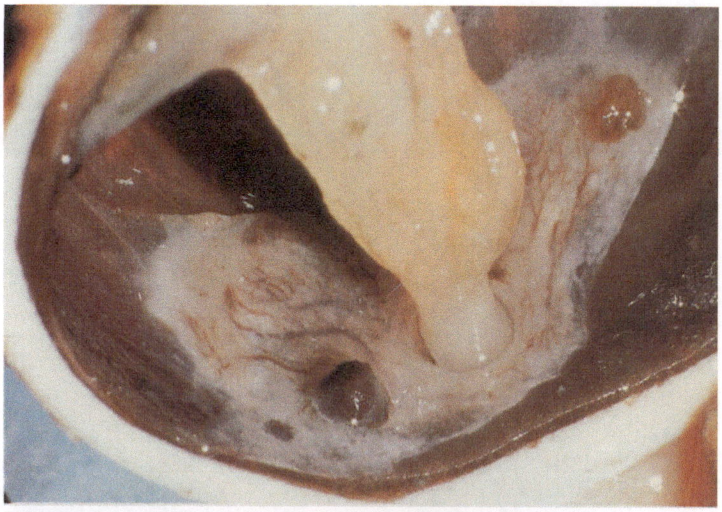
5.43

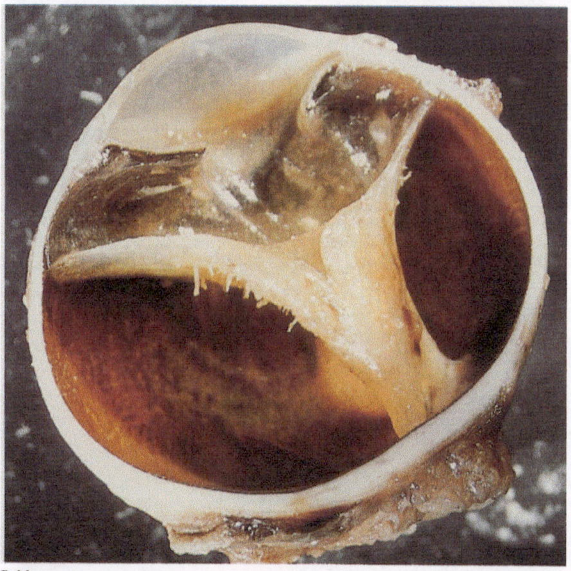
5.44

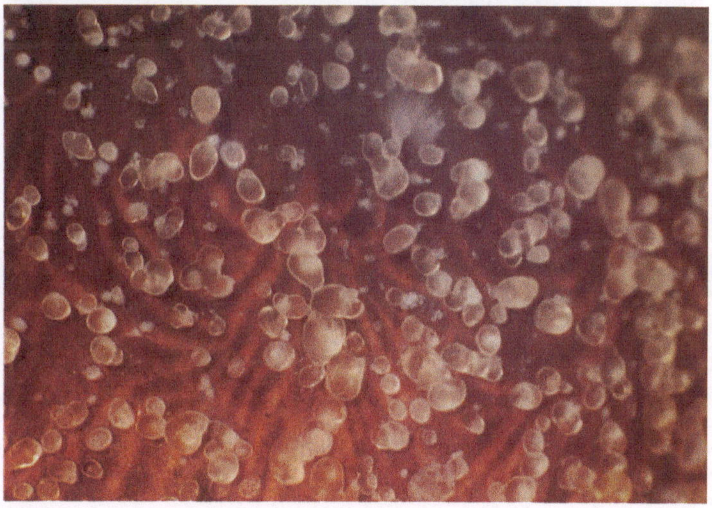
5.45

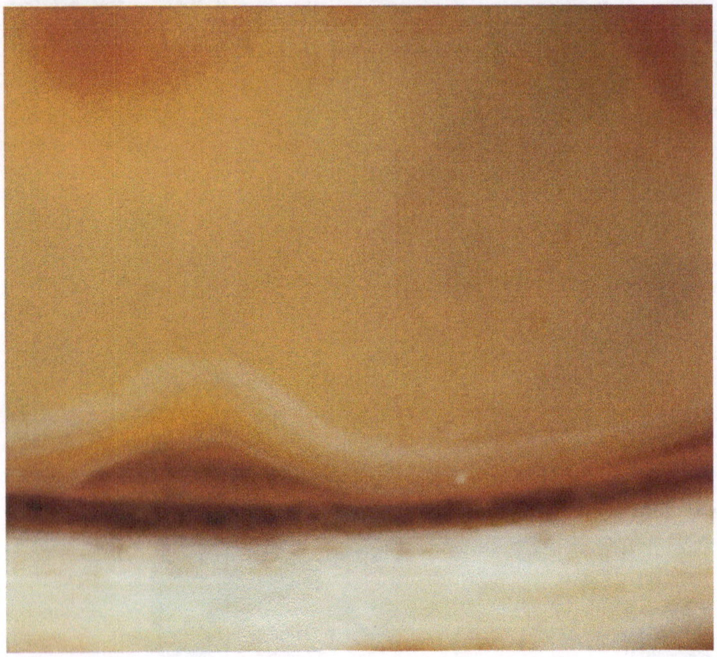

5.46

Isolated Serous Detachment of the Macula

Isolated serous detachment of the macula signals a localized barrier dysfunction at the site of Bruch's membrane and of the retinal pigment epithelium allowing a fluid accumulation beneath the central retina. This may occur idiopathically in younger adults and in focal ischemic and inflammatory disease of the choriocapillaris and choroid (see chapter 4). The enlarged macular choroidal oxygen diffusion distance will eventually result in cystoid degeneration of the detached macula, thus leading to permanent reduction of visual acuity.

Idiopathic Central Serous Retinopathy (Choroidopathy)

Idiopathic, self-limiting, central serous retinopathy occurring predominantly in young males is a localized noninflammatory and nonischemic retinal detachment. The etiology is unknown as is that of the somewhat similar condition of idiopathic serous detachment of the retinal pigment epithelium.

Fig. 5.46. Secondary circumscribed central retinal detachment in choroidal malignant melanoma. It is not unlike that of idiopathic central serous retinopathy. M 79/85: 47-year-old man with choroidal malignant melanoma and secondary retinal detachment.

Age-related Macular Degeneration (ARMD) Senile Macular Degeneration (SMD)

Age-related macular degeneration (ARMD) or senile macular degeneration (SMD) has become one of the major causes of legal blindness in the aging population. Its cause is not entirely clear. Older people showing drusen are predisposed to develop age-related macular degeneration. It either presents with progressive atrophy of the RPE and the overlying photoreceptors (age-related (senile) atrophic (dry, areolar) macular degeneration) or with subretinal neovascularization. In (senile atrophic (dry, areolar) macular degeneration) visual acuity is gradually reduced due to degeneration of the macular photoreceptors and secondary cystoid macular degeneration. Even macrocystoid degeneration may occur. With subretinal neovascularization ARMD (SMD) is accompanied by subretinal exudation (exudative phase), recurrent hemorrhage (hemorrhagic phase), and reparative reactions (scarred phase, macular pseudotumor) in a disease process termed senile disciform degeneration of the macula. Visual acuity is lost not only because of photoreceptor cell loss but also due to an enlarged oxygen diffusion distance. This again leads to cystoid macular degeneration. The etiology of ARMD (SMD) is unknown. An inflammatory immune process has been postulated. Following focal choroiditis a similar secondary reaction may develop.

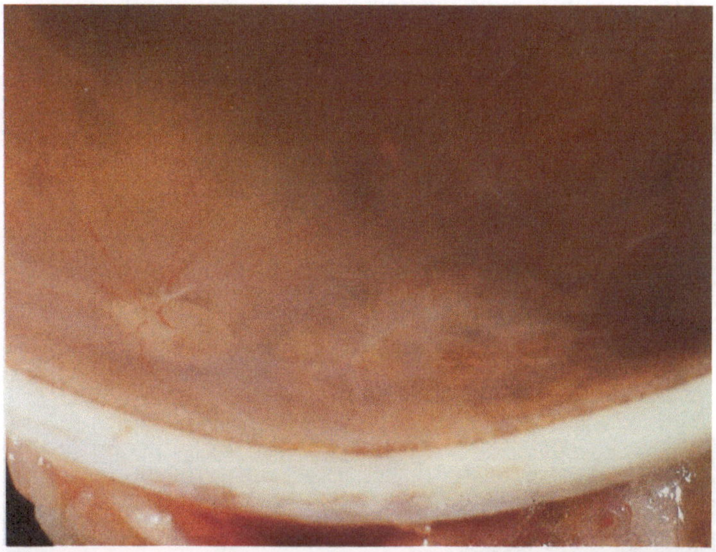

5.47

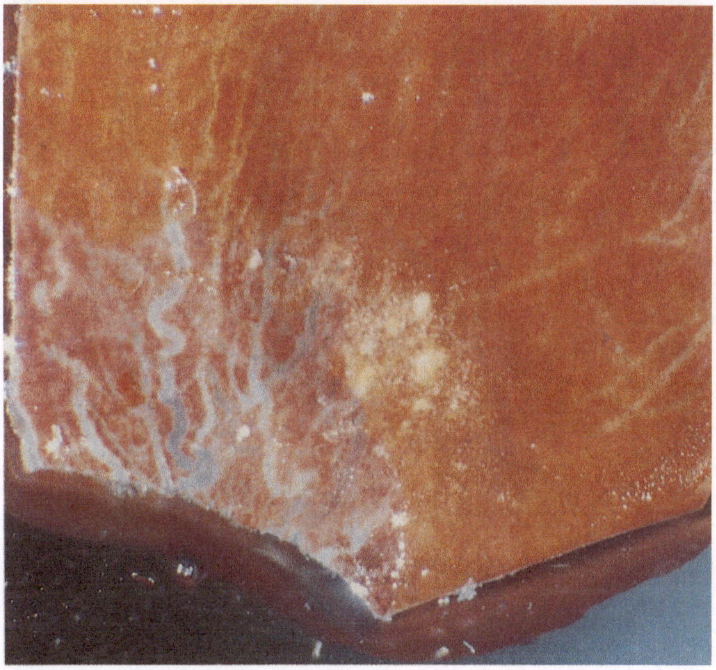

5.48

Age-related Atrophic (Dry, Areolar) Macular Degeneration (Haab Disease)

Fig. 5.47. Posterior pole showing a circumscribed, somewhat depigmented central area with thick choroidal blood vessels shining through. M 774/84: 85-year-old male with age-related atrophic (dry, areolar) macular degeneration in his right eye and age-related disciform (wet, exudative) macular degeneration in the left eye.

Fig. 5.48. Same specimen as in Fig. 5.47. The sensory retina has been removed. There are yellow granular deposits (drusen) of the retinal pigment epithelium beneath the fovea. Adjacent to these drusen, the retinal pigment epithelium has been removed showing the coarse grayish thick choroidal blood vessels.

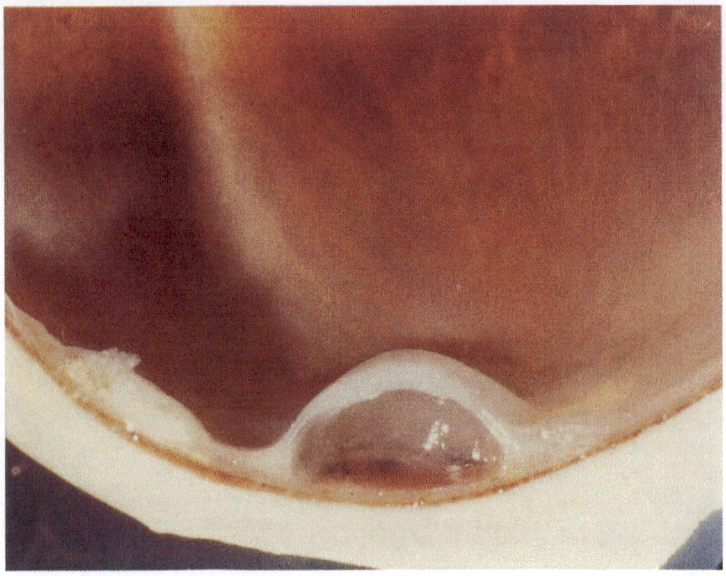

5.49

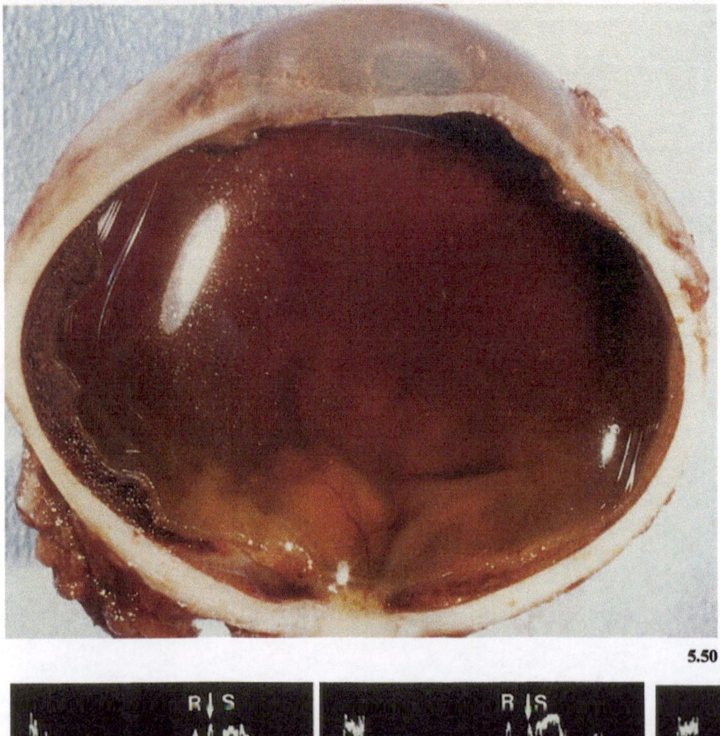

5.50

Age-related Disciform (Wet, Exudative) Macular Degeneration (Junius-Kuhnt Disease)

Exudative Phase

Fig. 5.49. Elevated sensory retina in the exudative phase of age-related disciform macular degeneration. The retinal pigment epithelium shows focal hyperplasia. M 1089/82: Autopsy eye of a 78-year-old male without clinical history. Death due to myocardial infarction.

Hemorrhagic Phase

Fig. 5.50. Unusually pronounced hemorrhagic elevation of the posterior retina and some hemorrhagic imbibition of the vitreous in age-related degeneration of the macula. M 343/72: 80-year-old man with sudden loss of visual acuity in one eye. Vitreous hemorrhage obscured any view of the fundus. Ultrasonography revealed a marked choroidal thickening incompatible with typical age-related macular degeneration. Enucleation because of suspected malignant melanoma of the posterior choroid.

Fig. 5.50 A. Age-related macular degeneration. A-scan echograms of different stages of age-related macular degeneration: **a–c** initial examination with retinal detachment (*R*), partly organized subretinal hemorrhage (*thin long arrows*) and a solid underlying layer (*short arrows*). **d** Follow-up examination after 5 months with decreased elevation of the area of age-related macular degeneration due to resorption of the subretinal hemorrhage; the retina lies directly over solid tissue indicating subretinal membrane, which comprises the area of degeneration (*S* = sclera).

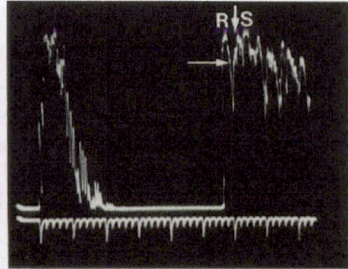

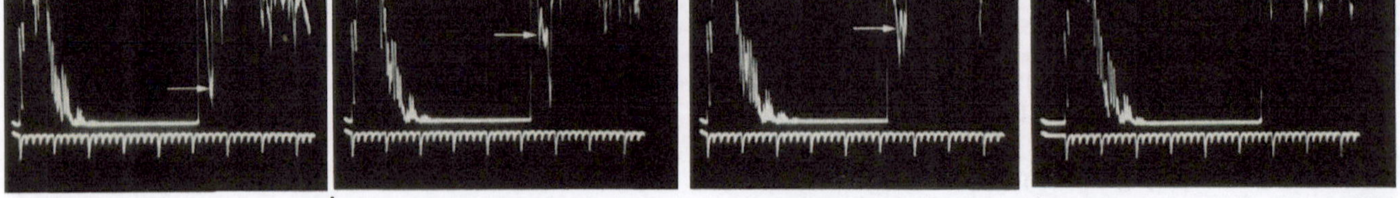

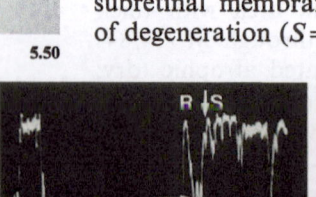

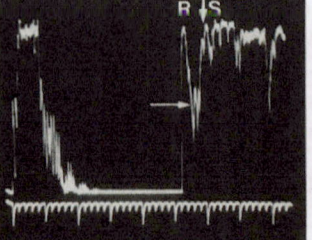

a b c d 5.50 A

Fig. 5.51. Higher magnification of previous figure showing coagulated blood in the subretinal space.

Fig. 5.52. Elevated central retina showing macrocystoid degeneration. Beneath the surrounding retina there are yellow deposits which represent remnants of previous subretinal hemorrhage. M 1089/82: Same patient as Fig. 5.49.

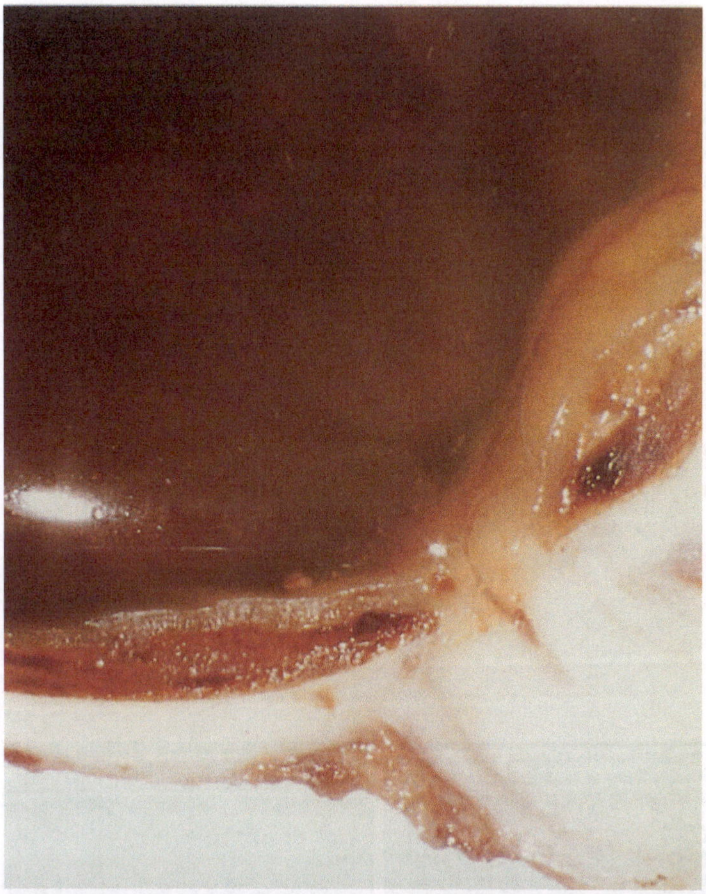

5.51

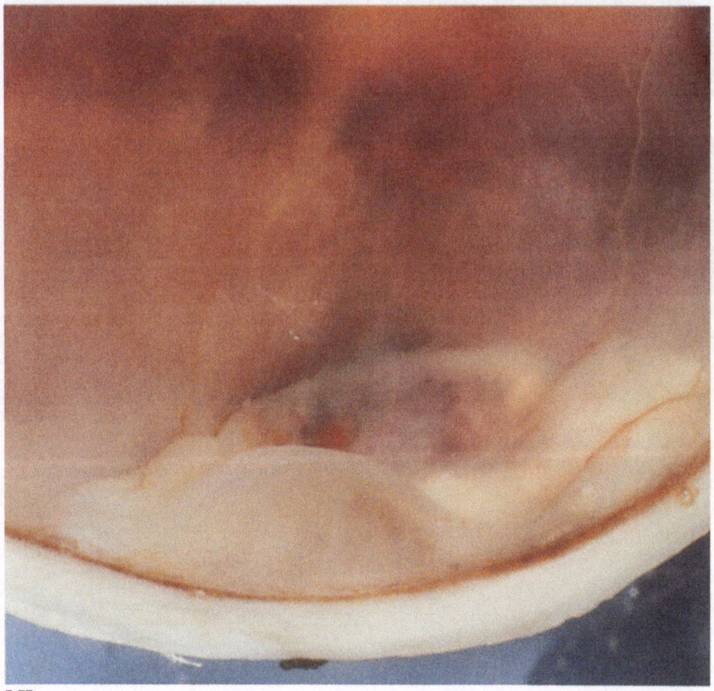

5.52

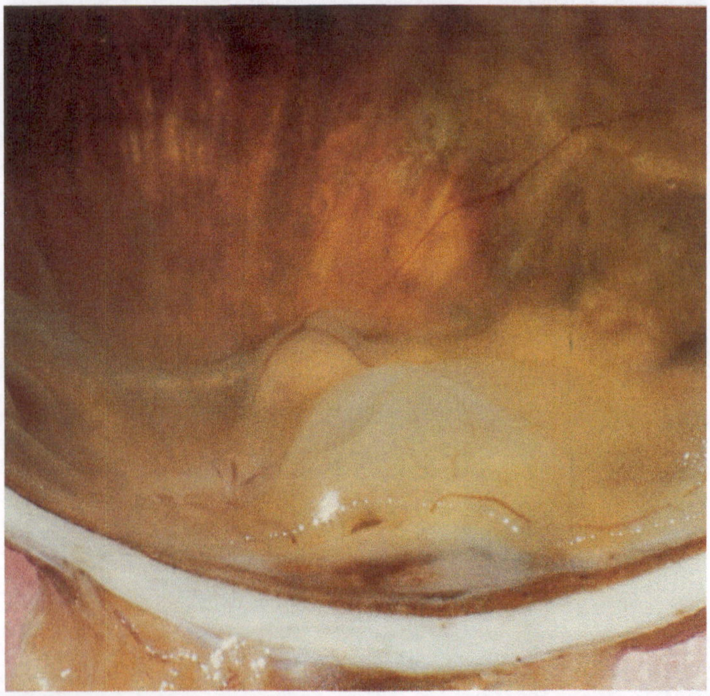

5.53

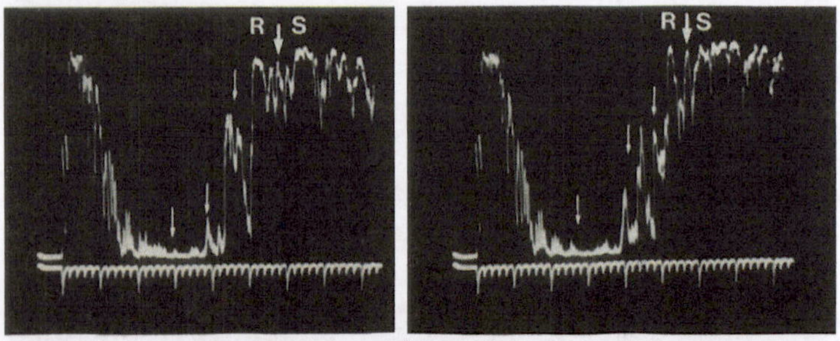

a b

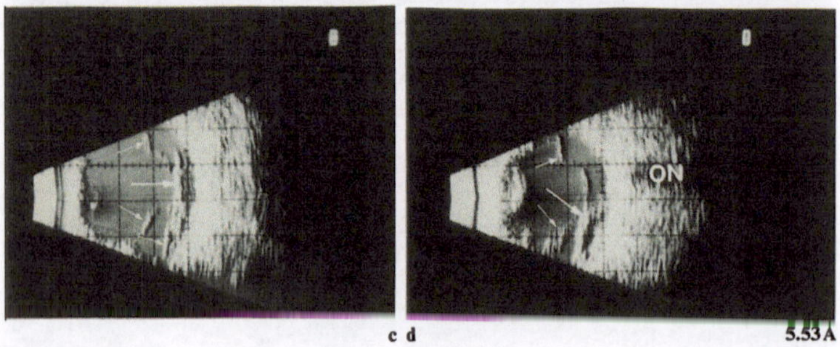

c d 5.53A

Scar Phase (Macular Pseudotumor)

Fig. 5.53. Grey scar tissue underneath the central thickened retina with some surrounding fresh (red) and old (yellow) subretinal hemorrhage. M 7/76: 68-year-old male with bilateral age-related disciform macular degeneration.

Fig. 5.53A. Age-related macular degeneration (macular pseudotumor). A-scan echograms (**a, b**) and contact B-scan echograms (**c** vertical section, **d** horizontal section at the posterior pole) of vitreous opacities (*thin short arrows*) and age-related macular degeneration/pseudotumor of the macula (*R*/*long arrows* = overlying retina; *S* = sclera; *ON* = optic nerve). Note the membranous heterogeneous structure (*thick arrows* in a, b) of the area of age-related macular degeneration in the A-scan echograms.

Fig. 5.53B. Age-related macular degeneration (macular pseudotumor). A-scan echograms of age-related macular degeneration at different stages of the disease representing the pseudotumorous appearance at the initial examination **(a, b, c, d)** with varying but mostly high reflectivity and heterogeneous structure of the internal echo signals between overlying retina (*R*) and sclera (*S*). Follow-up examination after 6 months **(e, f)** note the decreased elevation of the lesion.

Fig. 5.53C. Thickening of the retinochoroid layer. A-scan echograms of thickened retinochoroid layer that may represent macular or eccentric disciform degeneration (*R* = retina; *S* = sclera; *arrow* = choroid). **a, b** at "tissue-sensitivity" setting, **c** at low "measuring-sensitivity" setting of the standardized A-scan instrument (see Table 1/Preface).

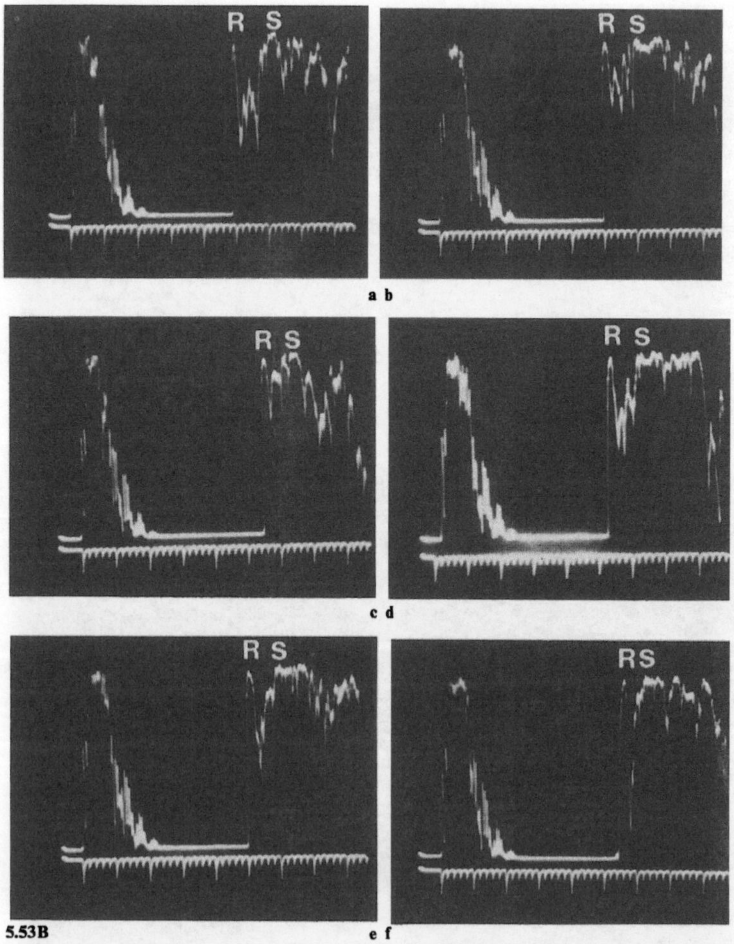

5.53B e f

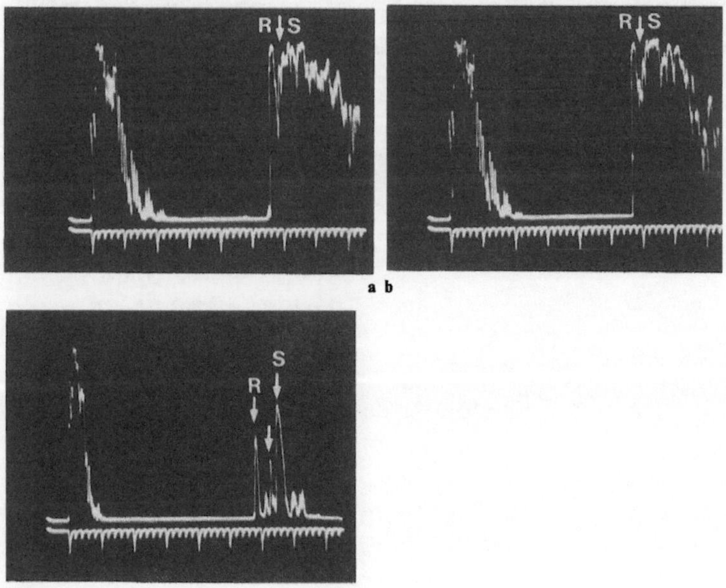

5.53C c

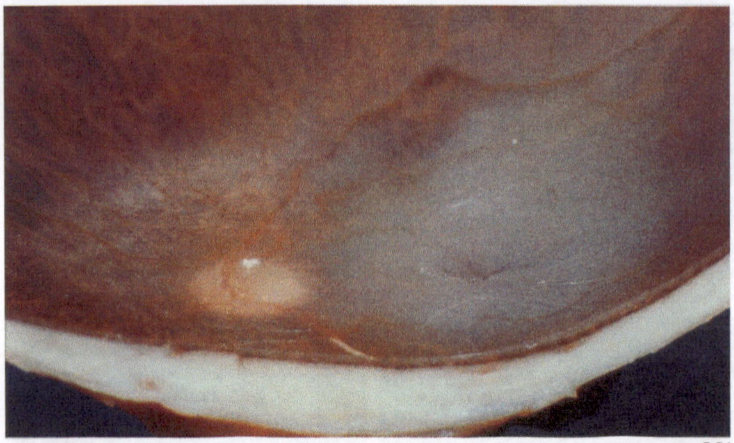

5.54

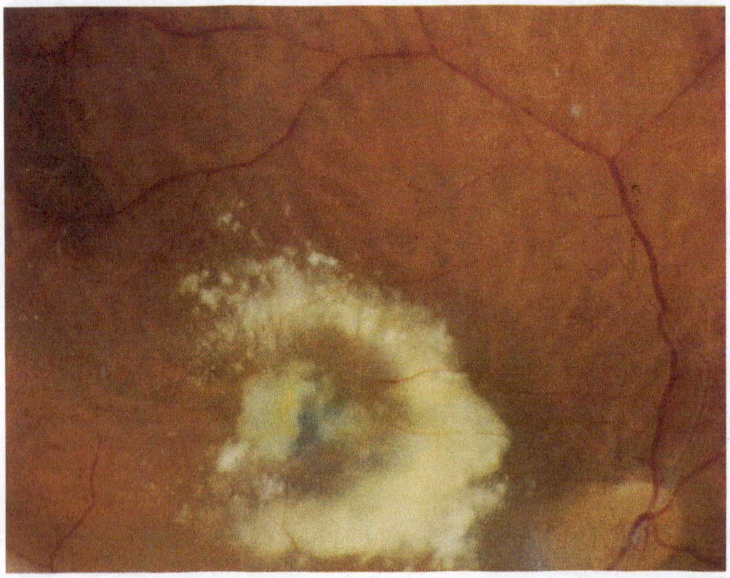

5.55

Secondary Macular Degeneration

Secondary changes of the central sensory retina may develop in various conditions (ischemic, inflammatory, traumatic, toxic, metabolic). Chronic cystoid macular edema following cataract extraction (Irvine-Gass syndrome) and in postirradiation retinopathy are only two examples. In time, chronic cystoid macular edema will eventually lead to a degenerative macular hole.

Irvine-Gass Syndrome

Fig. 5.54. Thickening and internal folding of the central retina. M 831/84: 74-year-old aphakic male with bullous keratopathy. Cataract extraction 5 years prior to enucleation.

Postirradiation Retinopathy

Fig. 5.55. Stellate pattern of accumulated intraretinal exudate around the fovea which displays defects of the retinal pigment epithelium. M 377/75: 52-year-old male with painful eye and mature cataract 5 years after surgery and postsurgical radiation for an adenoid cystic carcinoma of the parotid gland.

6. Vitreous

Developmental anomalies · Inflammation · Hemorrhage · Proliferation · Degeneration

Changes in the vitreous are among the commonest of ocular conditions. The transparent avascular vitreous body gel is rich in liquid and consists only of 1% proteinaceous elements (hyalocytes, collagen, and hyaluronic acid). Its outer collagenous surface is in contact with the inner limiting membrane of the retina (posterior vitreous cortex), the structure around the ora serrata (vitreous base), the posterior chamber and lens (anterior vitreous cortex). Cloquet's canal represents a remnant of the primary vitreous. The changes in the vitreous body consist either of disturbances of the vitreous gel structure or of secondary vitreous opacities. The patient with changes in the vitreous body may complain of muscae, blurred vision, or photopsia. Clinical examination of the vitreous is made easily possible using a slit-lamp through clear cornea and lens. If dense vitreous opacities are present, ultrasonography is an important technique providing data on the intraocular pathology. The vitreous is an excellent culture medium for microorganisms, and its collagen structure offers an excellent matrix for proliferating cellular (vascular, fibrous, glial) elements. With modern technical devices it is now possible to perform vitreous surgery and thus to prevent the complications of intravitreal proliferation and reparative processes.

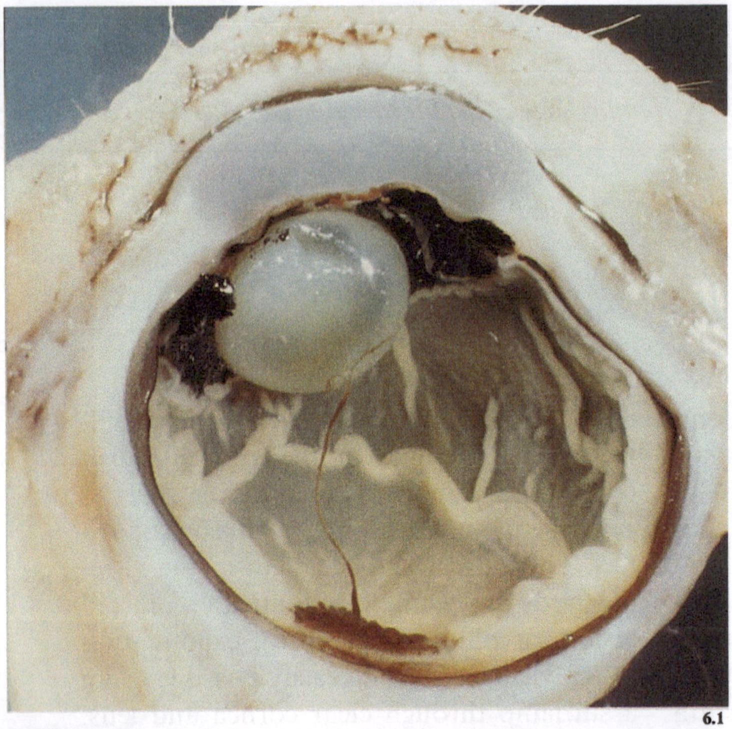

6.1

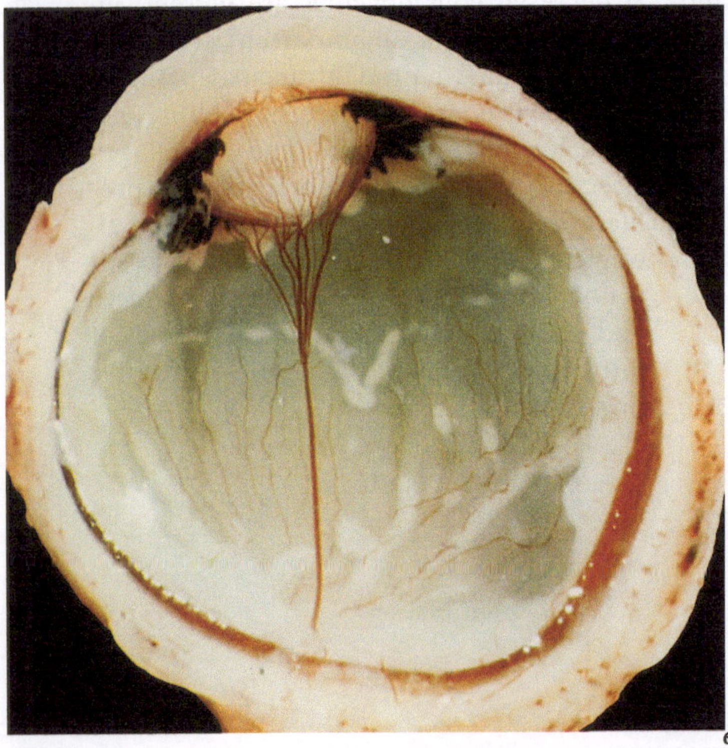

6.2

Developmental Anomalies

Most developmental anomalies of the vitreous are related to the primary vitreous with its blood vessels. In prematurity, elements of the primary vitreous are usually present. Normally these regress up to birth leaving only Cloquet's canal between the nasal back of the lens and the optic disc. But remnants of the primary vitreous may persist after birth as persistent hyaloid artery, Mittendorf's dot at the nasal back of the lens, Bergmeister's papilla, or persistent hyperplastic primary vitreous (PHPV).

Persistent Hyaloid Artery

Fig. 6.1. Autolytic folding of the avascular retina. Accumulation of vessels with some hemorrhage around the optic disc. Persistent hyaloid artery between the back of the lens and the optic disc. M 1045/82: Autopsy eye of a premature baby.

Fig. 6.2. Persistent hyaloid artery and tunica vasculosa lentis and the as yet incompletely vascularized peripheral retina. Disciform opacity of the posterior lens cortex in an otherwise normal-shaped lens. M 812/75: Eye of a male abortus with Lowe's syndrome at the 26th week of gestation.

Fig. 6.2 A. Persistent Hyaloid Artery. A-scan echogram (**a**) and contact B-scan echograms (**b, c**) of a persistent hyaloid artery (*arrows*) with circumscribed traction detachment of the retina at the posterior pole (*long arrows* in **c**; *ON* = optic nerve). Note the small globe diameter (microphthalmos) (**a**).

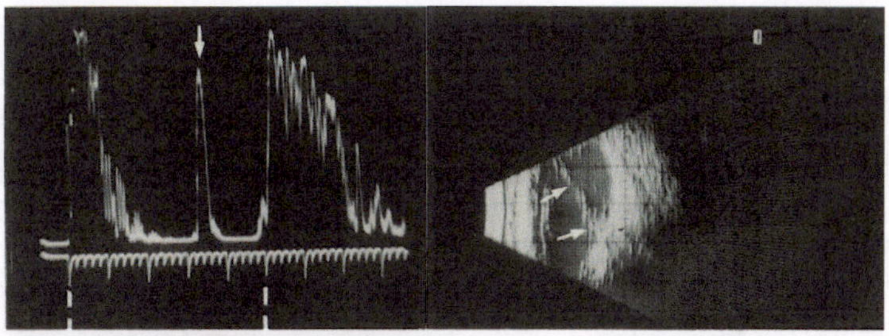

a b

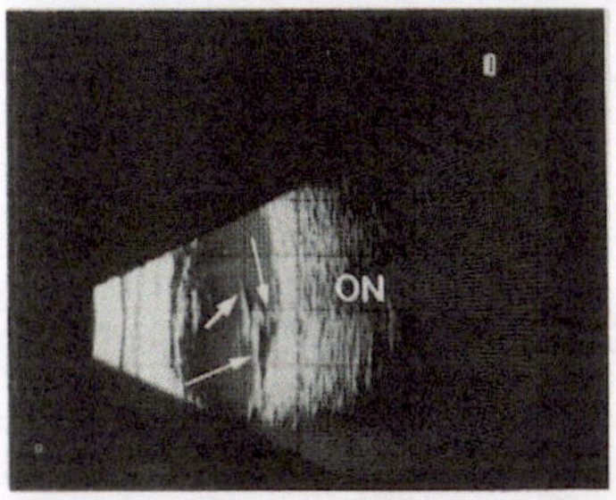

6.2 A c

Remnants of Hyaloid Artery

Fig. 6.3. Remnants of the hyaloid artery with coiling at the site of regression. M 642/79: Autopsy eye of a mature newborn baby with iris coloboma.

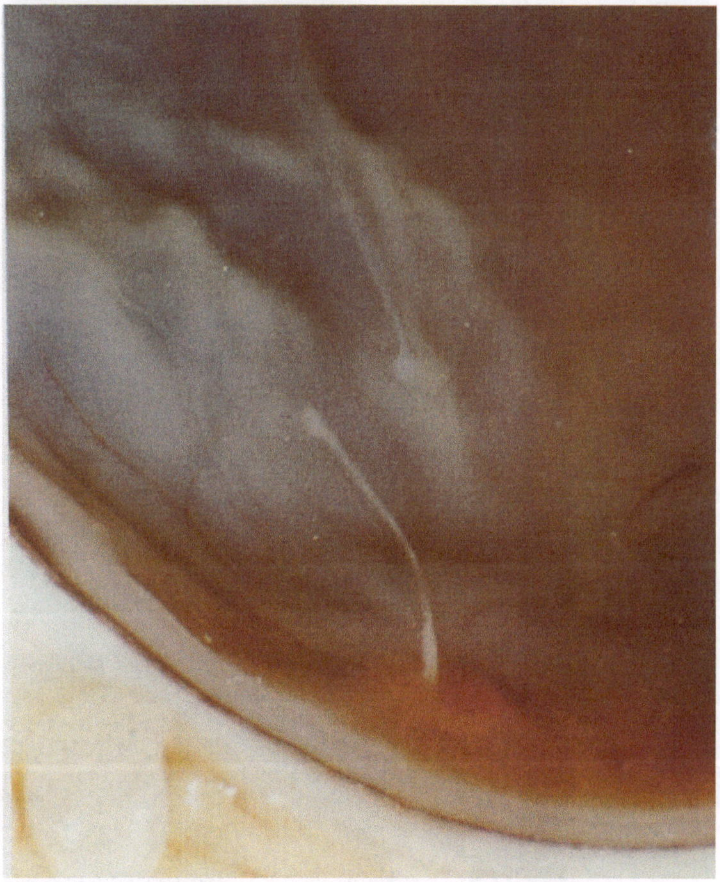

6.3

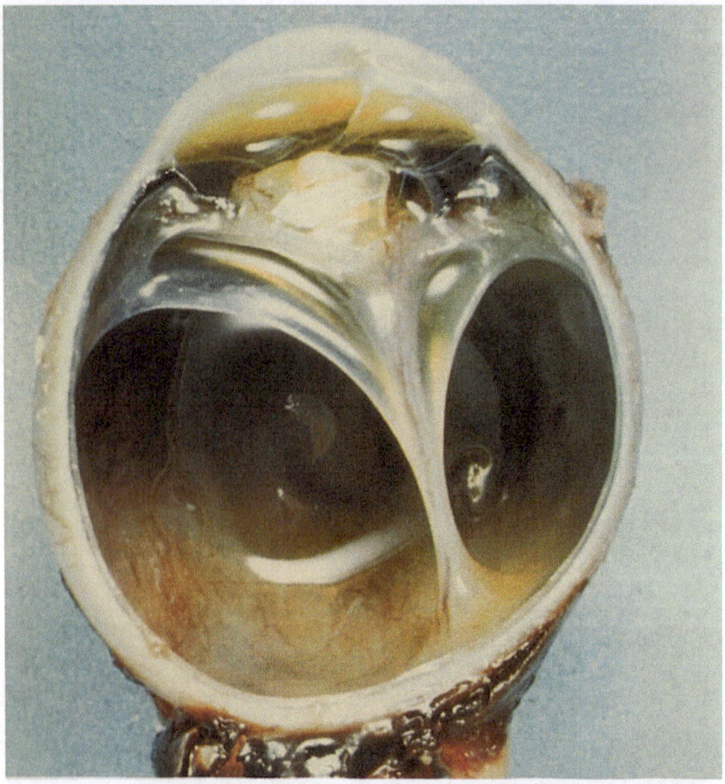

6.4

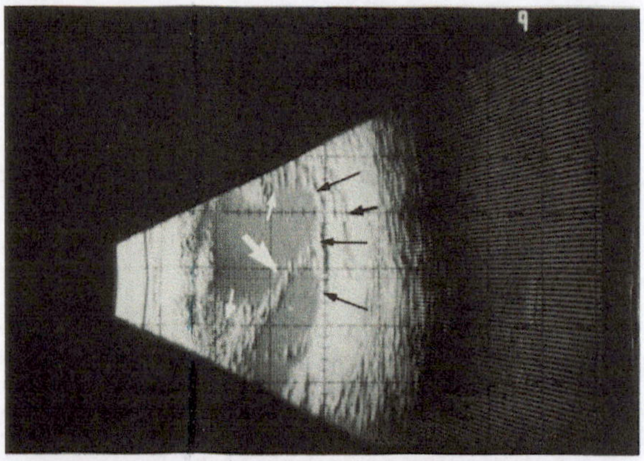

a

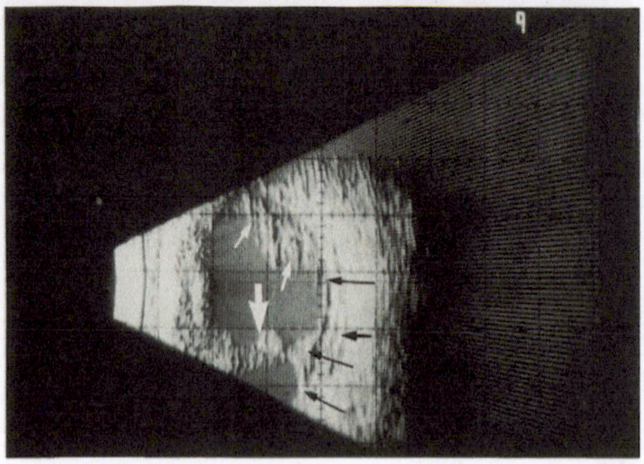

b 6.4A

Persistent Hyperplastic Primary Vitreous (PHPV)

Fig. 6.4. Enlarged globe with enlarged cornea. Grey vitreous strand and retrolental tissue (PHPV), small cataractous lens, hypoplastic iris, and thickening of the opaque central retina due to a defect in Descement's membrane. M 265/73: 4-week-old newborn baby with congenital glaucoma, congenital hydrophthalmos, enlarged corneal diameter, ring-shaped central corneal opacity, and suspected cataract.

Fig. 6.4A. Persistent Hyperplastic Primary Vitreous (PHPV). Contact B-scan echograms of a persistent hyperplastic primary vitreous demonstrating a (fibrovascular) strand (*thick white arrow*) inserting at the posteronasal fundus, traction and elevation of the ciliary body (*short white arrows*), and either diffuse or more localized thickening of the retinochoroid layer with a shallow retinal detachment at the point of attachment of the strand (*black arrows*).

Inflammation

The vitreous may become increasingly infiltrated by inflammatory cells in uveoretinitis whether infectious or noninfectious, or in reaction to intraocular or intravitreal microorganisms (posttraumatic, postoperative). The degree of infiltration varies from mild opacities to massive endophthalmitis (vitreous abscess). Cellular elements may aggregate on the collagen fibres or sometimes form round, floating, so-called snowballs. If inflammation is marked, there is protein leakage into the vitreous, liquefaction and shrinkage of the vitreous, and finally a healing process starting from the ciliary pars plana and the optic disc and resulting in a cyclitic membrane, vitreous strand formation, and eventually retinal detachment. In some traumatic or degenerative conditions, a marked macrophage response may simulate an inflammatory reaction.

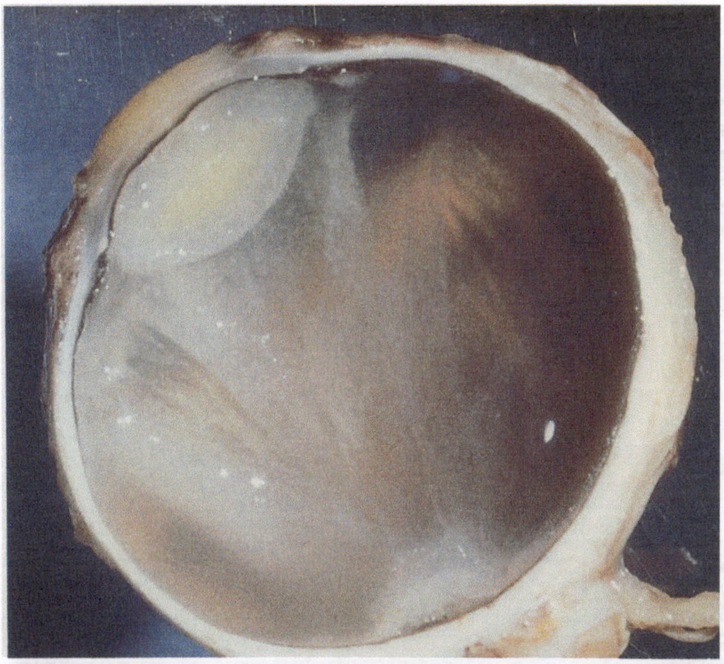

6.5

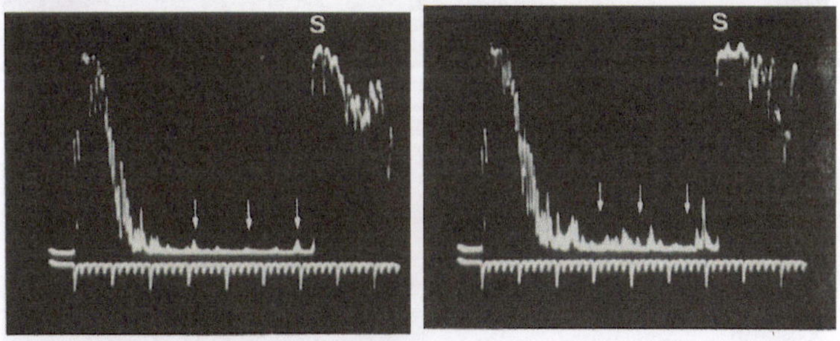

a b

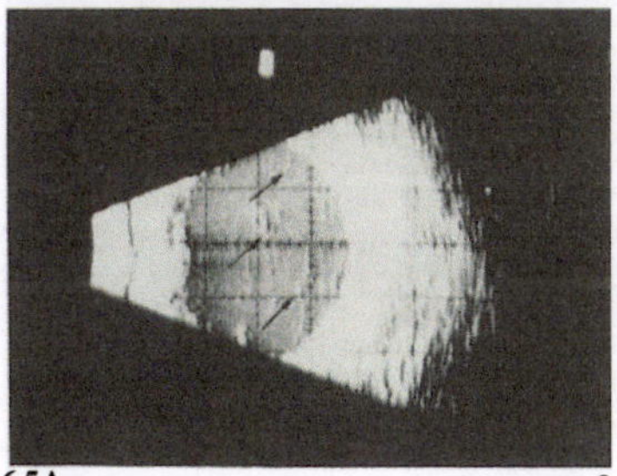

6.5A c

Fig. 6.5. Fibrillary and granular appearance of the cellular infiltrated opaque vitreous. Vitreous collagen spans from the vitreous base to the optic disc (posterior vitreous detachment). M 70/84: 76-year-old male with absolute glaucoma, keratitis, and secondary iridocyclitis.

Fig. 6.5A. Vitreous opacities. A-scan echograms of diffuse, mild vitreous opacities at tissue sensitivity setting (**a**) and at an increased sensitivity setting (**b**). Note that at increased sensitivity (**b**), the opacities (*arrows*) displayed are more pronounced and the density of the opacities can be judged (*S* = sclera). The contact B-scan echogram (**c**) nicely demonstrates the topographic distribution of the opacities within the vitreous cavity (*black arrows*).

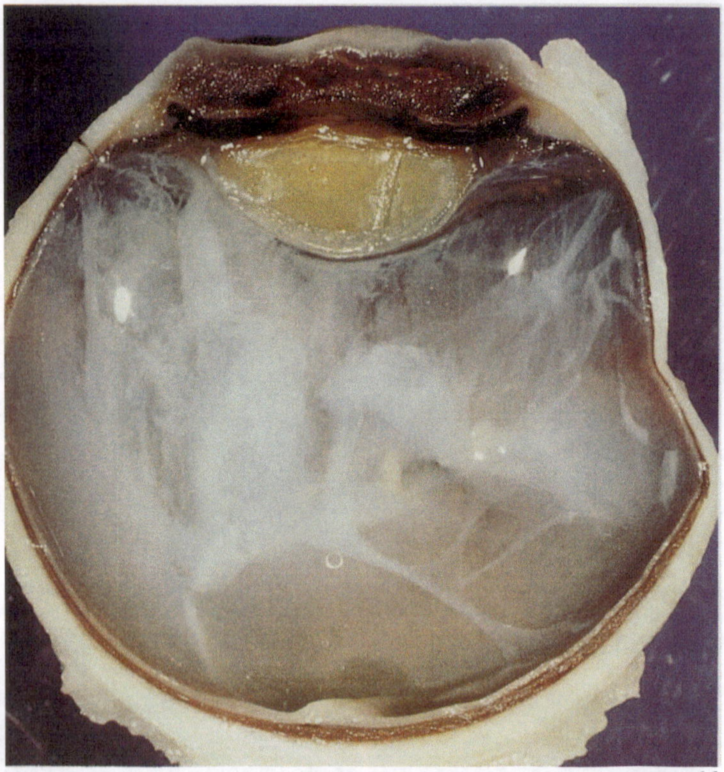

6.6

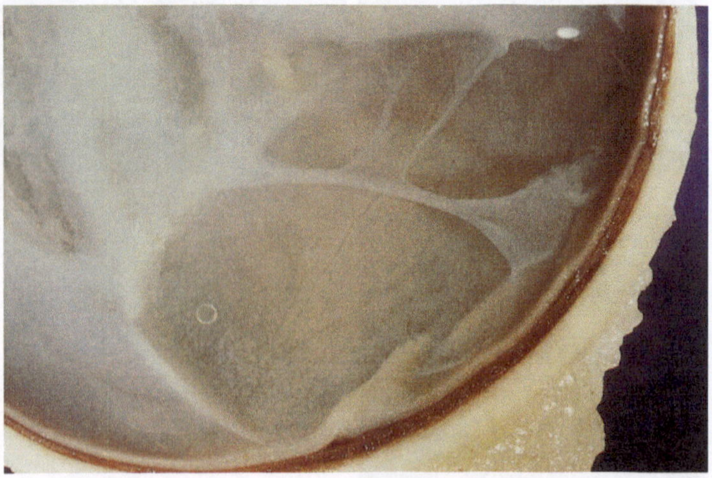

6.7

Fig. 6.6. Densely infiltrated grayish-white opaque vitreous with liquefaction and condensation of vitreous. M 68/85: Autopsy eye of a 68-year-old man who died of septicemia.

Fig. 6.7. The vitreous is partially adherent to the retina. In the area of vitreous detachment, the gray granular appearance of the inner retina surface is due to cellular aggregates.

Fig. 6.8. Opaque infiltrated vitreous with markedly increased protein content. At the vitreous base are large, round, inflammatory aggregates with fungal foci. M 144/85: 58-year-old diabetic man with metastatic Aspergillus endophthalmitis from venous infusion device.

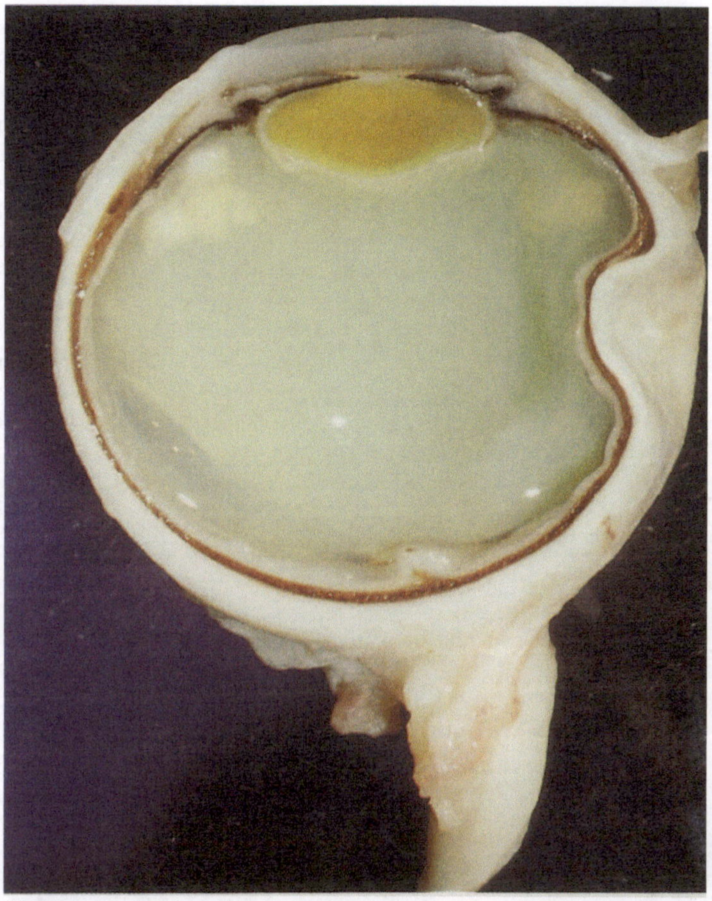

6.8

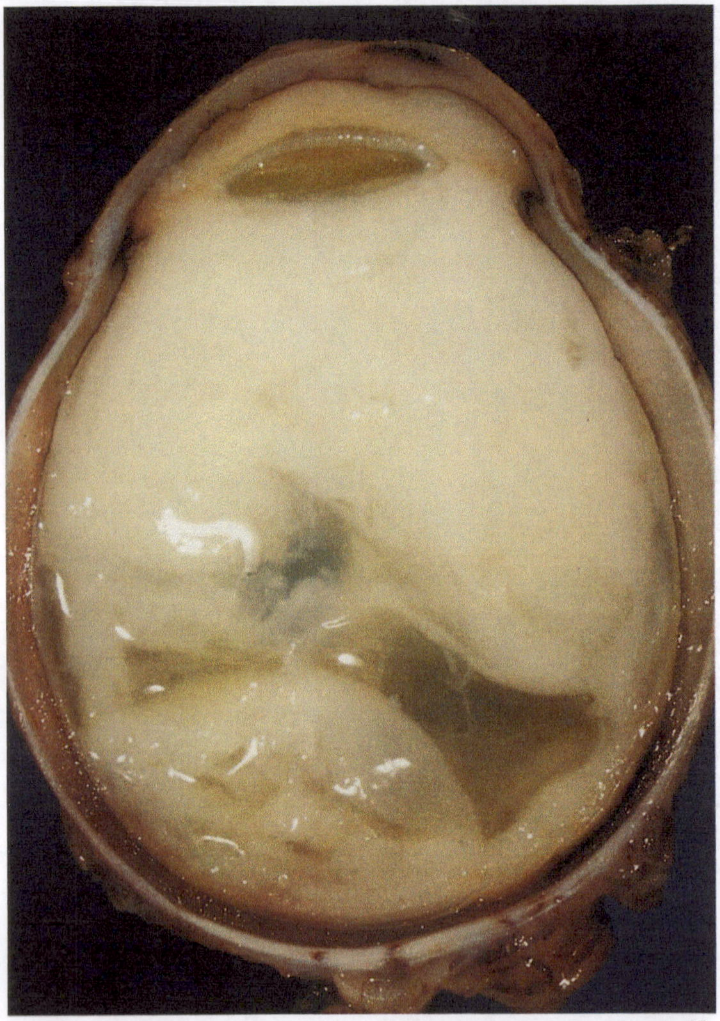

6.9

Fig. 6.9. Massive endophthalmitis with suppuration in the vitreous, posterior and anterior chamber. Some liquefaction in the posterior vitreous. The swollen uvea shows reactive exudation and hyperemia. M 513/83: 5-year-old boy with late postoperative endophthalmitis after keratoplasty for corneal teratoma.

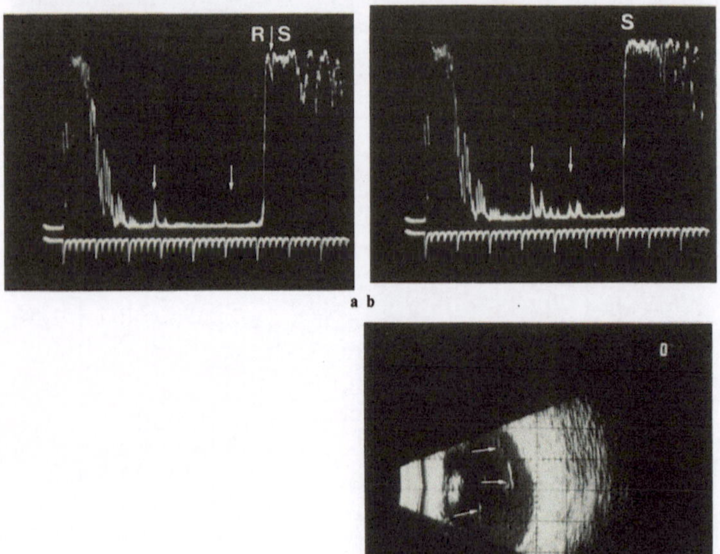

a b

c 6.9A

Fig. 6.9A. Endophthalmitis. A-scan echograms in two sections (**a, b**) with different highly reflective vitreous opacities (*arrows*). Single low to medium high echo spikes indicate vitreous infiltrates (**b**). In some areas of the fundus, a circumscribed shallow thickening of the retinochoroid layer is displayed (**a**). (R = retina; S = sclera). **c** Contact B-scan of a patient with endophthalmitis showing the distribution of the vitreous opacities.

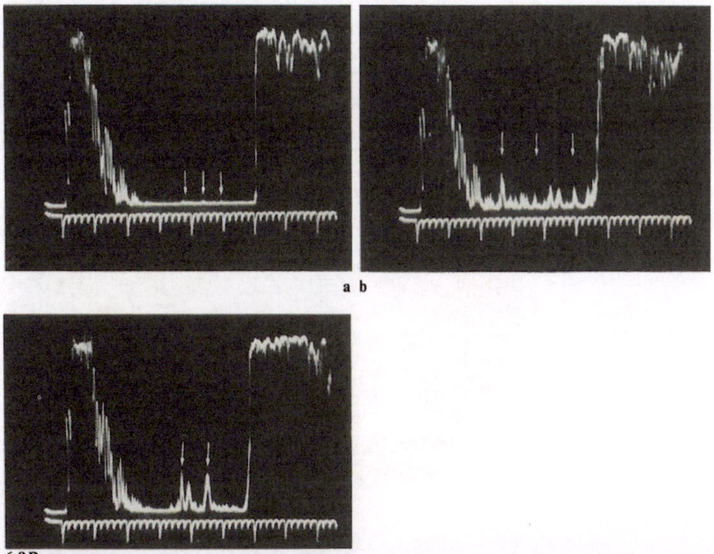

a b

6.9B c

Fig. 6.9B. Endophthalmitis. A-scan echograms of the development of vitreous opacities and vitreous infiltrations in endophthalmitis over a period of time. **a** first examination, **b, c** after 6 hours. *Arrows* indicate the echo-spikes representing the vitreous opacities and infiltrates (**c**).

Intravitreal Hemorrhage

There are many clinical conditions (trauma, systemic disease such as diabetes mellitus, local pathology such as retinal break formation, proliferative retinopathy after central retinal vein occlusion or malignant choroidal melanoma) that may cause hemorrhage into the vitreous. The degree of hemorrhage varies and so does the reduction of visual acuity. Erythrocytes within the vitreous also accumulate along the vitreous collagen framework. They will undergo hemolysis (yellowish color) and cause some phagocytic vitreous infiltration. Finally posterior vitreous detachment and collapse of the vitreous framework develops.

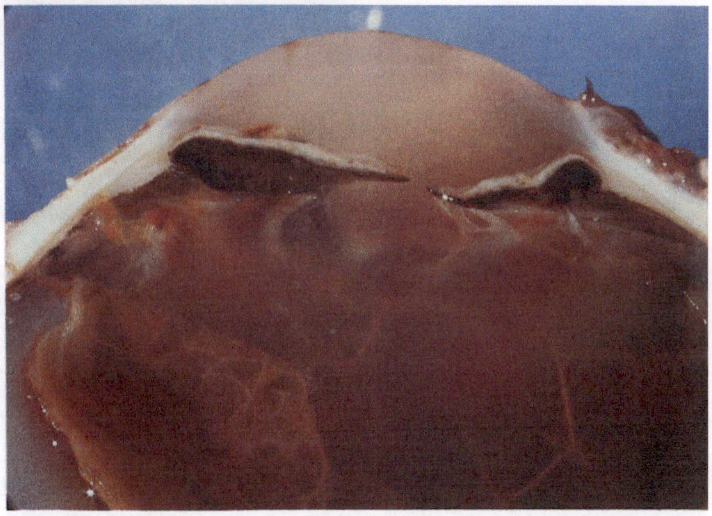

6.10

Fig. 6.10. Vitreous hemorrhage with a ring of fibrin behind the iris. Peripheral anterior synechias with obliteration of the chamber angle. The luxated lens is not visible. Retinal detachment. M 280/84: 74-year-old man with proliferative diabetes mellitus, recent vitreous hemorrhage, and absolute glaucoma due to rubeosis iridis with peripheral anterior synechias. The lens is luxated into the vitreous.

Fig. 6.11. Vitreous hemorrhage with advanced hemolysis (yellowish color), partially detached posterior vitreous and aphakia. M 720/75: 38-year-old male with untreatable glaucoma secondary to perforating corneoscleral injury, lens damage, and vitreous hemorrhage.

Fig. 6.12. Old vitreous hemorrhage with posterior vitreous detachment and granular accumulations of macrophages along retinal blood vessels. M 1055/76: 49-year-old man with untreatable secondary glaucoma and massive intravitreal hemorrhage 2 years after central retinal vein occlusion.

Fig. 6.12 A. Posterior vitreous detachment. Contact B-scan echograms of a posterior vitreous detachment (*arrows* = posterior vitreous surface) **a** before and **b** after an eye movement on instruction. Note the swaying movement of the freely mobile vitreous.

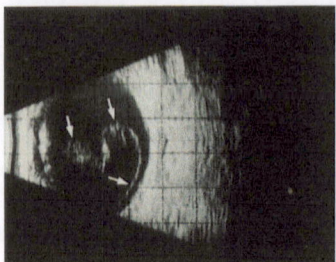

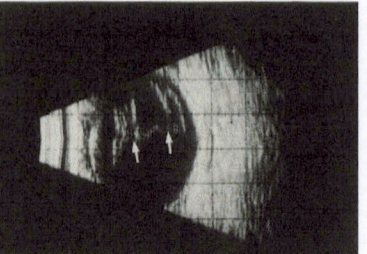

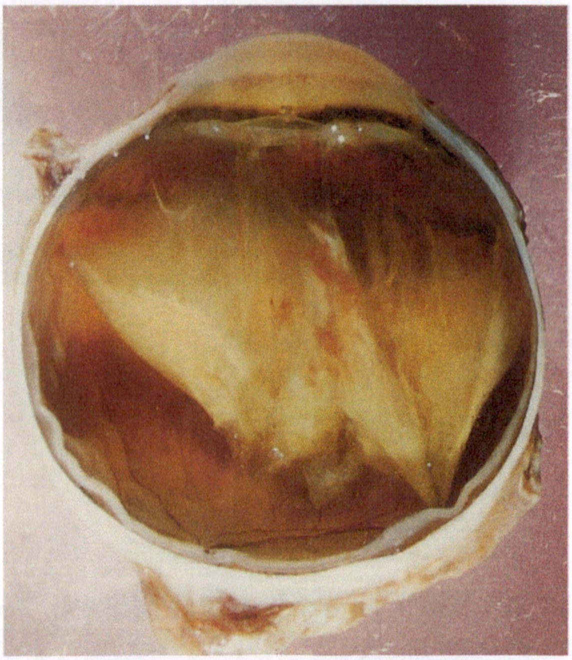

6.11

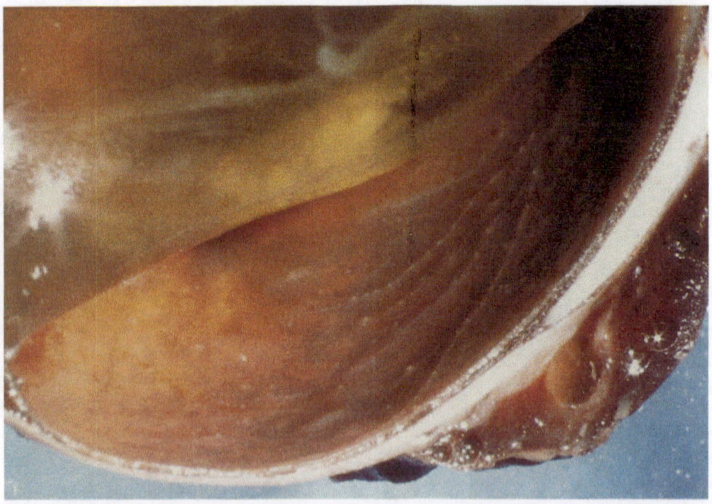

6.12

a b 6.12 A

Intravitreal Proliferation

Periretinal and intravitreal proliferation is stimulated by trauma, inflammation, hemorrhage, proliferative retinopathies, and long-standing retinal detachment. Cells of different origin arise within the vitreous, proliferate, and produce collagen which may shrink causing displacement of intraocular structures (mainly retina and ciliary body). Retinal "seafans"-shaped vasoproliferations develop in ocular and extraocular vascular and systemic diseases such as diabetes, sickle-cell disease, retrolental fibroplasia, and central retinal vein occlusion. Vitreal strands as well as periretinal membranes are increasingly removed at surgical vitrectomy.

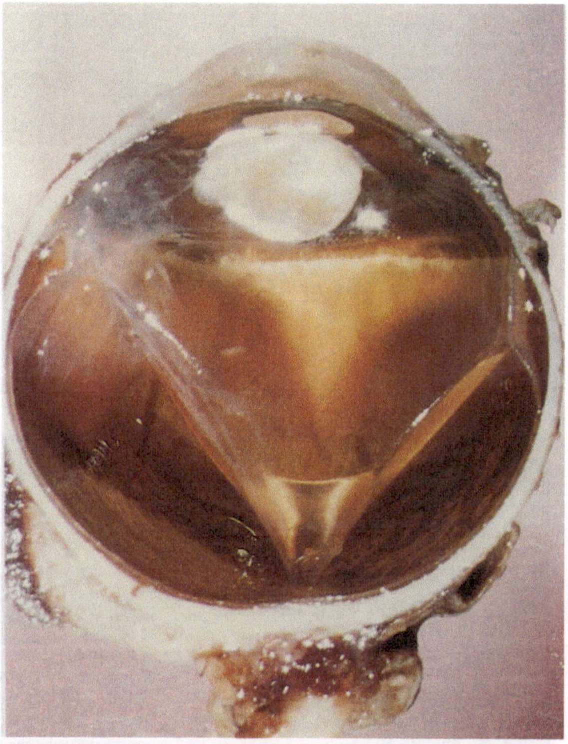

6.13

Fig. 6.13. Posterior vitreous detachment. Dense vitreous strands from the temporal vitreous base. Tractional peripheral retinal detachment. Hypermature cataract. M 480/75: 34-year-old man with cataract and painful blind eye 25 years after penetrating injury.

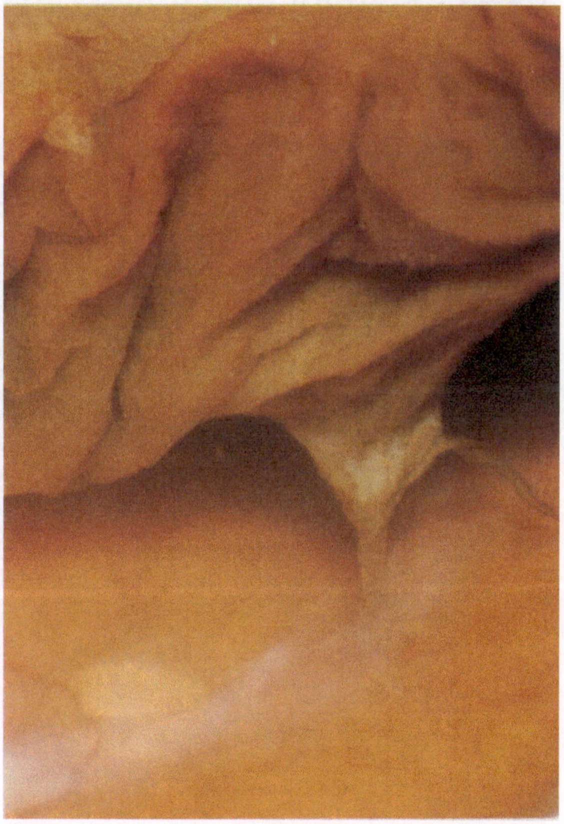

6.14

Fig. 6.14. Fibrous periretinal membrane adjacent to the optic disc. Old massive vitreous hemorrhage with posterior vitreous detachment and vitreoretinal adhesion. Fibrous proliferation into the vitreous at the adhesion site. M 358/72: 47-year-old man with spontaneous massive vitreous hemorrhage probably due to retinal vein occlusion.

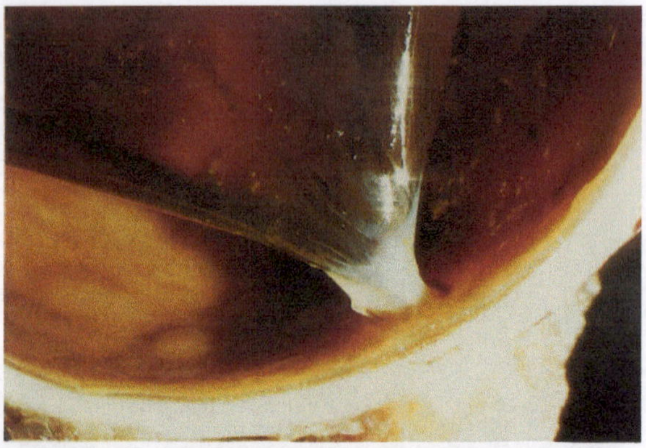

6.15

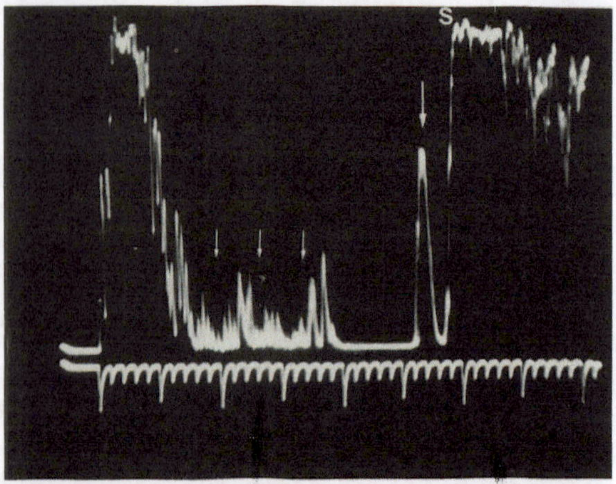

a

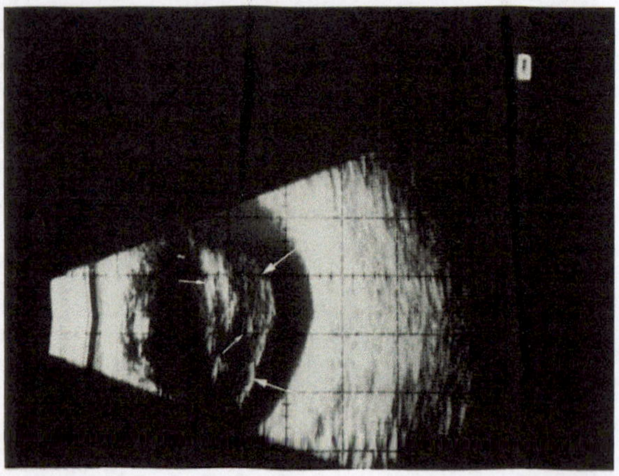

b 6.15A

Fig. 6.15. Posterior vitreous detachment. Connective tissue proliferating into the vitreous from the optic disc. M 718/77: 83-year-old man with painful blind eye after retinal vein occlusion, intravitreal hemorrhage, and subsequent glaucoma.

Fig. 6.15A. Posterior vitreous detachment/vitreous opacities. A-scan (**a**) and contact B-scan (**b**) echogram of a total posterior vitreous detachment (*long arrows* = detached posterior surface of the vitreous) and diffuse moderate to dense opacities (*small arrows*).

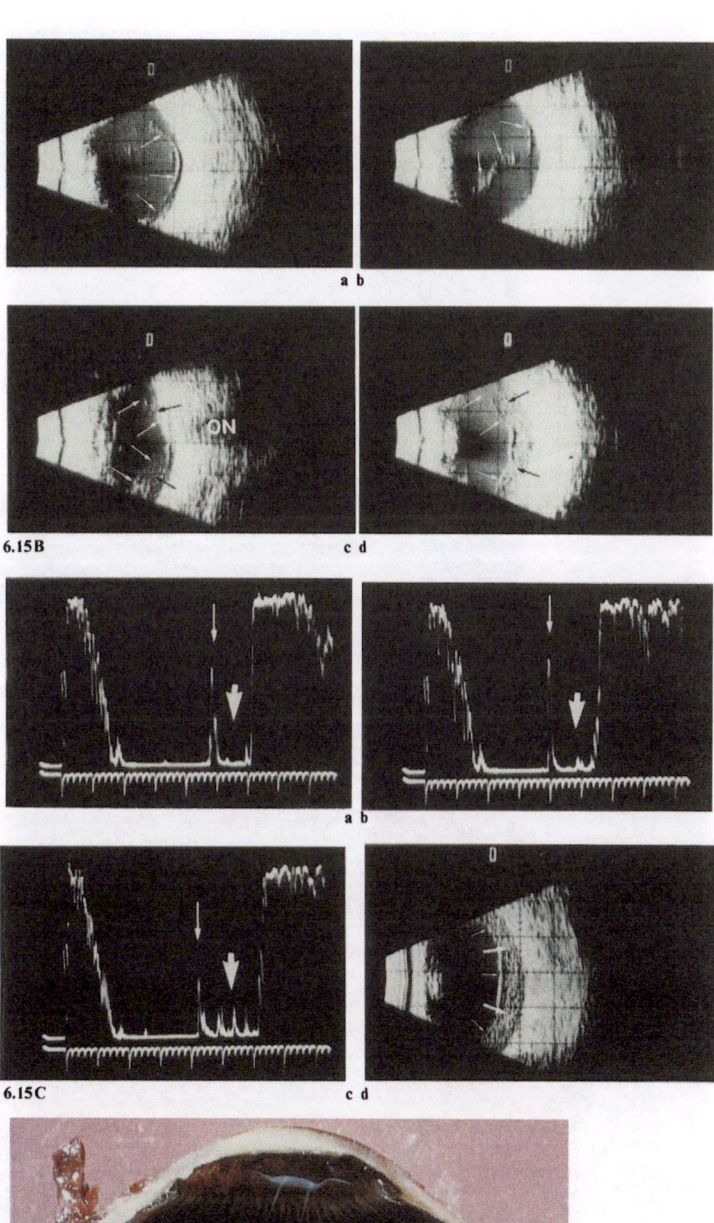

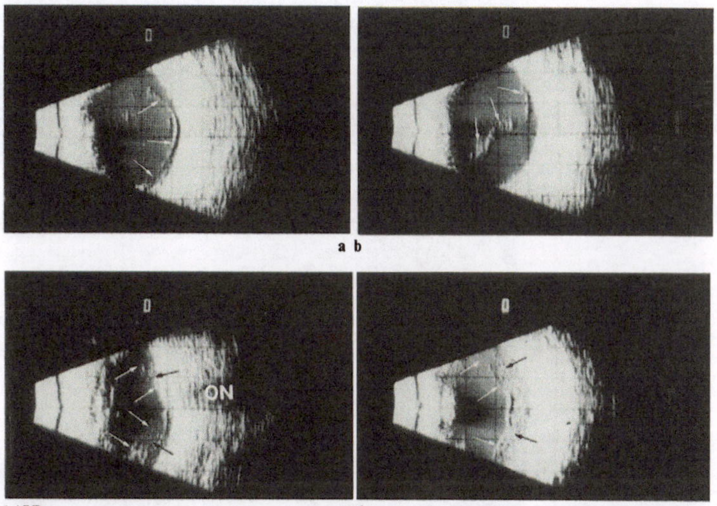

6.15B

Fig. 6.15B. Posterior vitreous detachment/Subvitreal opacities. Contact B-scan echograms of a freely mobile posterior vitreous detachment: **a** before and **b** after an eye movement. *Arrows* indicate the posterior vitreous surface. **c** mild diffuse opacities and dense peripapillary membranes (*black arrow*) and **d** moderate to dense diffuse opacities (*black arrows*) in the subvitreal space (*white arrows* = posterior vitreous surface; *ON* = optic nerve).

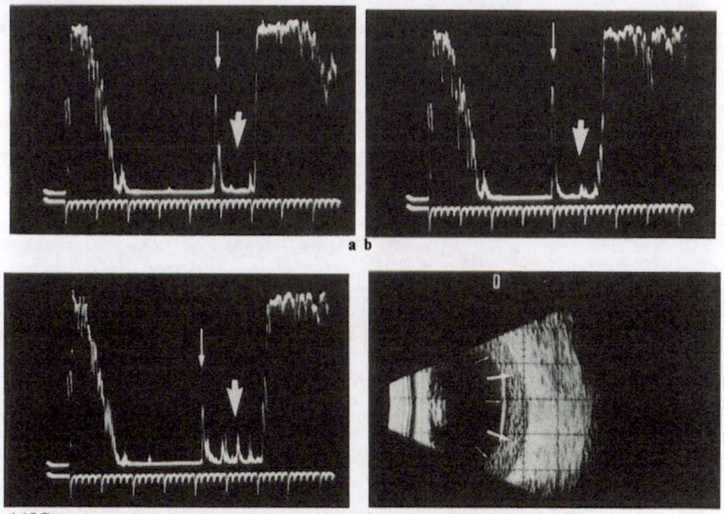

6.15C

Fig. 6.15C. Subvitreal opacities. A-scan echograms (**a–c**) and contact B-scan echogram (**d**) of a posterior vitreous detachment (*small arrows* = posterior vitreous surface) with moderate (**a, b**) to dense (**c, d**) subvitreal opacities (*big arrows*).

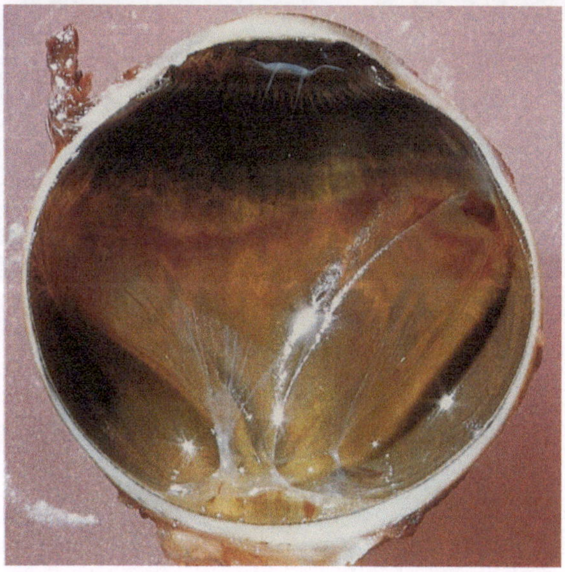

6.16

Fig. 6.16. Proliferative diabetic retinopathy with proliferation of newly formed blood vessels (gray lines) from the optic disc and the retina onto the detached posterior vitreous surface in a fan-like fashion. Vitreoretinal traction with secondary degenerative retinal changes. Some sedimented subretinal hemorrhage outlining the posterior aspect of the vitreous base. M 97/76: 76-year-old man with proliferative diabetes mellitus recognized for 13 years.

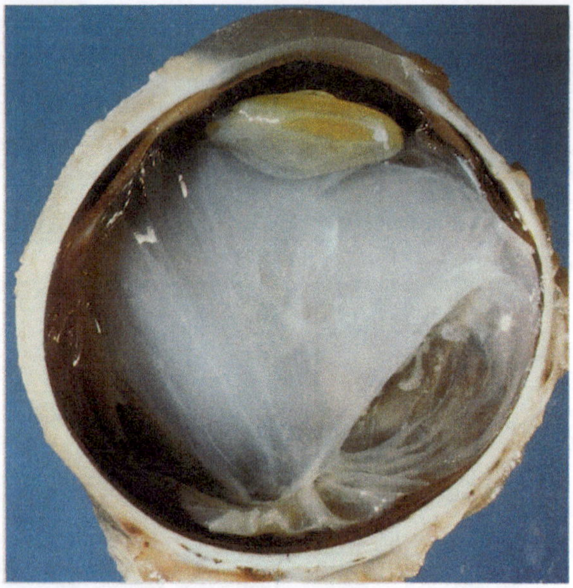

6.17

Fig. 6.17. Marked vitreous opacity with partial posterior vitreous detachment and periretinal proliferation from the optic disc. Tractional folding of the posterior retina. M 205/78: 21-year-old man who had had a traumatic avulsion of the optic nerve during a traffic accident 3 years earlier.

Degenerations

Liquefaction, collapse of the vitreous framework, and posterior vitreous detachment are typical degenerative changes occurring increasingly commonly with age and in association with a number of pathologic conditions. Localized vitreous liquefaction has been mentioned above with retinal degenerations. Asteroid hyalosis is a vitreous degeneration of unknown etiology.

Asteroid Hyalosis (Morbus Benson)

Unilateral asteroid hyalosis is a fairly uncommon condition with minute round glistening crystalloid deposits of phospholipids into the vitreous framework. It may occur in healthy eyes and in association with certain ocular diseases (diabetic retinopathy, malignant melanoma). Visual acuity is usually only little affected.

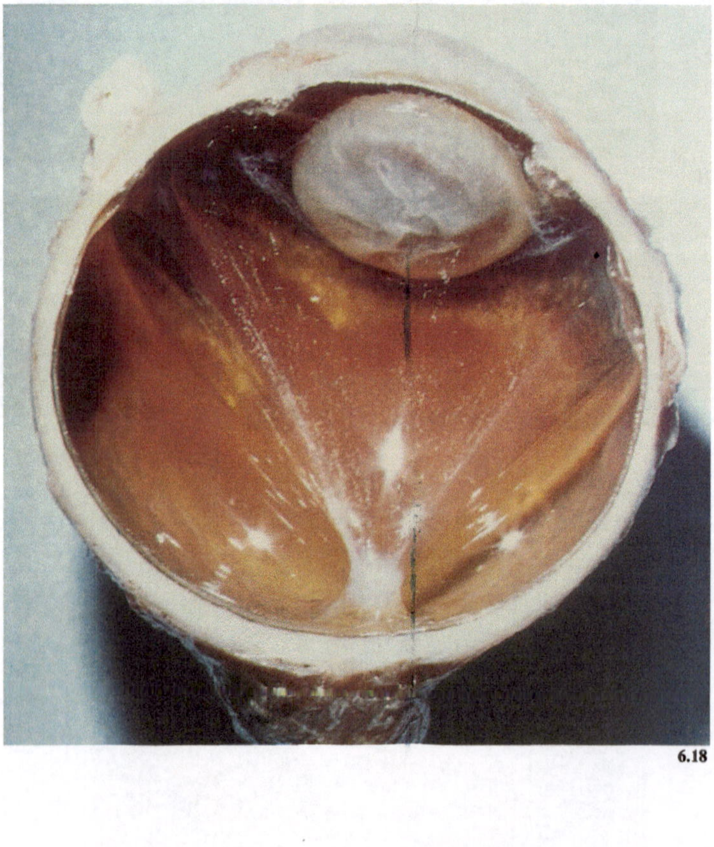

6.18

Fig. 6.18. Posterior vitreous detachment. Within the vitreous framework are whitish small round deposits. Some fibrovascular proliferation into the vitreous stalk from the optic disc secondary to central retinal vein occlusion. Cataract. M 800/76: 84-year-old man with pseudoexfoliative glaucoma for 13 years. Eleven years previously, he had had a concussion injury to this eye with central retinal vein occlusion.

Fig. 6.18A. Asteroid hyalosis. A-scan echograms (**a, b**) and contact B-scan echogram (**c**) of asteroid hyalosis. **a** echogram before eye movement, **b** echogram immediately after. Note the higher reflectivity of the asteroid bodies as compared to diffuse opacities (e.g., diffuse fresh vitreous hemorrhage), and the marked aftermovement seen in this condition (**b** blurred spikes in the A-scan echogram) and the typical clear space in front of the posterior ocular wall (*arrows*).

Fig. 6.19. High power view of the round vitreous deposits in asteroid hyalosis.

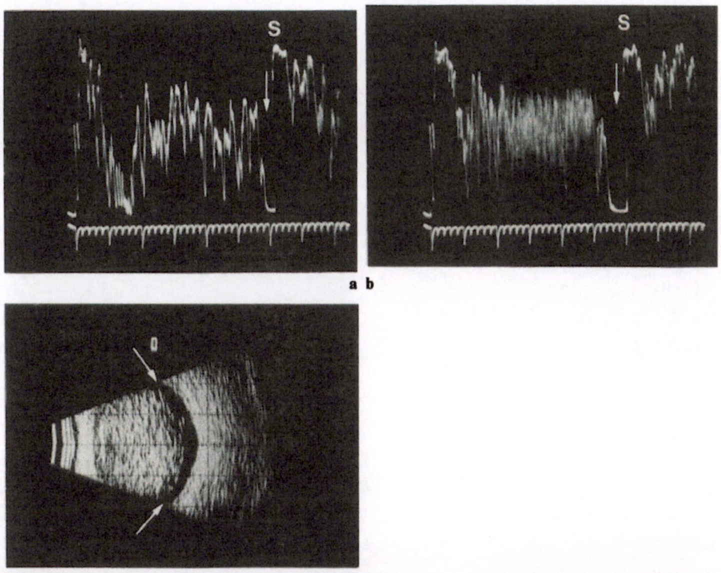

a b

c

6.18A

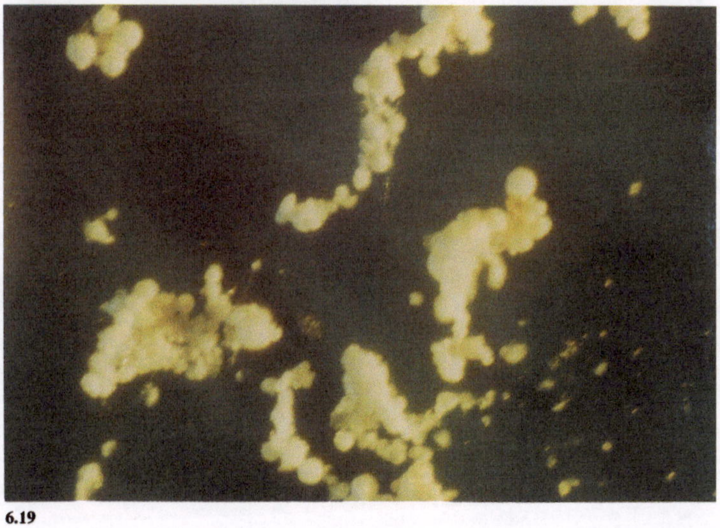

6.19

7. Lens

Congenital cataract · Age-related cataract · Secondary cataract · Phacolysis · Inflammation · Ring-shaped lens

Dislocation of the lens (see chapter 2), disconfiguration of the lens (see coloboma), and cataract (lens opacities) comprise the only pathology of this transparent avascular organ. The degree of of cataract varies as does the cause. Pigmentation of the lens nucleus is called nuclear cataract (sclerosis). Minor cortical opacities are termed incipient (incomplete) cataract. This may be so minor that it does not affect vision. Complete opacity of the lens is described as mature cataract, a swollen opaque lens known as intumescent cataract, and, finally, dehydration and shrinkage leads to a hypermature cataract. The most common general cause of blindness in the world is bilateral age-related (senile) cataract. Less common is bilateral congenital cataract from a number of metabolic disorders, maternal virus infection (rubella), or remnants of the tunica vasculosa lentis. Congenital opacities from remnants of the tunica vasculosa lentis are known as posterior or anterior polar cataract. Secondary cataract may develop in association with ocular disease such as uveitis, degenerative retinitis pigmentosa, or trauma. A plaque of proliferating fibrous lens epithelium may develop after trauma or intraocular inflammation forming an anterior subcapsular cataract. Toxic lens opacities may develop with the use of cortisteroids. Cataract may be associated with systemic disease as in diabetes mellitus. A lens capsule defect will lead either to phagocytosis of lens proteins or to lens-induced (phacoanaphylactic or phacotoxic) endophthalmitis.

The macroscopic appearance of the lens at grossing is markedly influenced by the fixative. Lesser degrees of cataract are better studied in vivo with the slit-lamp. Here, only some examples of marked cataract are demonstrated.

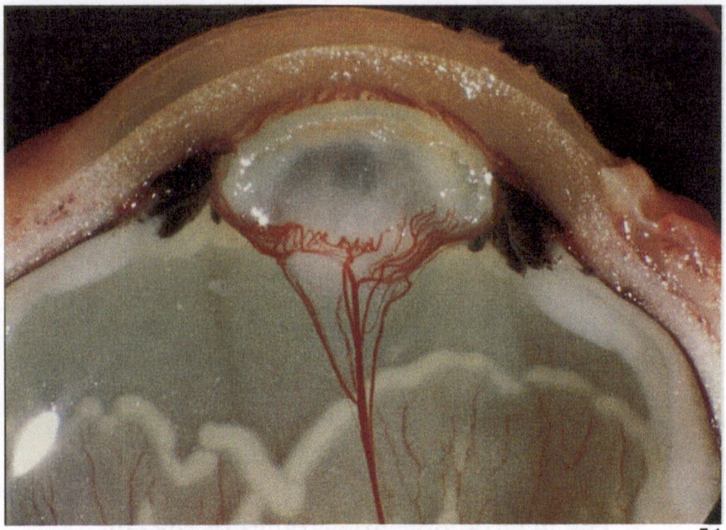

7.1

Congenital Cataract

Congenital cataracts are fairly common, usually bilateral, and of great clinical importance. They are caused by various anomalies interfering with cell metabolism. When the opacity is very dense, surgery is required to prevent amblyopia during the formative phase of the macula and the CNS (during the first few months of life).

Fig. 7.1. Cross section through the lens with persistent hyaloid artery and tunica vasculosa lentis. The posterior lens shows an opacity and backward protrusion of lens material. Histologically there is a posterior lens capsule defect and some macrophage reaction around the lens swollen fibres. There is as yet no pars plana of the ciliary body and retinal blood vessels have developed only to the equator. M 812/75: Male abortus 26th week of gestation with suspected Lowe's syndrome.

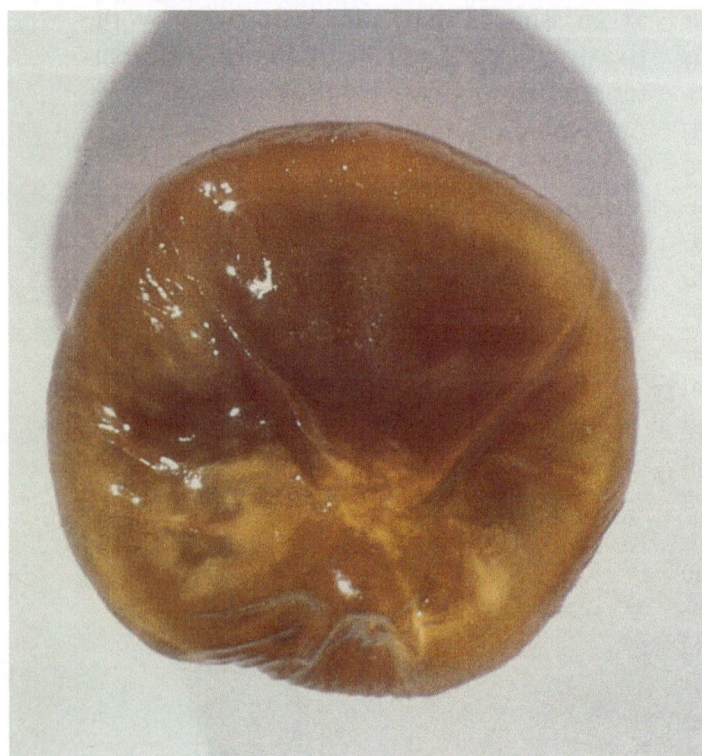

7.2

Age-related (Senile) Cataract

Age-related cataract is a slowly progressive opacification of the lens causing increasingly blurred vision. It starts rather early in life with increasing nuclear pigmentation (sclerosis); later cortical opacities develop. It is a multifactorial type of secondary cataract.

Nuclear Sclerosis

Fig. 7.2. Marked nuclear sclerosis with brownish pigmentation of the lens nucleus. Surgically extracted lens of a 100-year-old man.

Fig. 7.3. Black lens nucleus. Marked peripheral uveal scarring. M 406/72: 64-year-old man with painful blind eye due to secondary glaucoma. Posterior polar iron foreign body retained for 27 years.

Posterior Subcapsular Cataract

Fig. 7.4. Posterior subcapsular cataract. M 1187/80: Autopsy eye without clinical history.

Hypermature Cataract

Fig. 7.5. Shrunken lens with white cortical opacities and brown nuclear sclerosis. M 323/76: 78-year-old woman with hypermature age-related cataract.

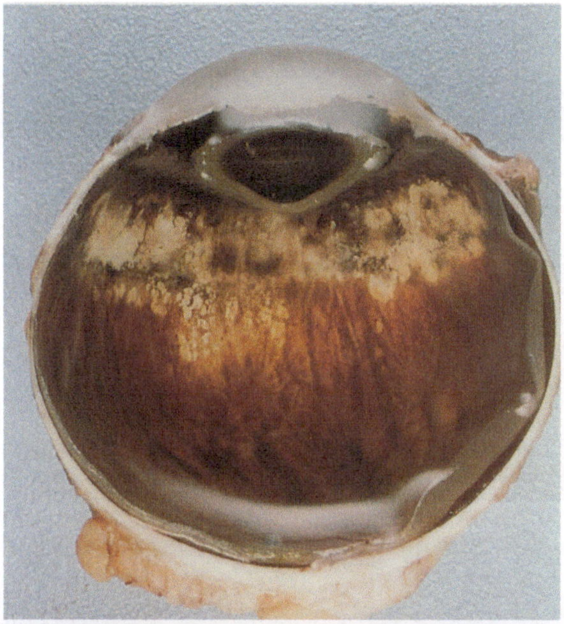

7.3

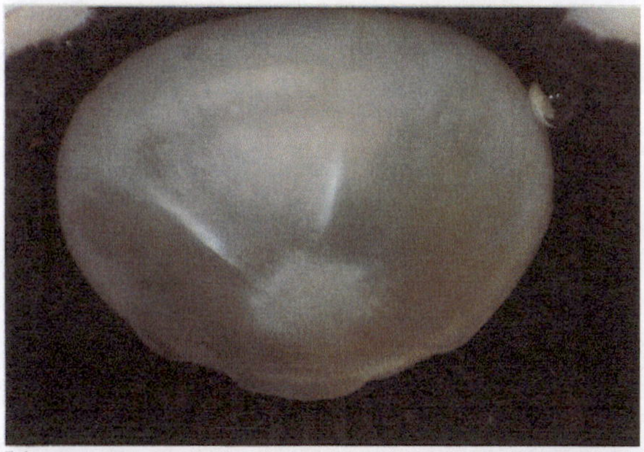

7.4

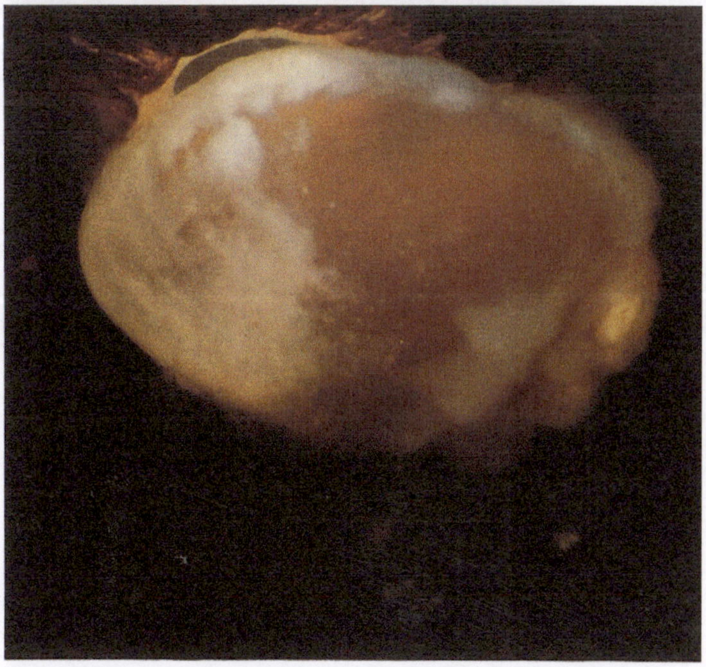

7.5

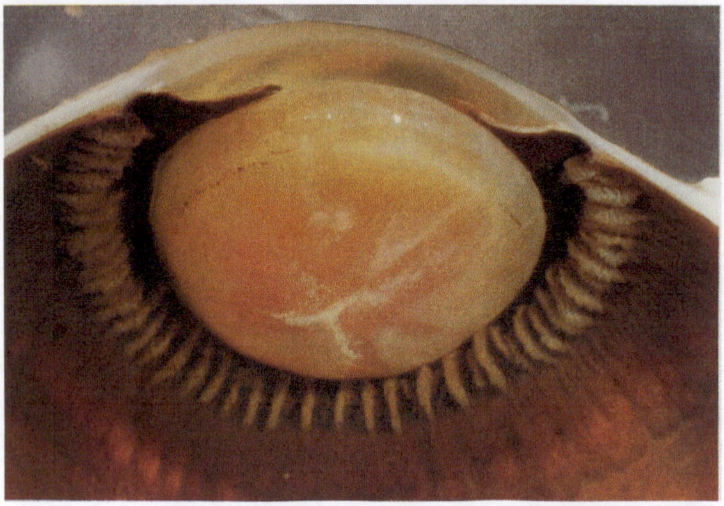

7.6

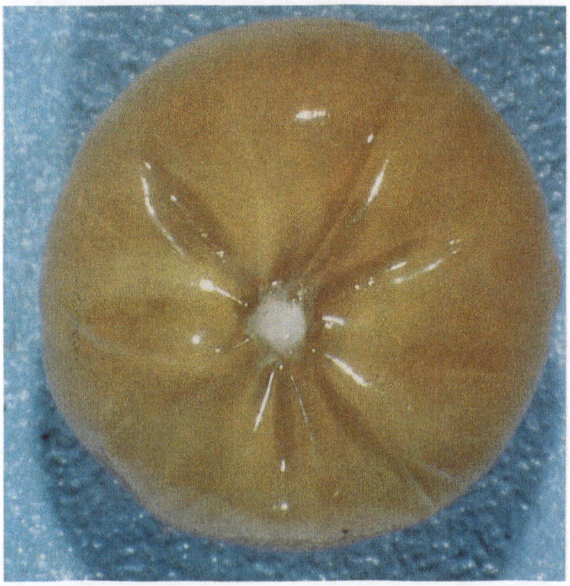

7.7

Secondary Cataract

Secondary cataracts develop in association with a known underlying condition which may be an ocular disease (uveitis, degenerative retinitis pigmentosa, trauma), a toxic reaction (corticosteroids), or systemic disease (diabetes mellitus). Principally they do not differ from age-related cataract although proliferating plaques of lens epithelial cells (polar cataract) are rare in the latter.

Fig. 7.6. Y-shaped opacity of the back of the lens. M 1013/79: 72-year-old man suffering from diabetes mellitus known for 12 years.

Anterior Polar Cataract

Fig. 7.7. Anterior polar cataract. M 589/74: 63-year-old myopic man who had suffered from severe sulfuric acid burn of the eye and dislocation of the lens into the liquefied vitreous.

Morgagnian Cataract

Morgagnian cataract is an advanced stage of cataract. The cortical lens fibres have disintegrated and liquefied so that the pigmented lens nucleus is mobile within the lens capsule.

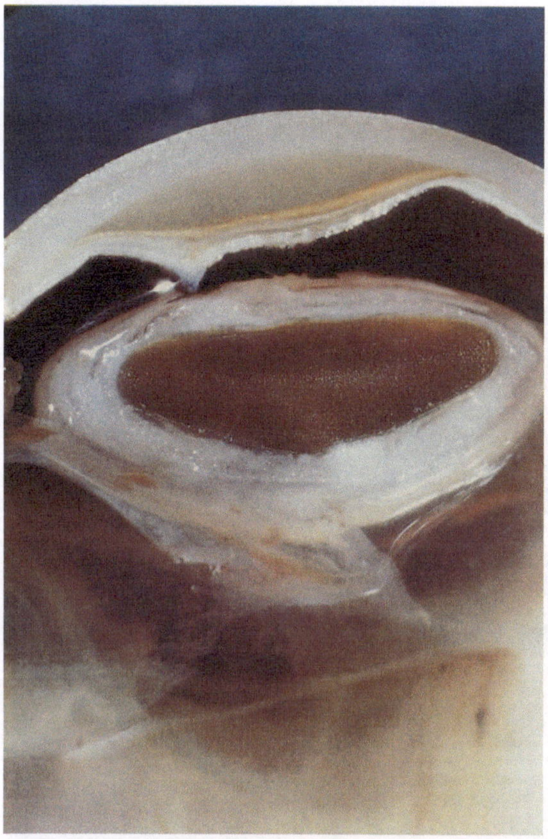

7.8

Fig. 7.8. Brown lens nucleus surrounded by white opaque liquefied cortical lens material. Opacities of the anterior vitreous and peripheral anterior synechias of the iris (goniosynechias). M 176/84: 77-year-old man with absolute postthrombotic neovascular glaucoma and secondary cataract.

Phacolysis

If a Morgagnian cataract is not operated, the lens may sometimes lose its fluid contents through the lens capsule and be absorbed. A macrophage reaction may then cause glaucoma. In rare instances the lens capsule in mature cataract may rupture, setting the lens matter free into the anterior or posterior chamber. This will result in either a macrophagic or leukocytic cellular response leading to lens-induced phacolytic glaucoma or endophthalmitis.

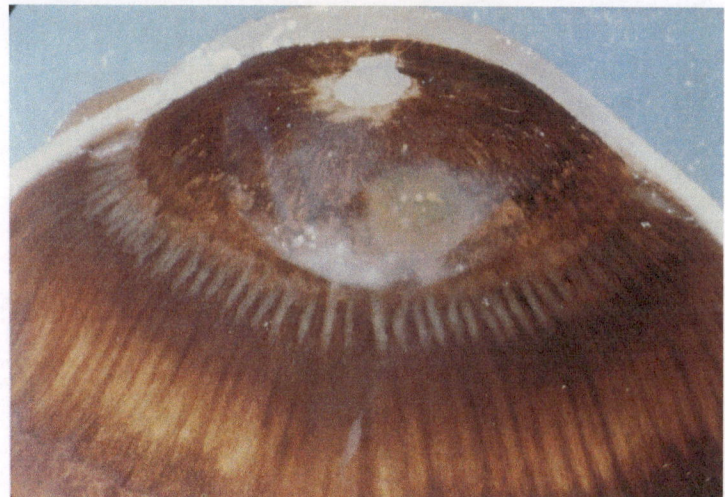

7.9

Fig. 7.9. Remnants of the lens behind the iris. The small lens nucleus contains round light-yellow oxalate crystals. There is a marked depigmentation of the iris pigment epithelium, possibly due to mechanical forces from a markedly swollen lens (mature cataract). M 15/80: 81-year-old man who had had mature cataract 4 years prior to enucleation for absolute glaucoma.

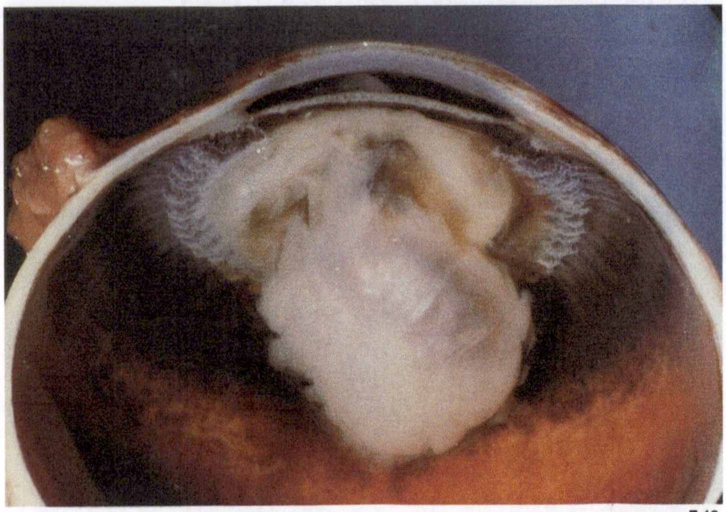

7.10

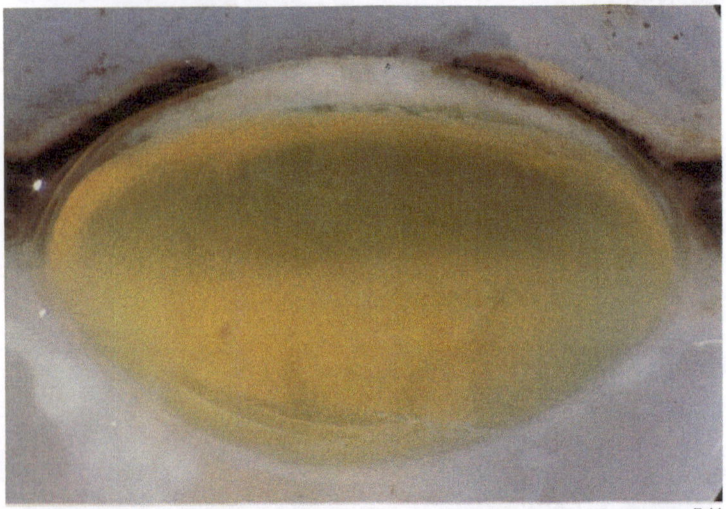

7.11

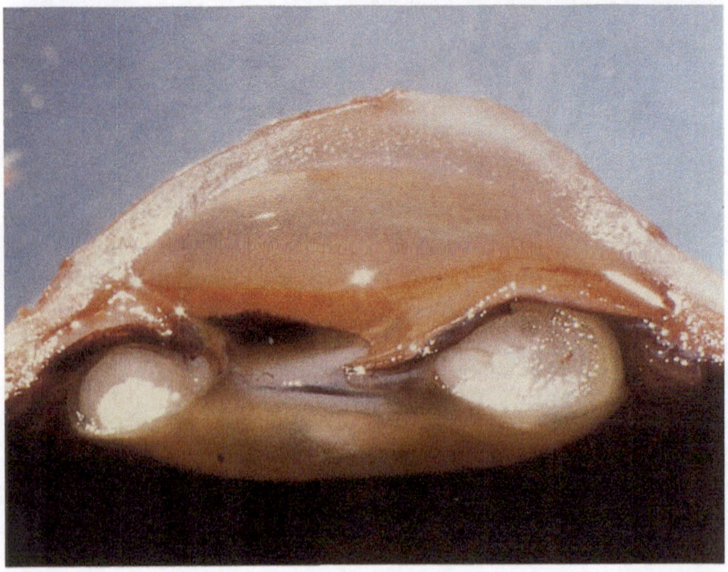

7.12

Fig. 7.10. Ruptured posterior lens capsule. Cortical lens material and the lens nucleus are displaced posteriorly. Whitish material on the ciliary processes (pseudoexfoliation). M 1187/82: 89-year-old man with absolute glaucoma and pseudoexfoliation syndrome.

Inflammation

A defect of the lens capsule (traumatic or spontaneous) with loss of lens protein (antigen) may cause a marked lens-induced hypersensitivity reaction (phacoanaphylactic endophthalmitis). Usually a granulomatous and more rarely a nongranulomatous reaction develops. Microorganisms enjoy an excellent culture medium in free lens protein. Rarely, a spontaneous rupture of the lens capsule may develop in bacterial endophthalmitis followed by intralental abscess formation.

Fig. 7.11. Marked intralental abscess formation in the anterior lens cortex. Opaque heavily infiltrated vitreous. M 341/76: Klebsiella sepsis and septic endophthalmitis from an intravenous tube.

Ring-shaped Lens

Congenital ring-shaped lens (Soemmering's ring cataract) is a rare occurrence. More frequently, a ring-shaped lens develops following trauma (accidental or surgical).

Fig. 7.12. Cross section through a ring-shaped lens remnant. Additionally, there are posterior synechias and fibrous proliferation adjacent to the synechias. M 7/81: 56-year-old man who had sustained an injury 30 years previously resulting in an intraocular metallic foreign body.

8. Optic Nerve

Coloboma · Elevated optic disc · Cupped optic disc · Optic atrophy · Hemorrhage

The optic nerve is a fascicle of the central nervous system and thus reacts like fascicles of the spinal cord. For example there is no axon regeneration. Its sheaths are a continuation of the intracranial meninges (dura mater, arachnoid, and pia mater) as is the subarachnoid space of the optic nerve.

Congenital anomalies such as aplasia or hypoplasia of the optic nerve and colobomas or pits of the optic disc are rare. A commonly encountered clinical entity is an elevated optic disc due to edema (papilledema), inflammation (papillitis), or deposits (drusen of optic disc). Papilledema develops from raised intracranial pressure (space occupying lesions, hydrocephalus, inflammation, cerebral vein thrombosis) and may be associated with hemorrhages at the optic disc or in superficial retina. Cupping of the optic disc is usually caused by increased intraocular pressure. Optic atrophy may result from a variety of diseases (vascular, degenerative, toxic) or may be secondary to papilledema, glaucoma or optic nerve inflammation. Tumors of the optic nerve or disc are mentioned in chapter 10.

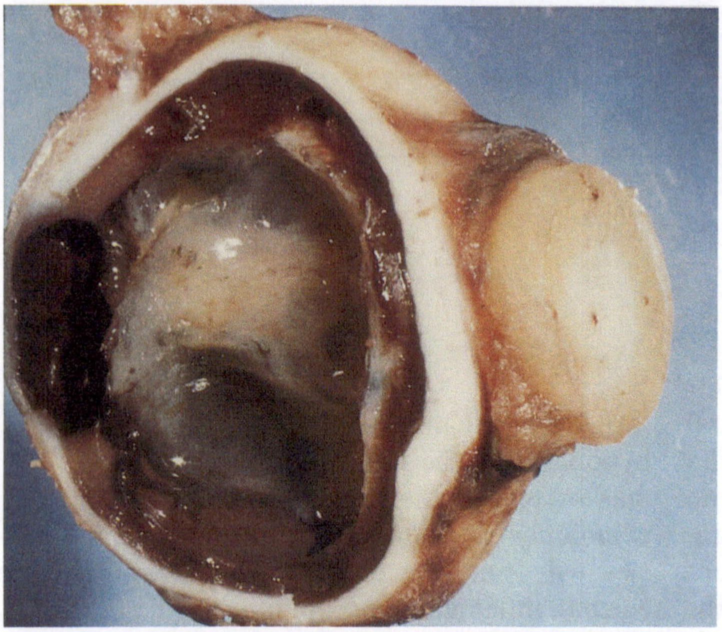

8.1

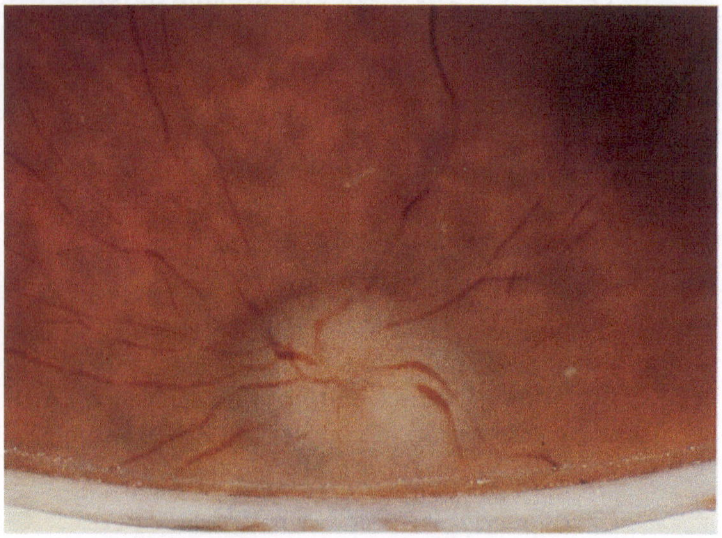

8.2

Coloboma of the Optic Disc

Optic disc colobomas are rare, usually unilateral, and often associated with other ocular abnormalities (retinal and choroidal coloboma, persistent hyaloid artery, retinal detachment). Within the coloboma, fat and muscle tissue may be found.

Fig. 8.1. Within the enlarged cross section of the optic nerve there is a white atrophic optic fascicle with central retinal blood vessels surrounded by yellowish fat tissue. Marked disorganization of intraocular structures. M 1108/80: 30-year-old man with blind microphthalmic eye since birth.

Elevated Optic Disc

Normally the round optic disc has distinct borders and is not elevated above the level of the retinal surface. Elevation and loss of its distinct edge are seen with papilledema, papillitis, and drusen (calcareous laminated deposits) of the optic nerve head.

Fig. 8.2. Elevated optic disc without hemorrhages into the optic disc or retina. Histology revealed drusen of the optic nerve head. M 343/76: 74-year-old female with metastatic adenocarcinoma. Orbital metastasis led to exposure keratitis and pain.

Cupped Optic Disc

A marked cupping of the optic disc with displacement of the central retinal veins to the nasal side is the characteristic finding in long-standing glaucoma. Some cupping of the disc usually without vessel displacement may develop in descending optic atrophy.

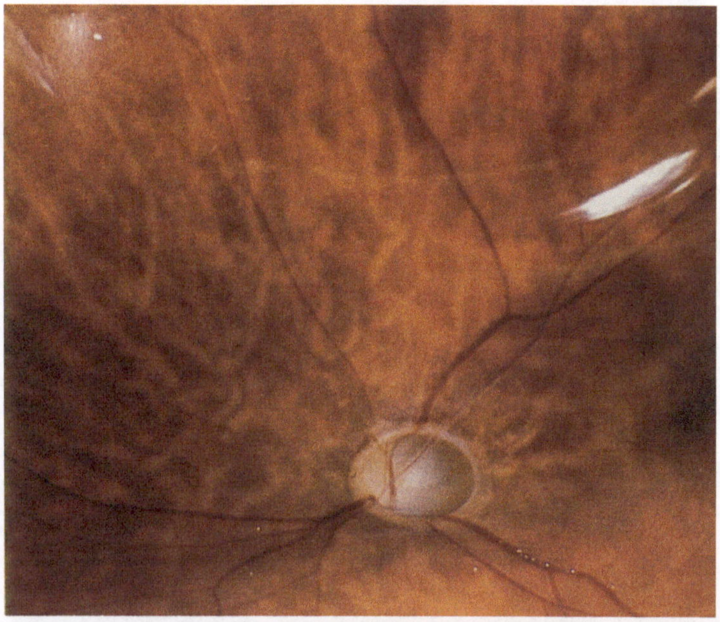

8.3

Fig. 8.3. Deep cupping (excavation) of the optic disc with nasal displacement of central retinal blood vessels. M 795/78: 31-year-old man who had suffered from bilateral alkali burn of the eye and secondary corneal scarring. A Strampelli-type keratoprosthesis had been implanted into one eye, which finally became blind and painful.

Optic Atrophy

Ascending and descending optic atrophy are differentiated. Both lead to a loss of myelin and axons, to glial proliferation and to thickening of connective tissue septae. This results in a shrinkage of the optic fascicle with widening of the subarachnoid space.

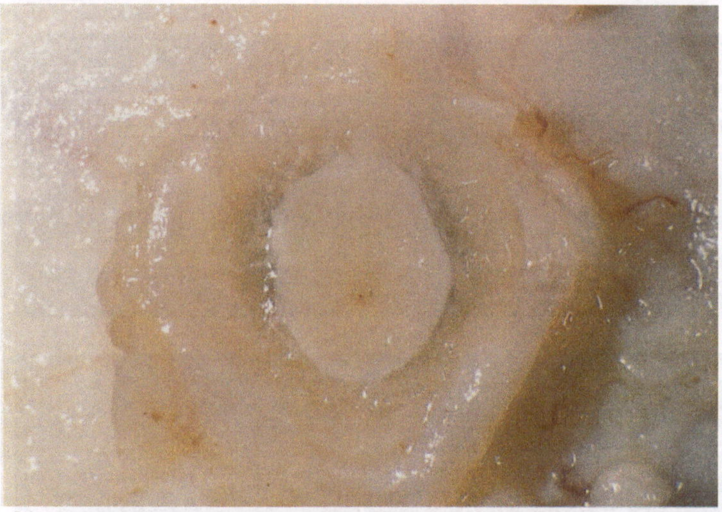

8.4

Fig. 8.4. Cross section of the optic nerve with atrophy of the optic fascicle and widened subarachnoid space. Autopsy eye without clinical history.

Subarachnoid Hemorrhage

Intracranial subarachnoid hemorrhage may extend into the subarachnoid space of the optic nerve. Sometimes there are associated retinal hemorrhages known as Terson's phenomenon.

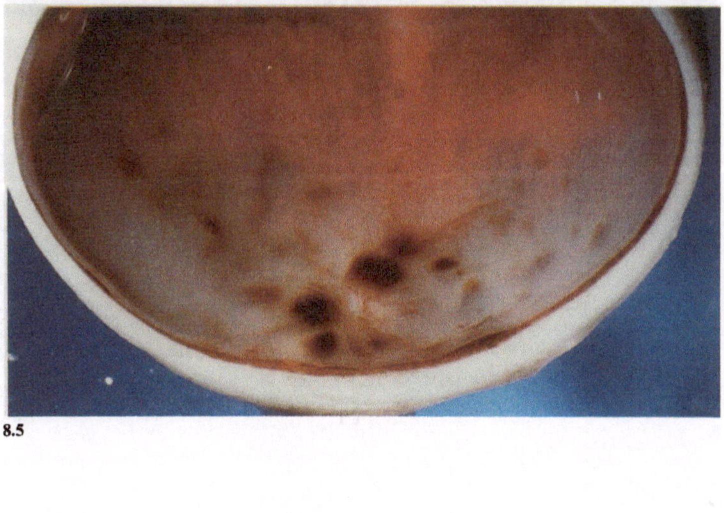

8.5

Fig. 8.5. Retinal hemorrhages (Terson's phenomenon). M 705/77: 53-year-old man who died from acute subarachnoid hemorrhage due to ruptured cerebral aneurysm.

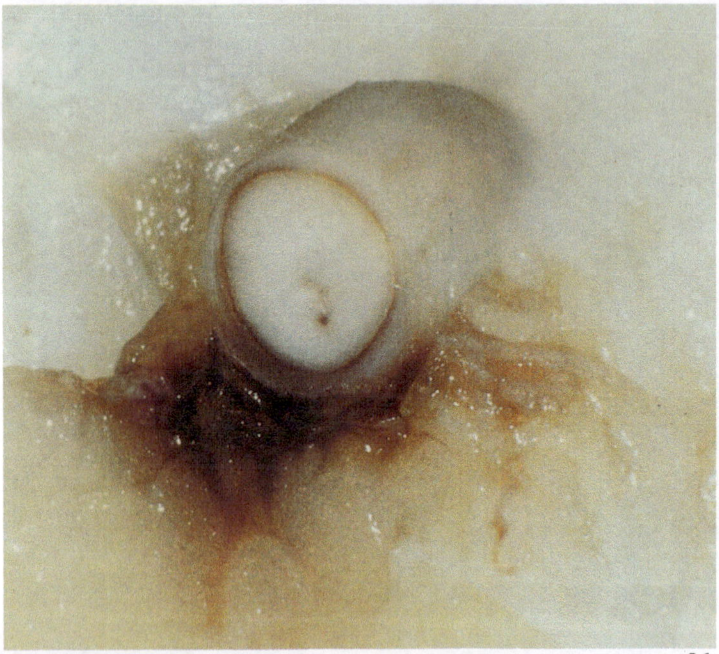

8.6

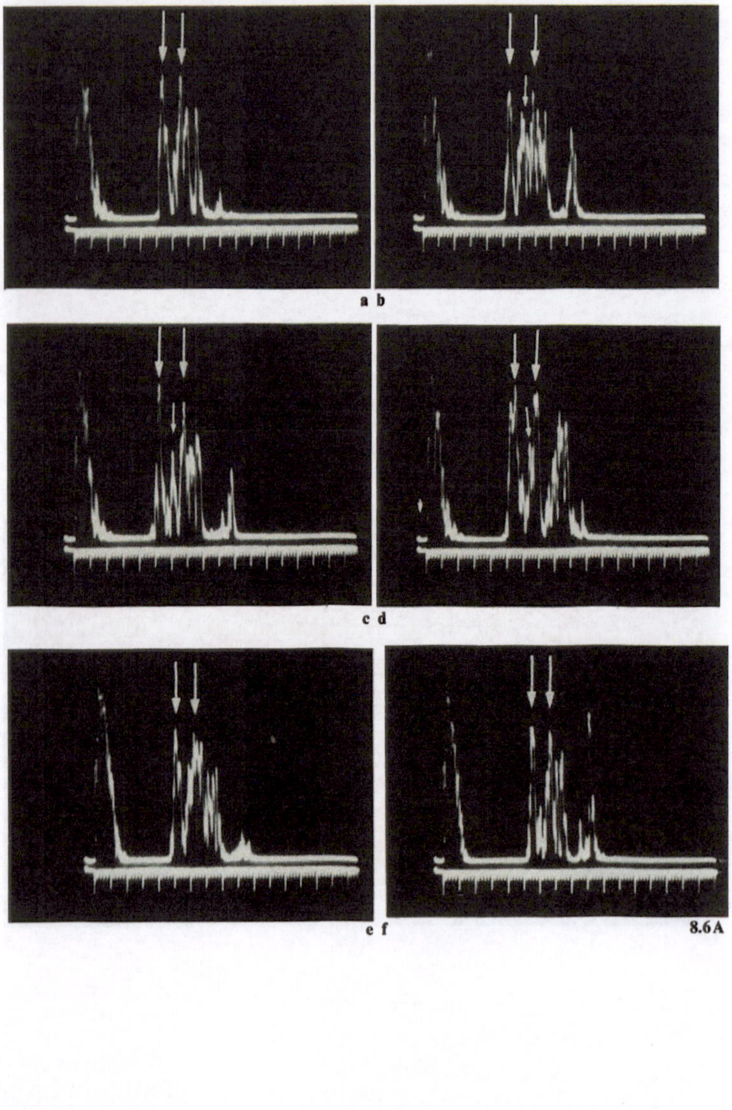

8.6A

Fig. 8.6. Subarachnoid hemorrhage of the optic nerve. M 1122/81: 17-year-old boy who died from traumatic skull fracture with subdural and subarachnoid hemorrhage.

Fig. 8.6A. Optic nerve/subarachnoid hemorrhage. A-scan echograms (cross sections) of a normal optic nerve (**a** arrows indicate temporal = left arrow and nasal = right arrow surface of the optic nerve/dura mater). The optic nerve is best displayed with the eye in the primary position by placing the sound probe on the temporal conjunctiva and angling it posteriorly. The medial rectus muscle serves as a landmark. Optic nerve with posttraumatic subarachnoid hemorrhage (**b, c** small arrow indicates optic nerve sheath widened by fluid. This may be verified by the so-called 45-degree test). **d** displaying the optic nerve using the 45-degree test; that is, the patient is asked to look about 45 degrees to the temporal side with the sound probe placed on the temporal conjunctiva. Note the decreased width of the subarachnoid space (small arrow). On follow-up examinations at two (**e**) and six (**f**) weeks the thickness of the optic nerve sheaths decreases.

9. Glaucoma

Congenital glaucoma · Open-angle glaucoma · Angle-closure glaucoma · Tissue reactions

Glaucoma is an elevation of intraocular pressure with consecutive ocular tissue and optic nerve damage, leading to visual field defects and blindness. Usually an increase in intraocular pressure results from impaired outflow. Hypersecretion is a rare cause. Congenital (developmental) glaucoma, primary glaucoma with open or closed chamber angle, and secondary glaucoma with open or closed angle due to intraocular inflammation, traumatic lesions, changes in the lens or uveal disease are differentiated. Absolute glaucoma denotes a blind, often painful eye with untreatable high intraocular pressure.

Clinically, glaucoma is of extreme importance because it is the leading cause of permanent blindness. Among primary glaucomas, open-angle glaucoma (chronic simple glaucoma) is far more common than closed-angle glaucoma. Macroscopy is only able to demonstrate tissue changes causing aqueous outflow obstruction and tissue reactions resulting from raised intraocular pressure. As many conditions with raised intraocular pressure are demonstrated elsewhere, only a few examples are presented here.

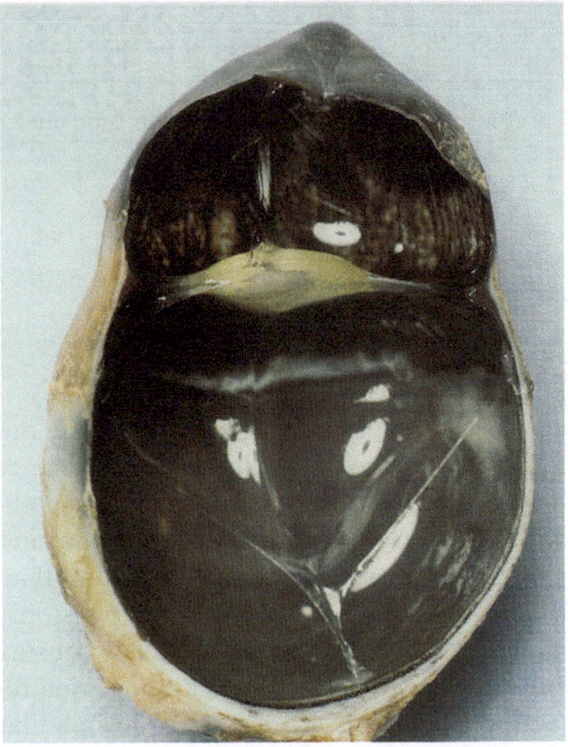

9.1

Congenital Glaucoma

Congenital glaucoma may be present at birth or develop shortly after. Often it is an inherited malformation of the angle structures associated with other ocular or systemic malformations. Chronically raised intraocular pressure results in enlargement of the eye (buphthalmos, hydrophthalmos) including the cornea. This results in a deep space anterior to the lens, and if the iris is in normal position, a deep anterior chamber. In cases with total anterior synechia, a large corneal staphyloma will be present.

Fig. 9.1. Marked corneal staphyloma, enlarged corneal and interciliary diameter, and less obvious enlargement of the posterior segment of the eye. Small lens. Vitreous liquefaction and posterior vitreous detachment. M 272/78: 8-year-old girl with congenital glaucoma, nystagmus, buphthalmos (hydrophthalmos), and corneal staphyloma.

Open-angle (Chronic Simple) Glaucoma

This is the most common type of primary glaucoma and its incidence increases with age (especially over the age of 40). It is usually bilateral and is initially asymptomatic. The only sign is an elevated intraocular pressure. The anterior chamber angle appears morphologically normal. These patients have a higher risk of central retinal vein occlusion. Late in the disease, the patient becomes aware of visual field defects and decreased visual acuity. Secondary open-angle glaucoma develops from structural elements (cells and its remnants, blood, pigment, pseudoexfoliative material) obstructing the aqueous outflow system. In some patients primary open-angle glaucoma is associated with pseudoexfoliation syndrome.

Pseudoexfoliation Syndrome

This is a deposition of fibrillar proteinaceous material of as yet unknown origin (basement membrane material has been suspected) on the structures lining the posterior and anterior chamber. This has been termed glaucoma capsulare when associated with open-angle glaucoma.

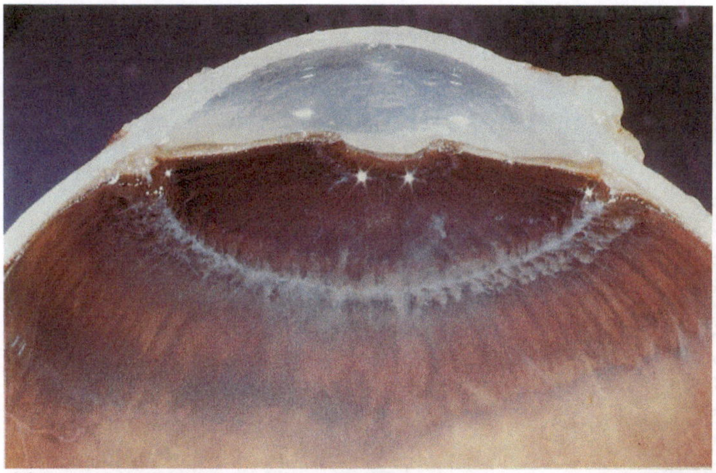

9.2

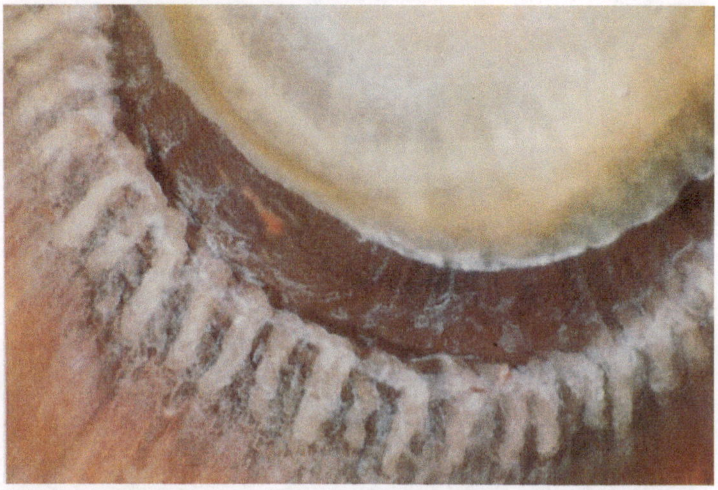

9.3

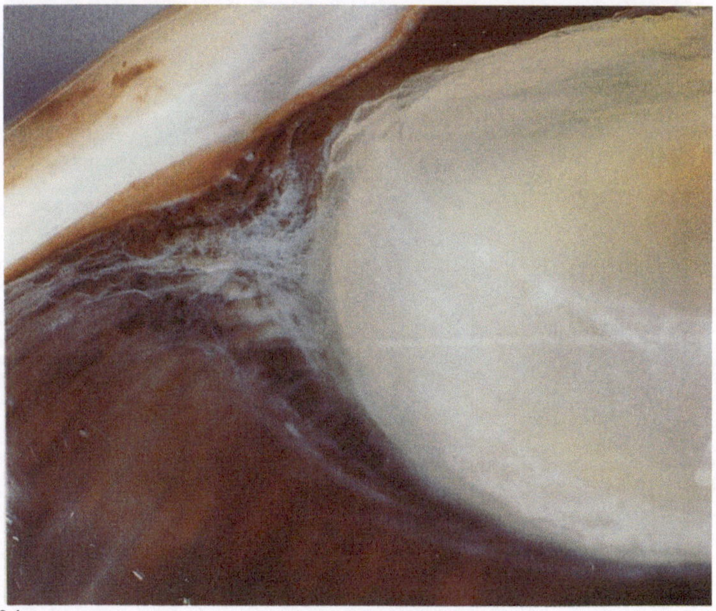

9.4

Fig. 9.2. Pseudoexfoliative material mainly covering the posterior aspect of the ciliary processes. The anterior chamber angle is open. The lens has been removed at grossing. M 280/84: 74-year-old woman with glaucoma capsulare.

Fig. 9.3. Pseudoexfoliative material on the ciliary body, the back of the iris, and the equator of the lens. M 411/73: 84-year-old man with glaucoma capsulare, bullous keratopathy and acute corneal ulcer.

Fig. 9.4. Pseudoexfoliative material on the zonules. M 1146/83: 72-year-old man with glaucoma capsulare and rubeosis iridis due to central retinal vein occlusion.

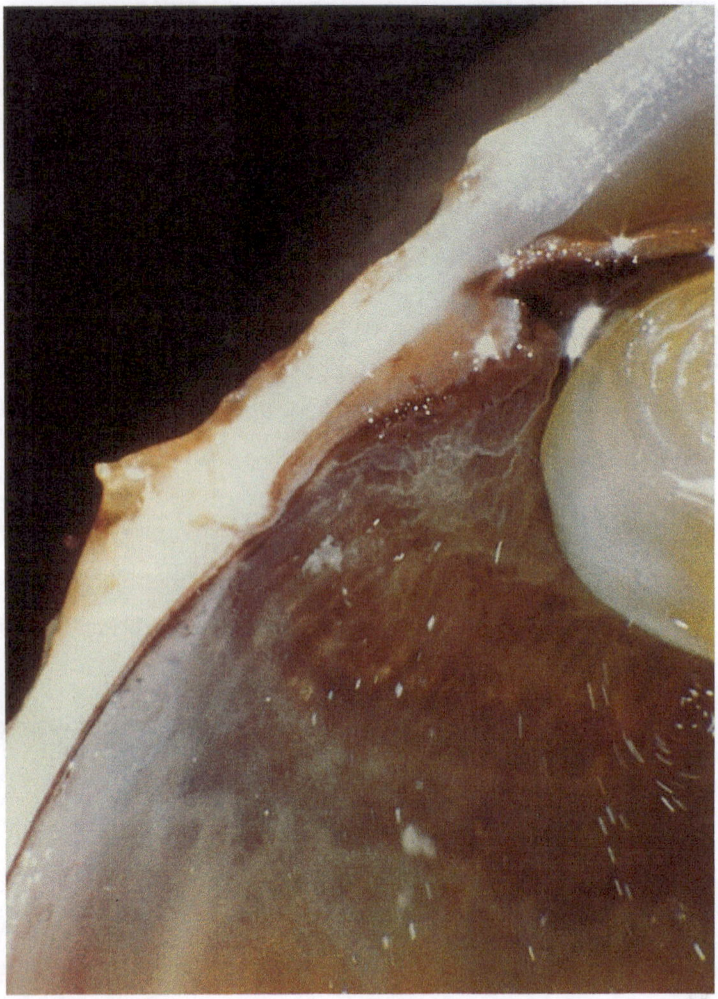

9.5

Closed-Angle Glaucoma

Primary closed-angle (acute congestive) glaucoma develops in predisposed eyes, especially small (hypermetropic) eyes, with a narrow anterior chamber angle.

Secondary closed-angle glaucoma is usually the result of postinflammatory, posttraumatic, or postthrombotic peripheral anterior synechias (goniosynechias) or anterior displacement of the iris-lens diaphragm (e.g., lens swelling or displacement, posterior synechias, tumors and others).

Neovascular Glaucoma

There are a variety of conditions which cause neovascularization of the anterior surface of the iris (clinically termed rubeosis iridis). Among the most important are proliferative diabetic and postthrombotic retinopathy, trauma, untreated retinal detachment, and tumors. Peripheral anterior synechias (goniosynechias) resulting from the neovascular tissue often lead to untreatable and finally absolute glaucoma.

Fig. 9.5. Peripheral anterior synechia (goniosynechia). The white dots in the vitreous are light reflexes. M 252/77: 73-year-old man with untreatable absolute postthrombotic neovascular glaucoma.

Glaucomatous Tissue Reactions

Acute as well as chronic elevation of intraocular pressure causes tissue damage. Acute congestive glaucoma produces hypoxic changes (glaukomflecken in the lens, infarcts of the iris, optic nerve edema) which are better observed by biomicroscopy or histopathology. Chronic tissue damage is macroscopically most obvious on the optic disc (cupping) and optic nerve (atrophy). In long-standing glaucoma, chorioretinal atrophy may develop. Peculiar radial scleral depressions with reactive changes of the overlying retinal pigment epithelium may be observed in absolute glaucoma.

Glaucomatous Optic Nerve

Fig. 9.6. Cupped optic disc and optic atrophy with widened subarachnoid space of the optic nerve. M 772/80: 69-year-old woman with untreatable absolute glaucoma.

Radial Scleral Depressions

Fig. 9.7. Radial hyperpigmented stripes between the ora serrata and the posterior pole. M 14/79: 58-year-old man with absolute glaucoma from secondary posttraumatic angle closure 41 years after penetrating injury.

Fig. 9.8. Cross section through the stripes at the equator showing depressions of the sclera.

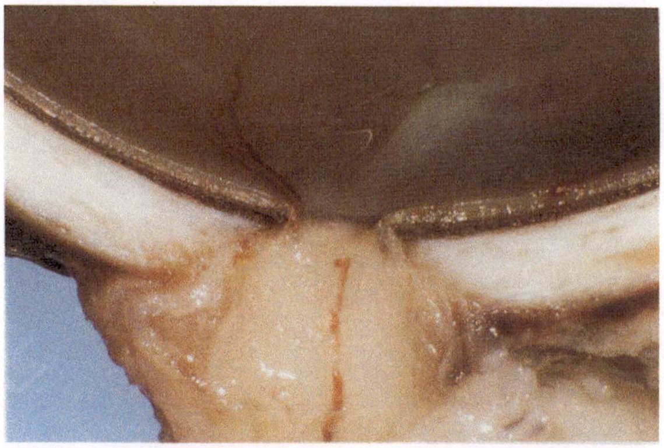

9.6

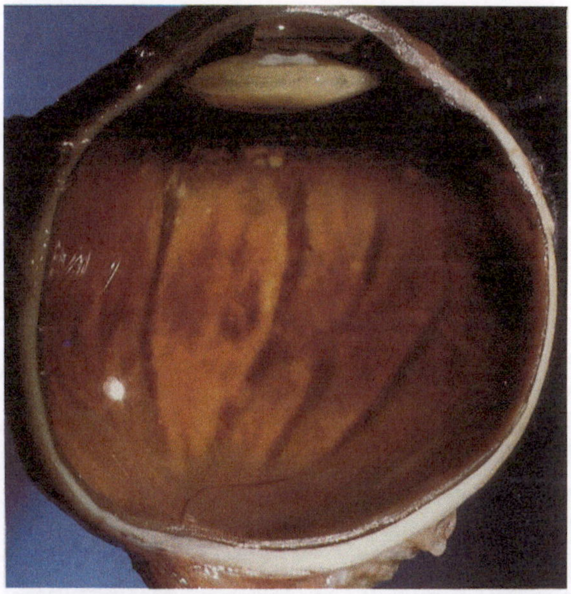

9.7

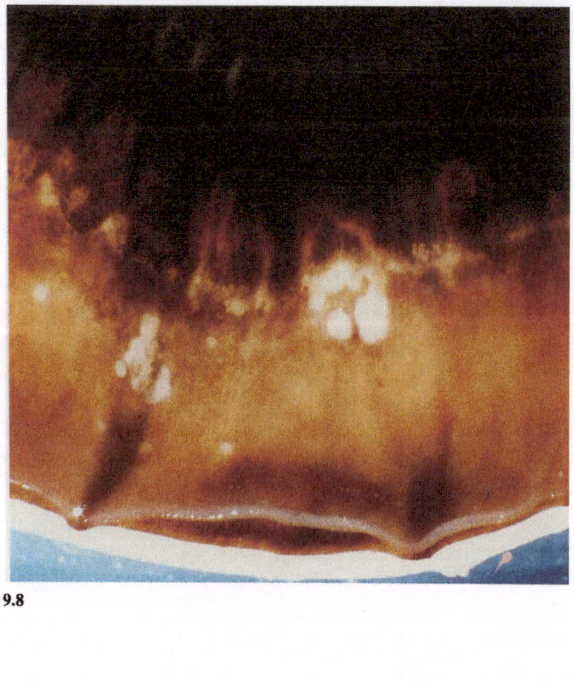

9.8

10. Tumors and Pseudotumors

Intraocular: *Nevi · Hemangioma · Angiomatosis · Malignant melanoma · Retinoblastoma Metastases · Pseudotumors*

Optic nerve: *Glioma · Meningioma*

Orbital: *Hemangioma · Cyst · Lymphoma · Metastases · Pseudotumors*

The eye and its adnexae may be the primary site of a variety of benign and malignant ectodermal, neuroectodermal, and mesenchymal tumors. Tumors of the lid and conjunctiva are not mentioned here. Tumors of the eye and the orbit usually cause fairly early symptoms and/or signs. Visual acuity, visual fields, and the normal position of the eye are often affected. Highly malignant intraocular and orbital tumors must be differentiated from benign space-occupying lesions. The indirect ophthalmoscope, fluorescein angiography, and ultrasonography are the most important diagnostic tools for differentiating intraocular masses. Ultrasonography and CT scanning have facilitated the examination of patients with suspected orbital tumors. The macroscopic appearance of malignant orbital tumors such as rhabdomyosarcoma adds very little to the understanding or orbital disease. They are therefore not included here.

Secondary ocular and orbital tumors may arise from adjacent structures or metastasize to the eye and orbit from distant primary tumors.

Nonneoplastic space-occupying lesions (inflammatory, degenerative, developmental) are often called pseudotumors because their symptoms and/or signs mimic a malignant growth.

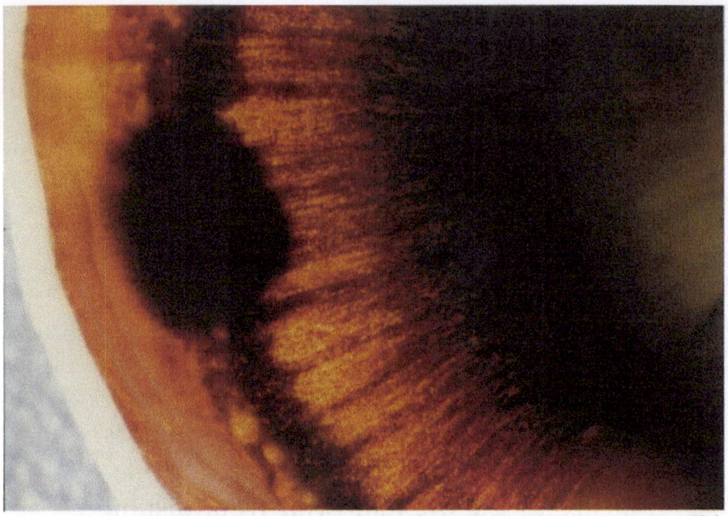

10.1

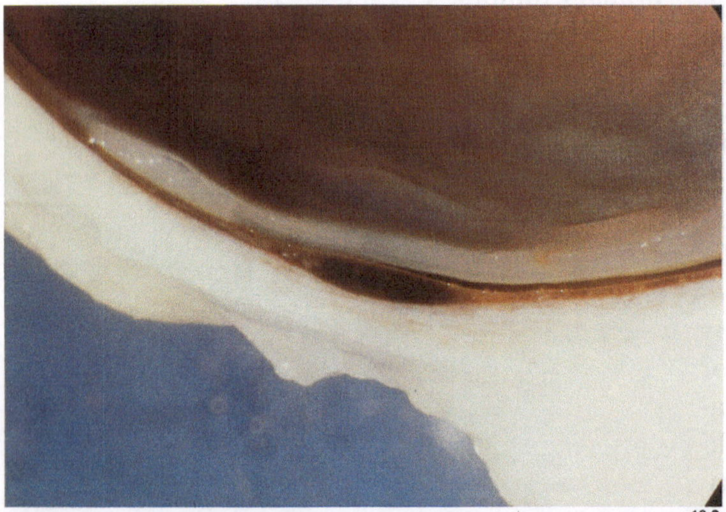

10.2

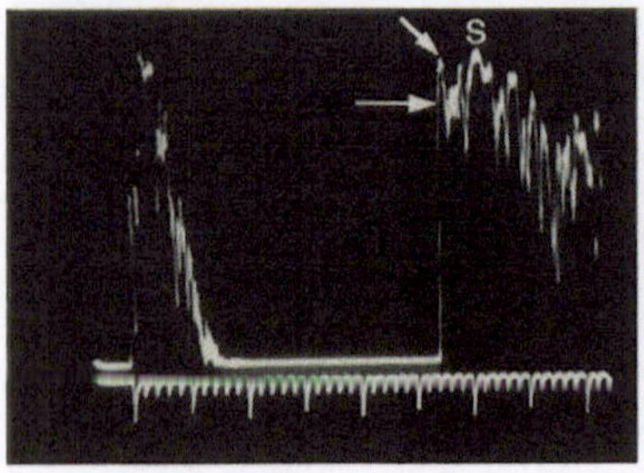

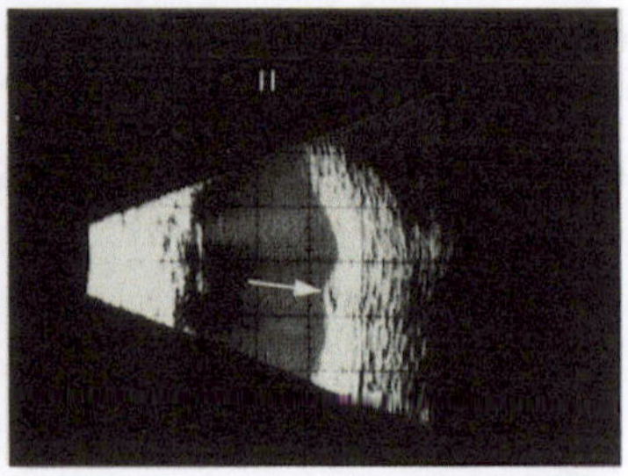

a b 10.2A

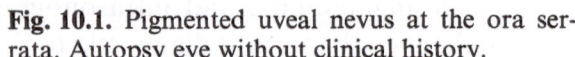

Primary Benign Intraocular Tumors

Common benign intraocular tumors are uveal nevi and Fuchs' adenoma of the ciliary body. Less common are angiomas of the choroid or retina, as well as glial tumors of the retina and optic nerve head. Benign intraocular neural, osseous, ciliary epithelial, or muscle tumors are very rare. All of them may play a role in the differential diagnosis of malignant intraocular tumors.

Uveal Nevi

Pigmented flat nevi of 1–2 disc diameters are a common finding throughout the entire uvea, but especially in the choroid. They usually do not cause symptoms and are an incidental finding during routine ophthalmoscopy. Larger nevi may be difficult to differentiate from small malignant melanomas.

Fig. 10.1. Pigmented uveal nevus at the ora serrata. Autopsy eye without clinical history.

Fig. 10.2. Cross section through a pigmented choroidal nevus at the posterior pole. The nevus fills the entire thickness of the choroid. The overlying retina is unaffected. M 379/82: Autopsy eye of a 41-year-old man without clinical history.

Fig. 10.2 A. Choroidal nevus. A-scan echogram (**a**) and contact B-scan echogram (**b**) of a choroidal nevus. Note the high reflectivity and mostly homogeneous structure (*thin arrow*) in the A-scan (*S*= sclera) and the flat to slightly dome-shaped appearance in the B-scan.

Hemangioma of the Choroid

Isolated Hemangioma of the Choroid

Isolated hemangioma of the choroid, not associated with Sturge-Weber syndrome may be difficult to differentiate from malignant melanoma of the choroid. Secondary intraocular tissue reaction such as cystoid degeneration of the retina with field defects, serous retinal detachment, and subretinal hemorrhage with scarring can, in fact, lead to the clinical appearance of solid retinal detachment.

Fig. 10.3. Engorged vessels within a thickened portion of the posterior choroid. Thickened retina of the posterior pole due to secondary cystoid degeneration of the macula. M 248/74: 67-year-old woman enucleated because of suspected malignant melanoma of the choroid.

Fig. 10.3A. Choroidal hemangioma. A-scan echograms (**a, b**) and contact B-scan echograms (**c, d**) of a small choroidal hemangioma (*R*=retina; *S*=sclera; *arrows*=hemangioma). Note the high reflectivity and the homogeneity of the structure (**a**). Follow-up examination showed little increased prominence.

Fig. 10.4. Serous detachment of the macula. Some subretinal hemorrhage and scarring. Hemangioma of the choroid between the optic disc and macula. Large pigmented nevus on the temporal side of the macula. M 152/76: 63-year-old man enucleated because of suspected malignant melanoma of the choroid.

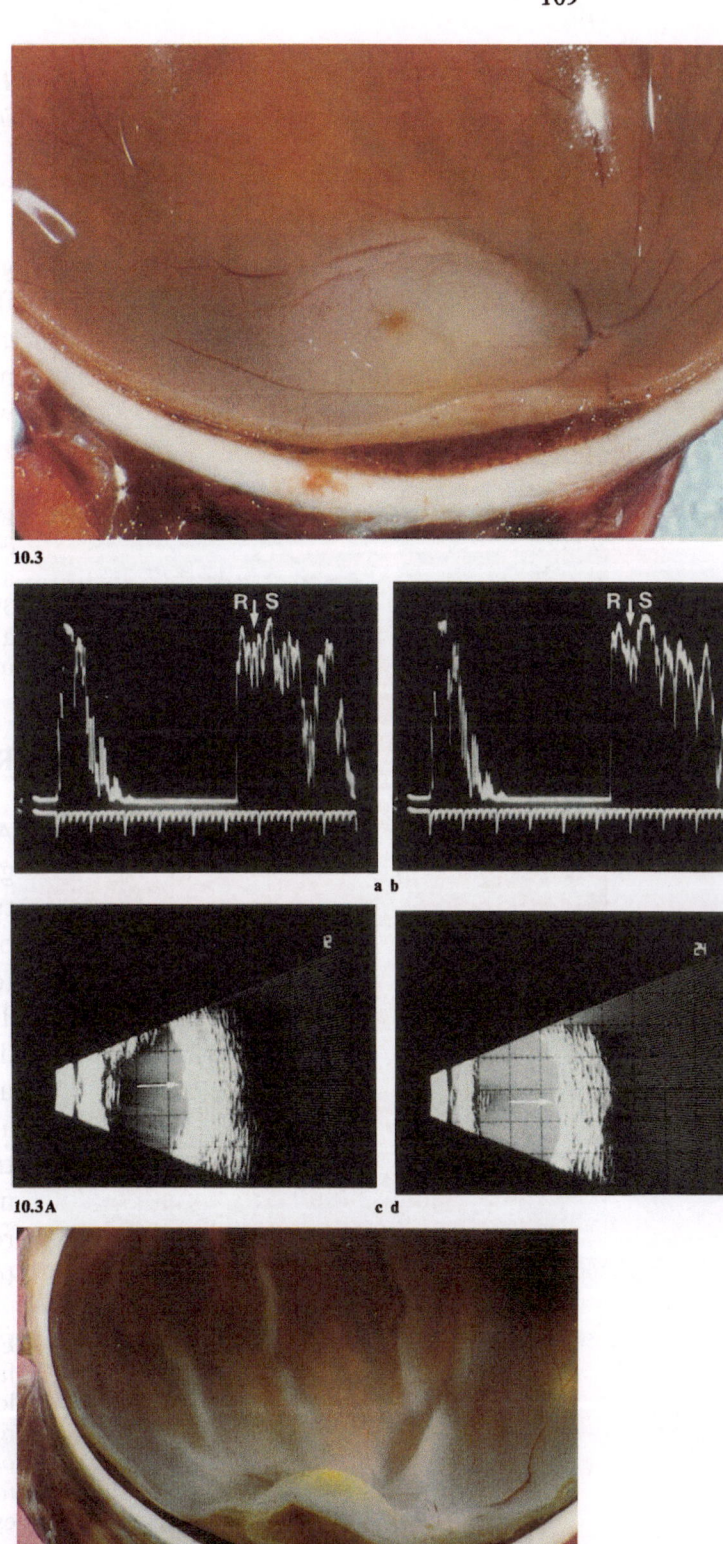

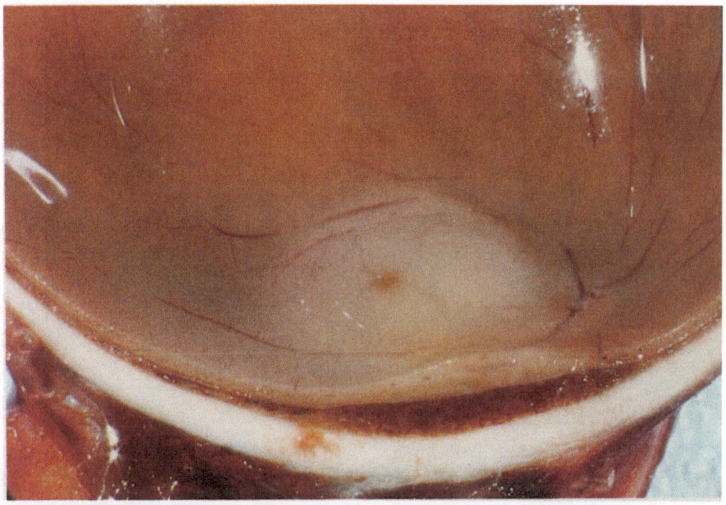

10.3

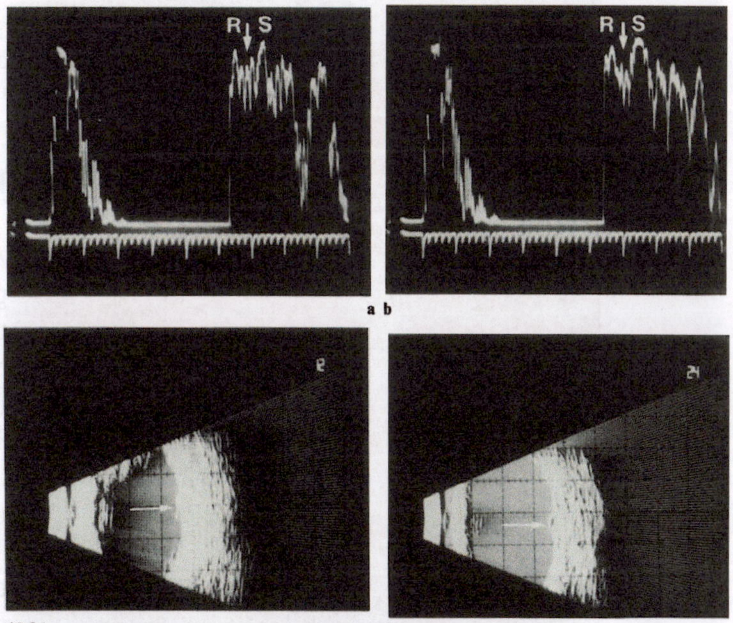

a b

10.3A c d

10.4

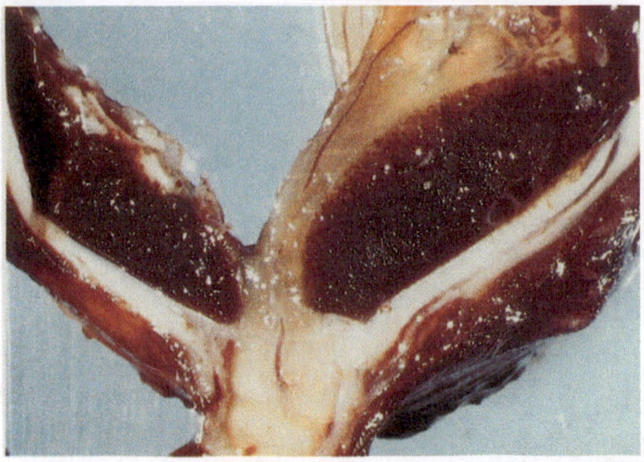

10.5

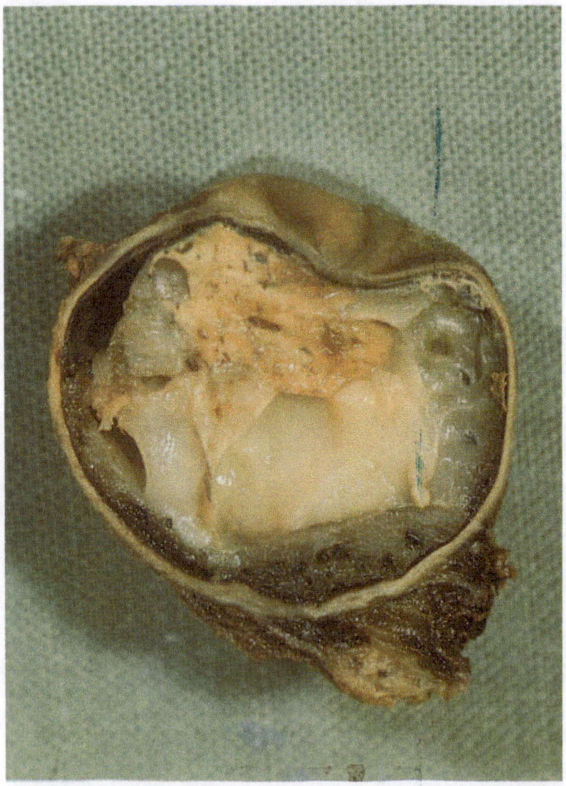

10.6

Hemangioma of the Choroid in Sturge-Weber Syndrome

Sturge-Weber syndrome (encephalotrigeminal angiomatosis, meningocutaneous angiomatosis) with unilateral facial nevus flammeus, cavernous hemangioma of the choroid, hemangioma of the meninges, and meningeal calcification is often associated with congenital or secondary glaucoma, seizures, and mental retardation.

Fig. 10.5. Large cavernous hemangioma of the central choroid around the optic disc with secondary degenerative changes of the retina. M 642/82: 39-year-old man with Sturge-Weber syndrome and absolute glaucoma. This eye had had a penetrating injury 10 years previously.

Retinal Angioma (von Hippel's Tumor)

Angioma of the retina (capillary hemangioma, angiomatosis retinae, von Hippel's tumor) may develop as an isolated tumor or in association with an hemangioblastoma of the cerebellum (Lindau's tumor). This association is called von Hippel-Lindau's disease. In early stages the small nodular retinal angioma with its feeder vessel are easily recognized clinically and are treated with light coagulation. Large angiomas result in secondary changes of the surrounding retina and finally the tumor leads to disorganization of intraocular structures.

Fig. 10.6. A nitric acid decalcified globe with artifactitious discoloration of the tissues. Opaque yellow tumorous mass in the anterior vitreous with retinal detachment (white subretinal fluid) and secondary ossification at the posterior pole (grayish mass). M 217/74: 23-year-old female with a blind eye for 11 years and glaucoma for 3 years.

Intraocular Malignant Melanoma

Malignant melanoma of the uveal structures is the most common primary intraocular tumor. The incidence is about one malignant melanoma of the uveal tract in population of 100,000 per year. This number has been constant over decades. Exogenous factors such as sunlight and endogenous factors such as pigmentation may play a role in the development of the tumor. The patient harboring an intraocular malignant melanoma is usually about 50 to 60 years old and has very little risk of developing a similar tumor in the fellow eye. Genetic transmission is extremely rare. Generally speaking, ophthalmologists are interested in treating a malignant melanoma before it becomes a risk to the patient's life and eye.

Malignant Melanoma of the Choroid

The most common site for a malignant melanoma is the choroid (posterior segment of the eye), where about 85% of the tumors

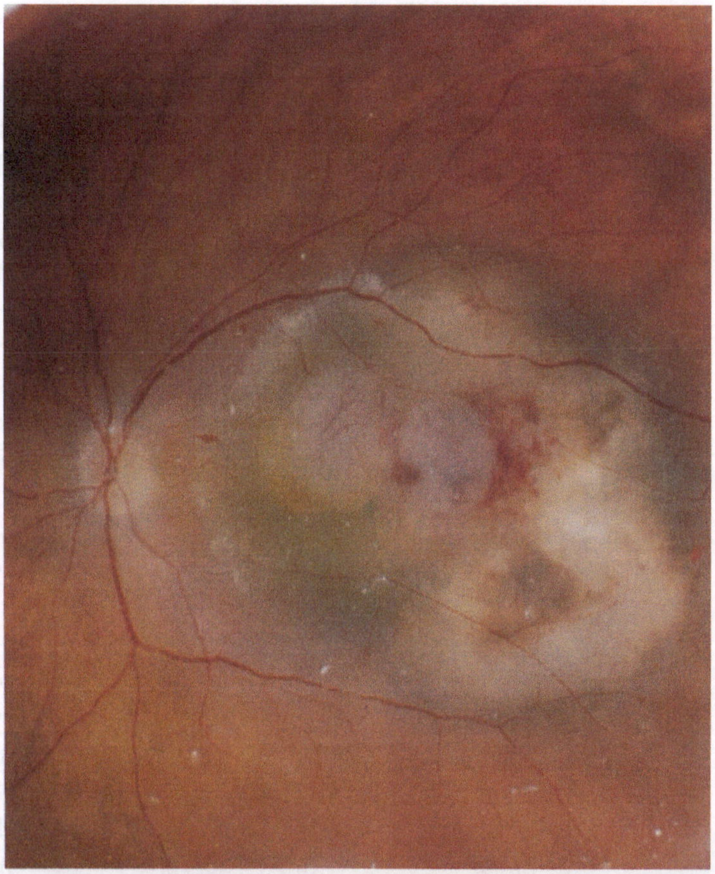

10.7

Fig. 10.7. Fairly small malignant melanoma at the posterior pole of the eye with some hemorrhages and secondary retinal degeneration. M 255/74: 62-year-old female with malignant melanoma of the choroid at the choroid at the posterior pole. The tumor was observed clinically for 2 years.

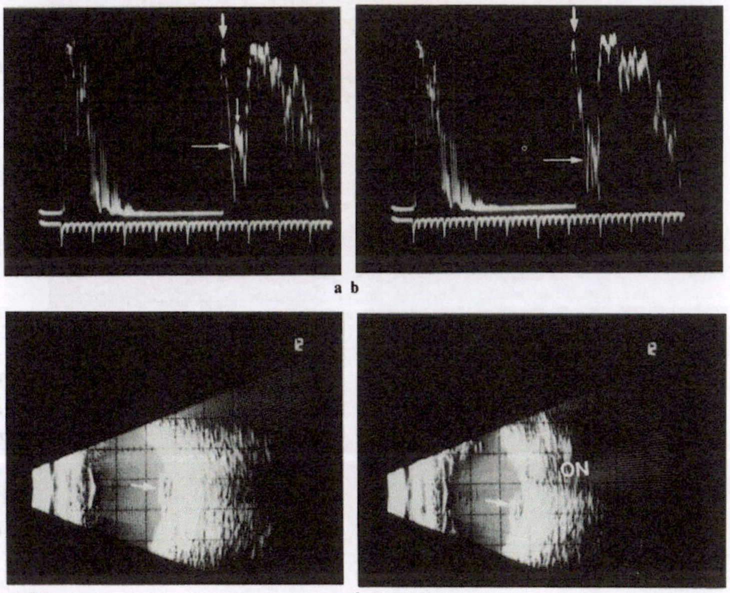

a b

10.7A c d

Fig. 10.7A. Malignant melanoma of the choroid. A-scan echograms (**a, b**) and contact B-scan echograms (**c, d**) of a small choroidal melanoma localized at the posterior pole. Note the very high surface signal (*short arrows*) and the low to medium high internal echo signals from the melanoma (*long arrows*) which are mostly homogeneous and typically show some fast flickering signals representing vessels within the melanoma (*small arrow*/**a**). Vertical (**c**) and horizontal (**d**) sections with the contact B-scan show a flat, dome-shaped appearance and its location at the posterior pole (*ON*=optic nerve).

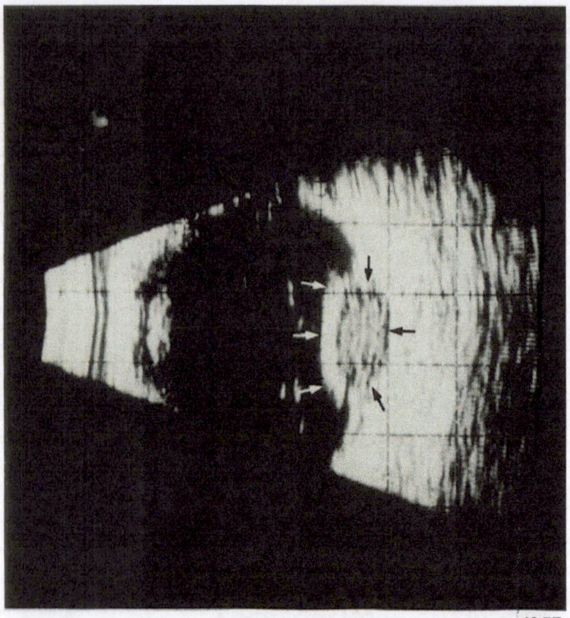

10.7B

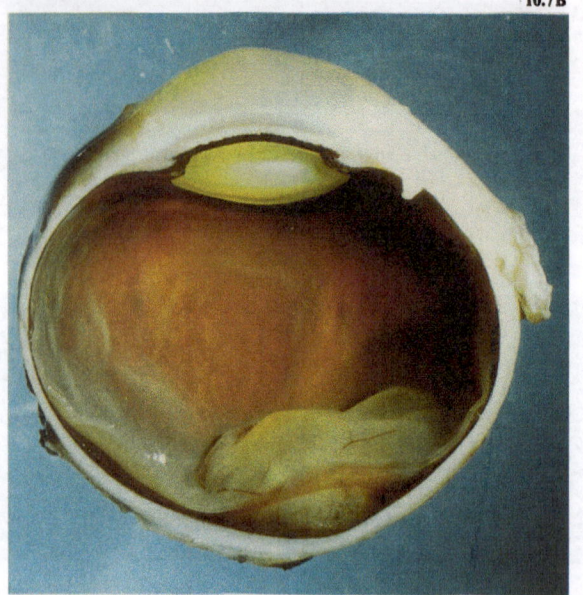

10.8

develop. The tumor grows in nodular fashion in most cases, leading to penetration of Bruch's membrane and a mushroom-shaped appearance. Growth may occasionally be flat (diffuse) and confined to choroid without showing any tendency to penetrate Bruch's membrane. Clinically the most reliable prognostic factor in malignant melanomas of the choroid is the tumor size. With increasing size the prognosis becomes poorer and secondary intraocular reactions (retinal detachment, vitreous hemorrhage, secondary glaucoma) may obscure a direct view of the tumor. Often it is these late secondary reactions which produce the first symptoms of an advanced lesions. However in routine ophthalmoscopic examination and in patients where the tumor is located beneath the macula thus causing early symptoms, a small malignant melanoma may be detected. Tumors measuring over 10 mm in diameter have a poorer prognosis than smaller ones. The tumor may be pigmented or nonpigmented (amelanotic). Marked pigmentation may signal a poorer prognosis. Another reliable prognostic factor is the tumor cell type. Tumors composed entirely of spindle-shaped cells have a better prognosis than those containing the larger epitheloid cell type. Spontaneous regression is extremely rare, but necrosis of the tumor may occur. Tumors with extra-

Fig. 10.7B. Malignant melanoma of the choroid. Contact B-scan echogram of a choroidal melanoma with pronounced "choroidal excavation" (*black arrows*), a diagnostic, although not pathognomonic echographic feature.

Fig. 10.8. Small malignant melanoma of 3 mm height and 9 mm diameter in the posterior choroid. There is a secondary retinal detachment around the tumor. M 557/77: 35-year-old female with malignant melanoma of the central choroid. A central lesion was classified as central choroiditis by several ophthalmologists 9 years previously.

ocular invasion (along the scleral emissaria, the optic nerve or along the trabecular meshwork and Schlemm's canal) will usually have metastasized and thus have a very poor prognosis. Blood-borne metastases are found mainly in the liver. The small malignant melanoma of the choroid may be destroyed locally with preservation of the eye by irradiation and/or coagulation.

Fig. 10.8A. Malignant melanoma of the choroid. A-scan echograms of three different malignant melanomas. Note the slightly different reflectivity of the internal echo signals (**a** low, **b** medium-high) and the low to medium sound attenuation within the melanoma (**c**). Measurements of the maximum elevation of the lesion are achieved by measuring the distance between melanoma surface and the sclera (*arrows*) at "measuring-sensitivity" setting of the standardized A-scan instrument (see Table 1/Preface).

Fig. 10.8B. Malignant melanoma of the choroid. Contact B-scan echograms of a choroidal melanoma (*black arrows*) with adjacent retinal detachment (*white arrows*).

Fig. 10.9. Large mushroom-shaped amelanotic malignant melanoma of the choroid which has penetrated Bruch's membrane. Retinal detachment at the central shoulder of the tumor. M 805/83: 60-year-old woman with malignant melanoma of the choroid and secondary retinal detachment.

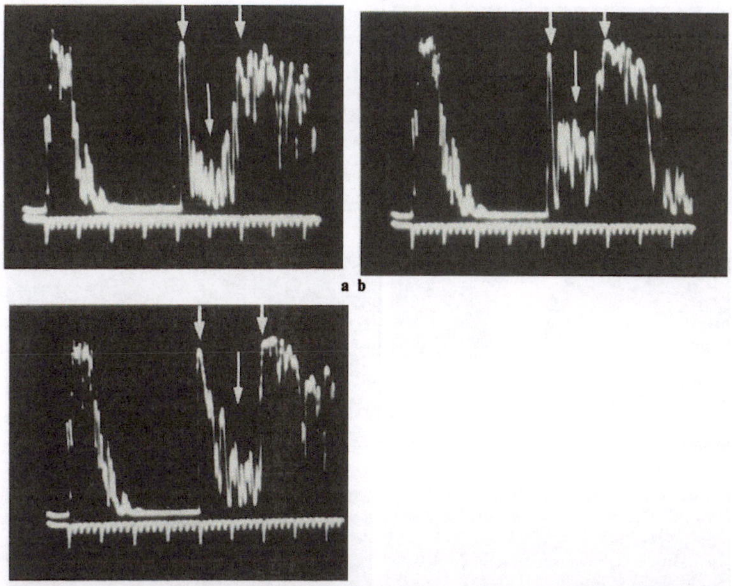

a b

10.8A c

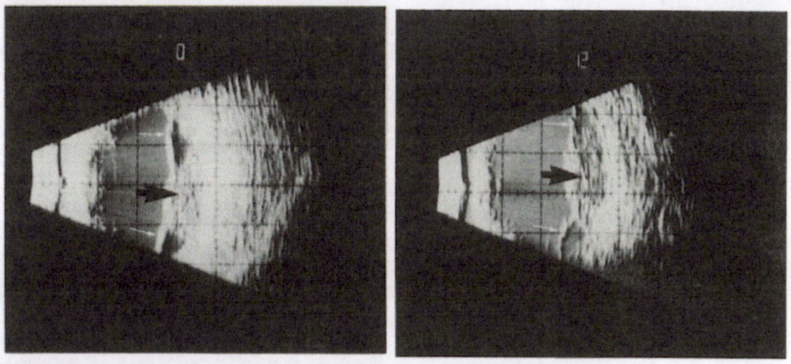

10.8B

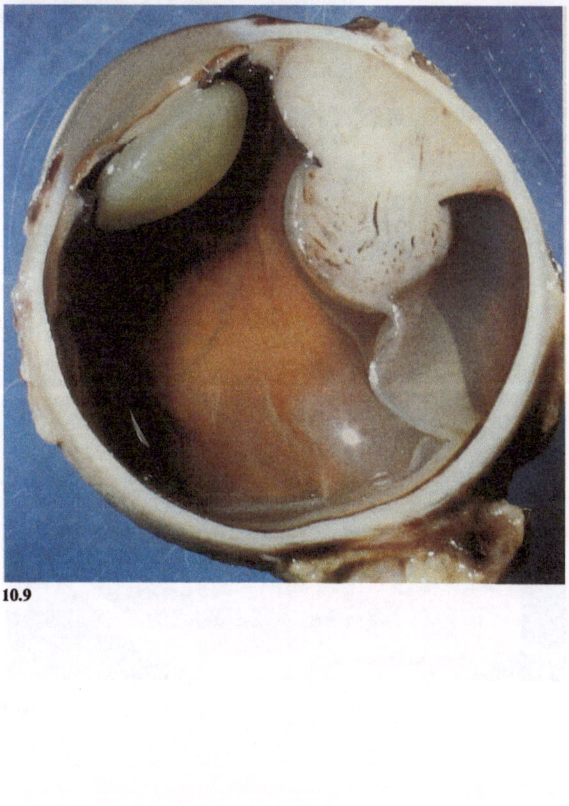

10.9

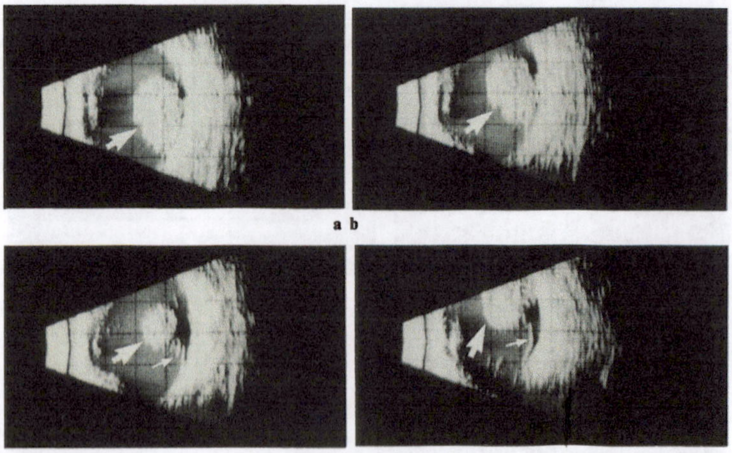

a b c d 10.9A

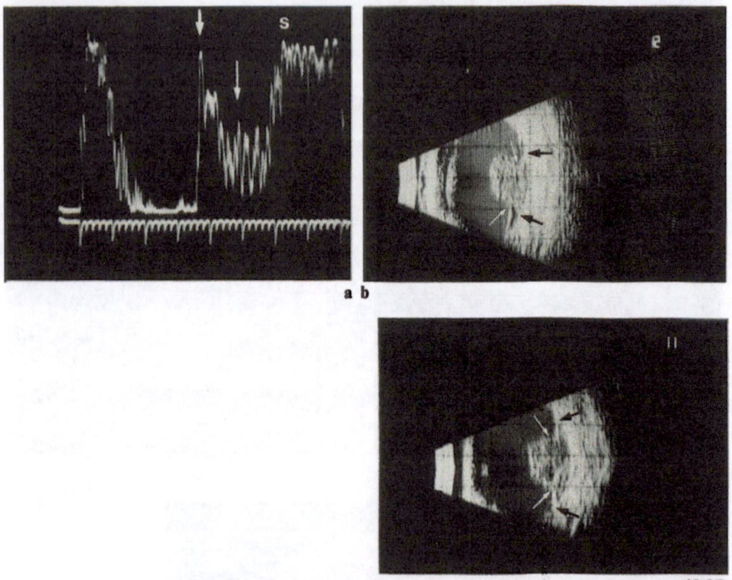

a b c 10.9B

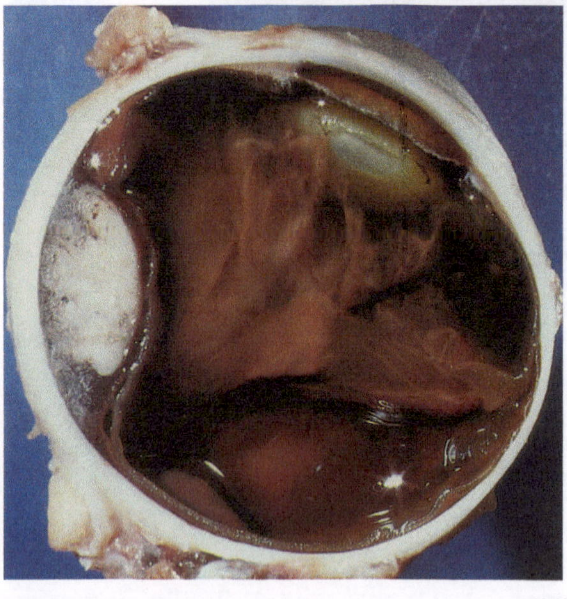

10.10

Fig. 10.9A. Malignant melanoma of the choroid. Contact B-scan echograms of four different sections of a choroidal melanoma. Note the mushroom-shaped or collar-button appearance representing a break in Bruch's membrane, and an adjacent retinal detachment (*small arrows*, **c**, **d**).

Fig. 10.9B. Malignant melanoma of the choroid. A-scan echogram (**a**) and contact B-scan echograms (**b**, **c**) of a choroidal melanoma. Note the relative homogeneity and low to medium-high reflectivity of the internal echo signals (**a**) and the mushroom or collar-stud shape documented with B-scan (**b**, **c**) indicating a break in Bruch's membrane (*white arrows*).

Fig. 10.10. Malignant melanoma of the choroid with vitreous hemorrhage and posterior vitreous detachment. The tumor had infiltrated into a sclera emissarium. M 1008/83: 60-year-old man with acute vitreal hemorrhage which arose 3 months previously. Ultrasonography revealed a tumor of the choroid.

Fig. 10.11. Close view of a highly pigmented mushroom-shaped malignant melanoma of the choroid with secondary retinal detachment. This tumor had invaded a scleral emissarium and extended extraocularly. M 806/81: 61-year-old woman suffering from visual disturbances for several weeks.

Fig. 10.12. Successfully photocoagulated small malignant melanoma of the posterior choroid with a ring of chorioretinal scarring. The central pigmentation consists of scar tissue with an accumulation of melanophages. M 1139/78: 54-year-old woman with high myopia and a small malignant melanoma of the posterior choroid. Photocoagulation of the tumor was performed over several session.

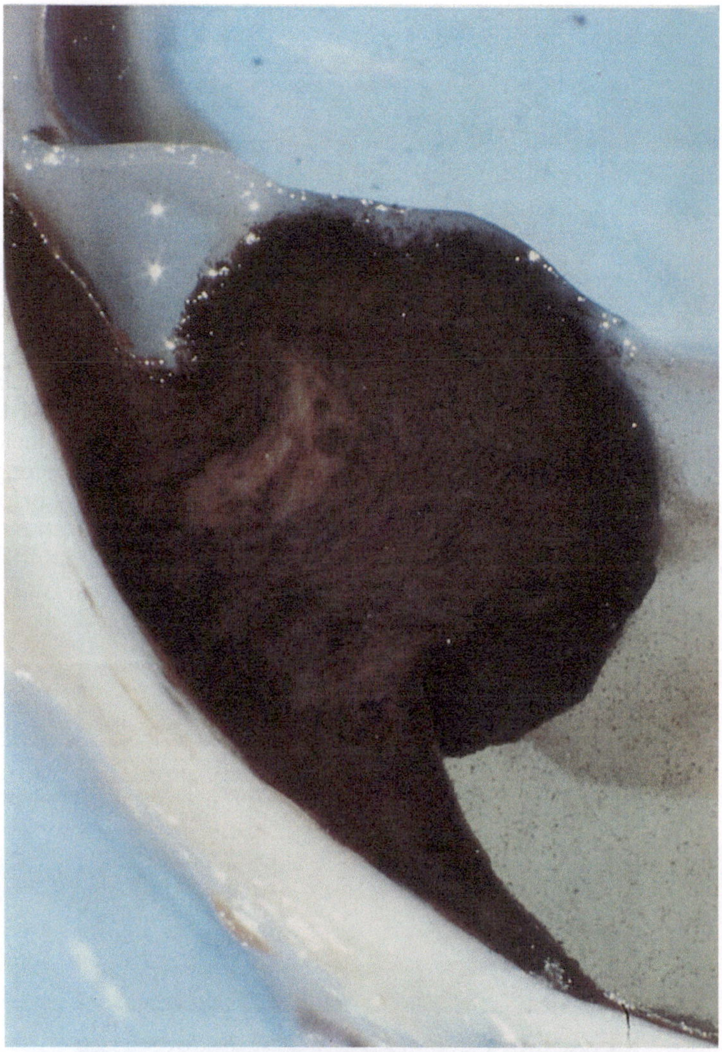

10.11

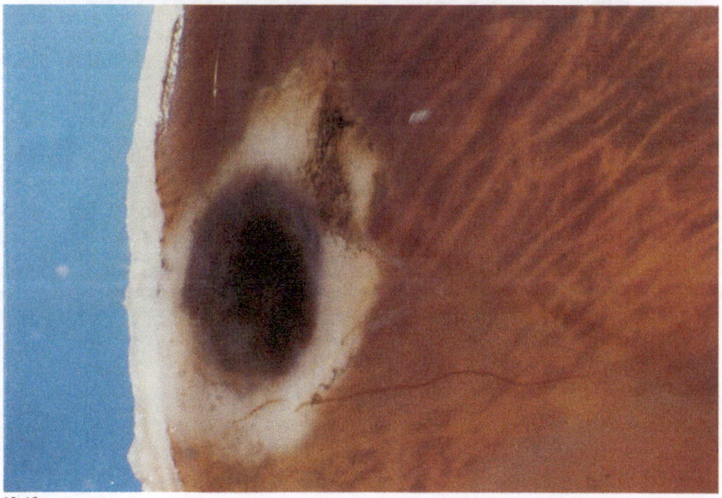

10.12

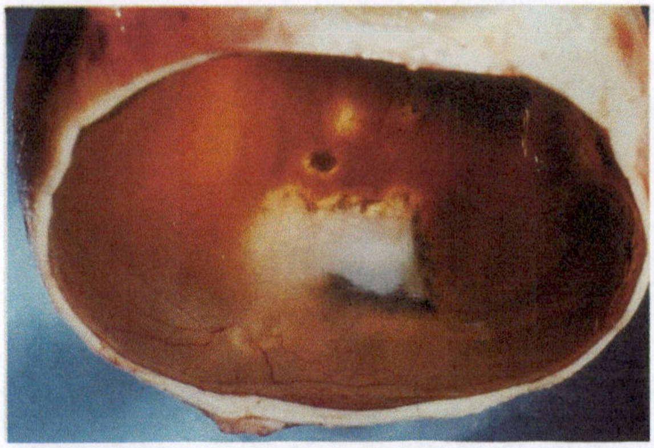

10.13

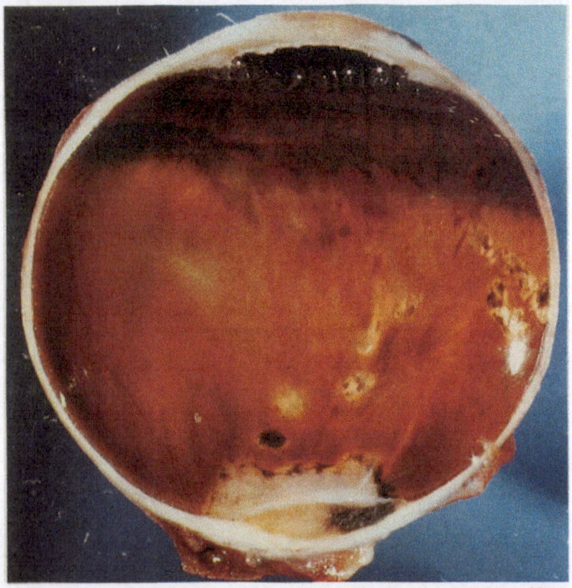

10.14

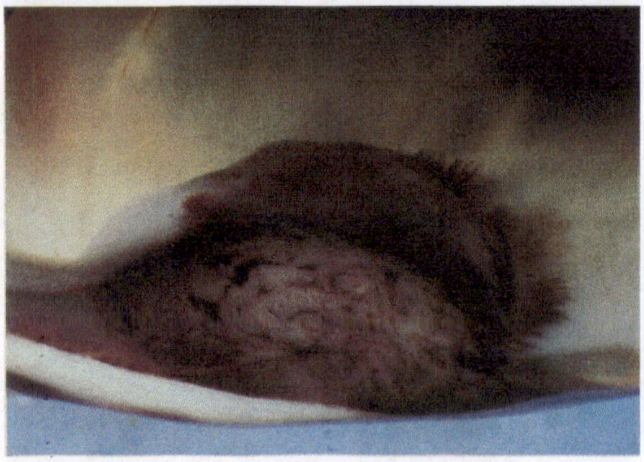

10.15

Fig. 10.13. Unsuccessfully photocoagulated malignant melanoma of the choroid. M 99/78: 42-year-old woman with small malignant melanoma of the choroid. Postoperatively she developed recurrent vitreous hemorrhages.

Fig. 10.14. Cross section through the lesion of Fig. 10.13 showing a malignant melanoma beneath the photocoagulation scar. No extraocular extension.

Fig. 10.15. Small mushroom-shaped malignant melanoma infiltrating the overlying retina. M 1066/83: 69-year-old man with small malignant melanoma known for 1 year. Unsuccessful photocoagulation had been performed 9 and 6 months prior to enucleation.

Fig. 10.16. Malignant melanoma of the choroid with nodular growth through the overlying retina into the vitreous space. M 243/85: 77-year-old man with malignant melanoma and retinal detachment.

Fig. 10.17. High magnification of the cut surface of a mushroom-shaped malignant melanoma of the choroid showing amelanotic areas within a fairly pigmented tumor. M 579/83: 50-year-old woman with acute hemorrhage into the vitreous. Ultrasonography revealed a tumor of the choroid.

Fig. 10.18. 3 mm thick flat (diffuse) pigmented malignant melanoma of the nasal choroid with retinal detachment. M 542/79: 78-year-old man who had noticed hyperemia of the conjunctiva and visual disturbances 2 weeks prior to enucleation.

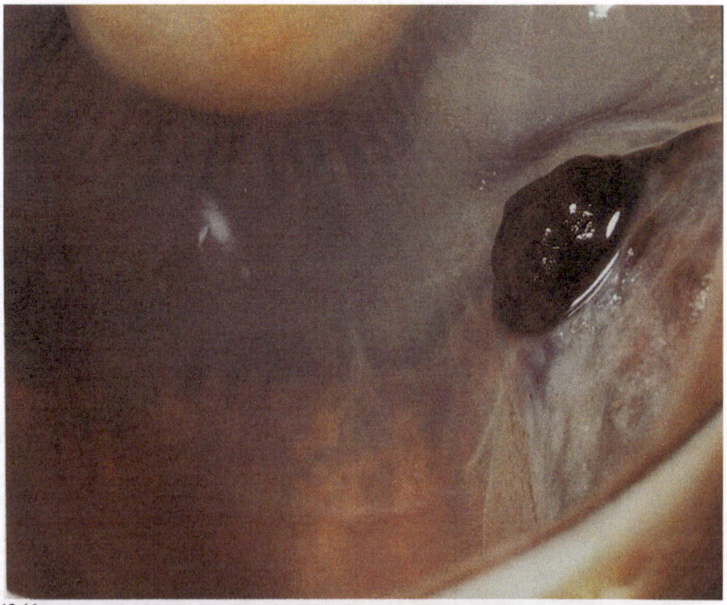
10.16

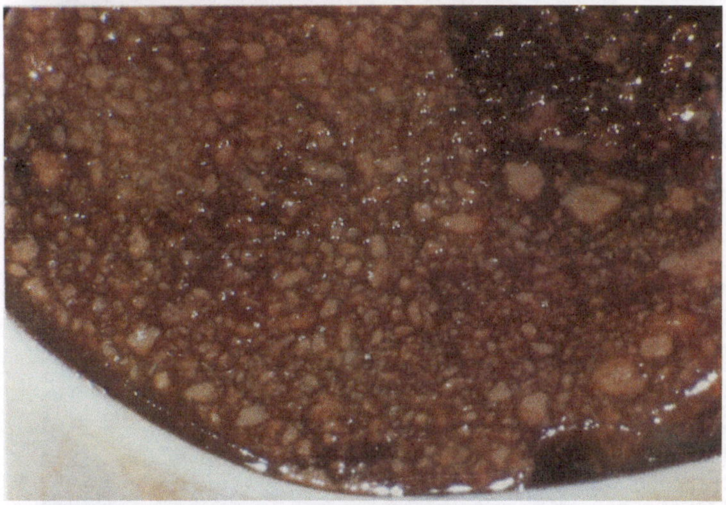
10.17

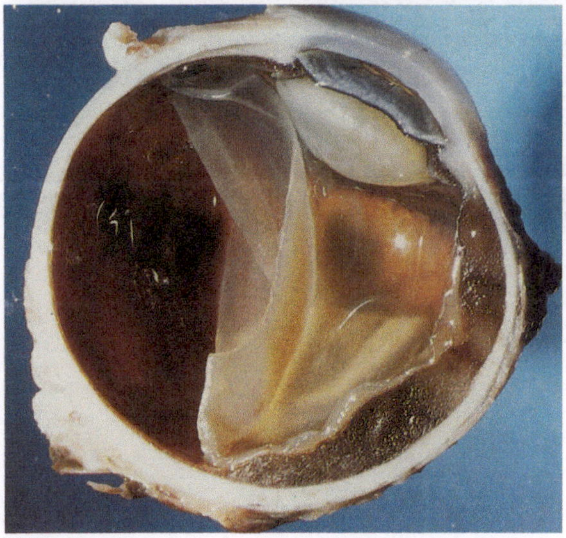
10.18

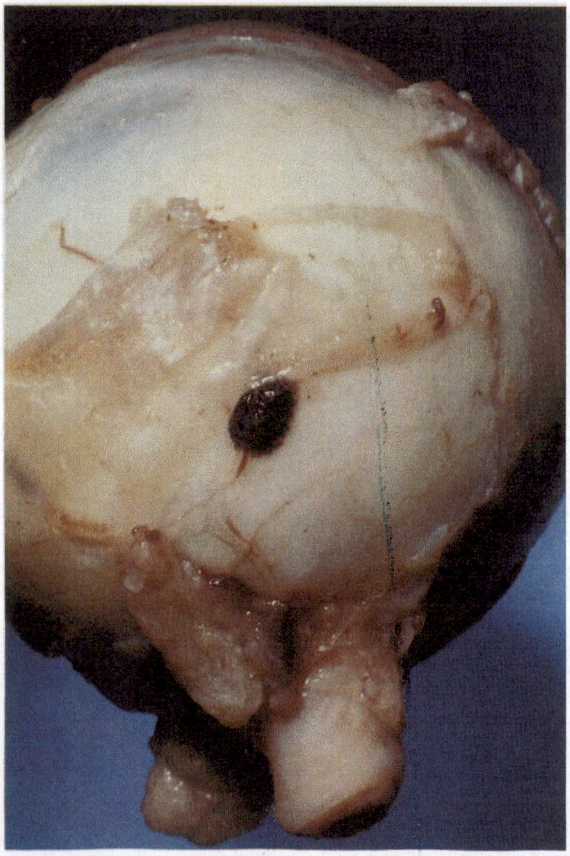

10.19

Fig. 10.19. Small extraocular extension of a 12-mm prominent pigmented malignant melanoma of the choroid measuring 17 mm in diameter. M 573/80: 75-year-old woman with solid retinal detachment.

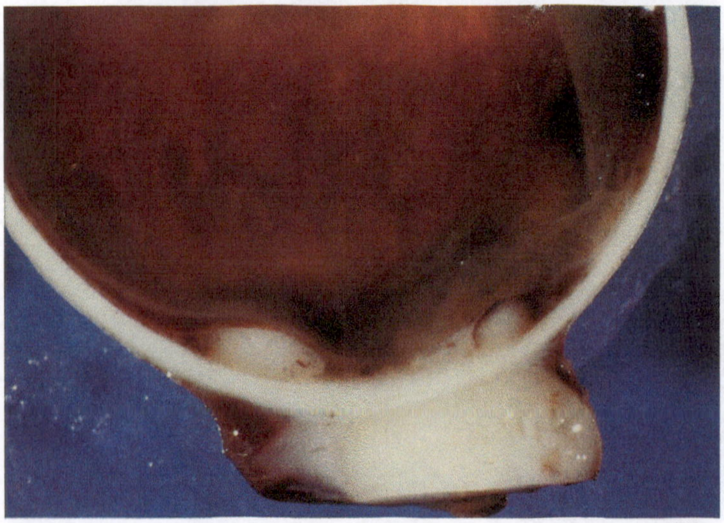

10.20

Fig. 10.20. 2.5-mm prominent amelanotic malignant melanoma around the optic disc with infiltration of the optic nerve and adjacent tissue. M 729/84: 76-year-old woman complaining of visual disturbances for a year. As a breast carcinoma had been removed 40 years previously, the initial diagnosis was that of a metastasis to the choroid. Irradiation of the eye and orbit were unsuccessful. After 9 months there were signs of extraocular extension of the tumor.

Fig. 10.21. Cross section through malignant melanoma of Fig. 10.20 with extraocular extension showing marked tumorous cuffing of the optic nerve.

Fig. 10.22. Pigmented malignant melanoma filling the entire globe and infiltrating the optic nerve and orbit. M 653/75: 77-year-old woman who had been treated for neovascular glaucoma for 1 year. She presented with a red protruding eye.

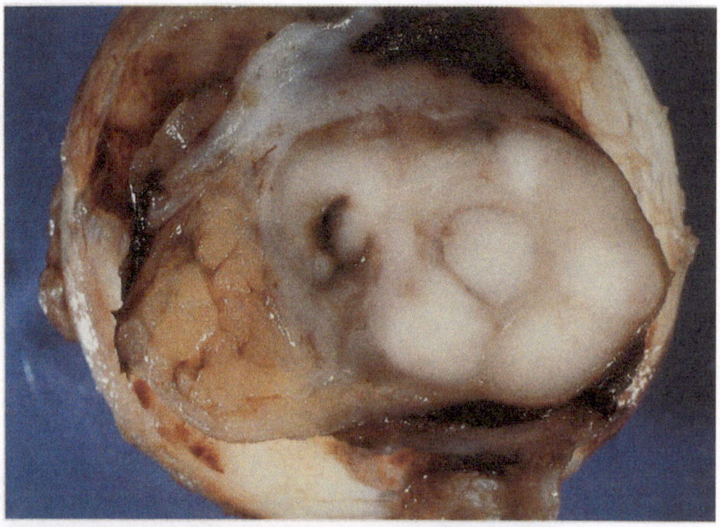

10.21

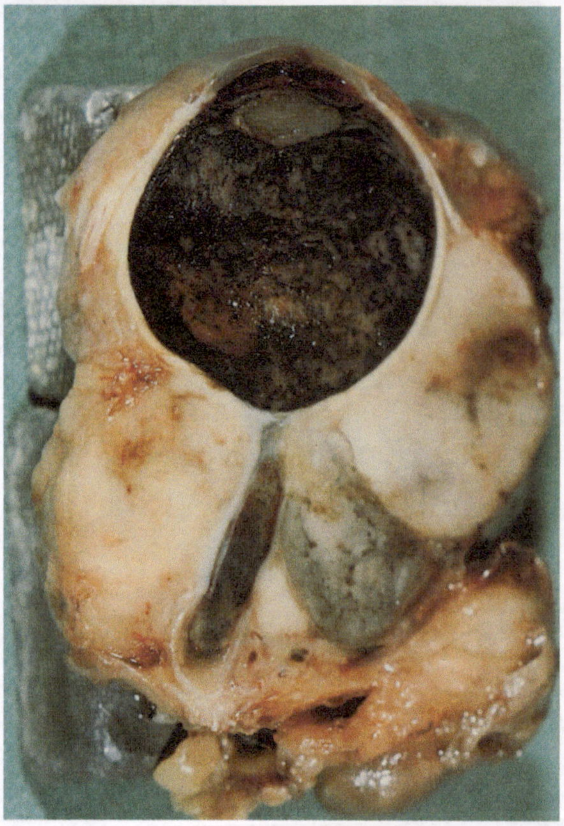

10.22

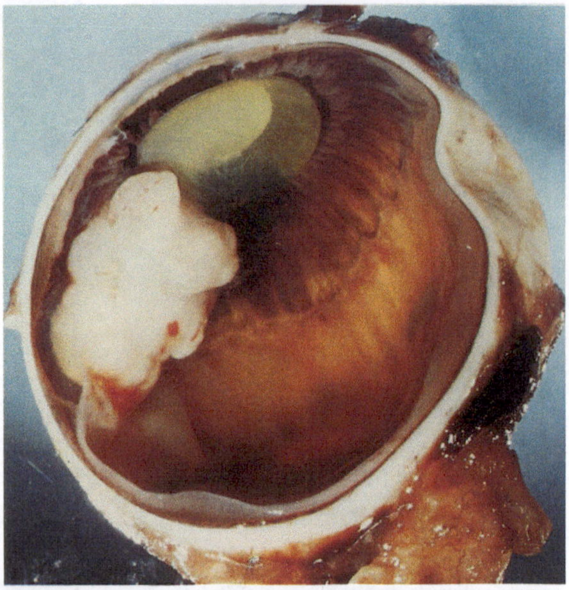

10.23

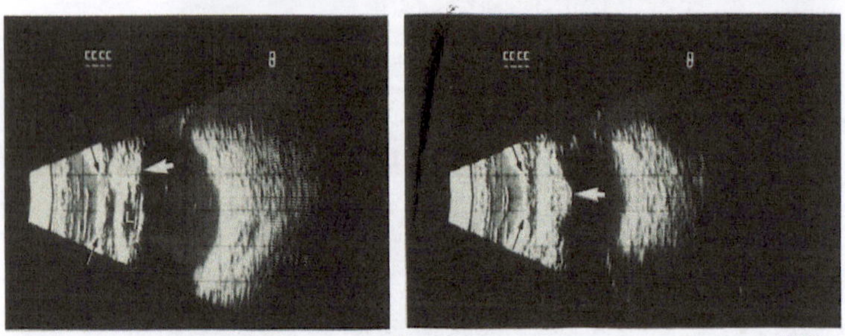

a b 10.23A

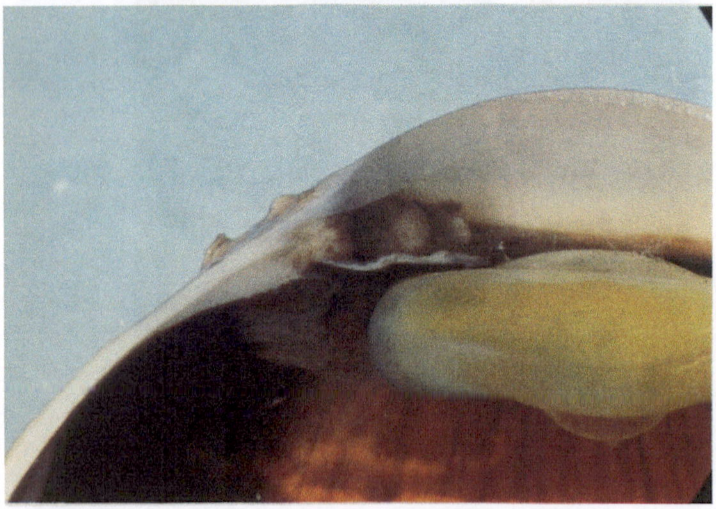

10.24

Malignant Melanoma of the Ciliary Body

Malignant melanomas of the ciliary body are hidden behind the iris and thus are usually not observed until a late prominent stage, leading to a poorer prognosis. At an early stage small melanomas of the ciliary body can be removed surgically by cyclectomy.

Fig. 10.23. Amelanotic malignant melanoma of the ciliary body and peripheral choroid touching the lens. Localized cataract at the site of tumor touch. Small hemorrhages on the inner surface of the tumor and at its central base. M 263/81: 43-year-old man who had noticed blurred vision for 4 weeks.

Fig. 10.23 A. Malignant melanoma of the iris and ciliary body. B-scan echograms obtained using the immersion technique (i.e., the sound probe is not placed directly on the conjunctiva but is held in a small water-filled cup positioned in the conjunctival sac; *black arrows* = edge of the base of the cup). **a** vertical axial section with display of the lens (*L*). **b** paraxial section, centered on the lesion (*white arrows*).

Malignant Melanoma of the Iris

Melanomas of the iris account for 5%–10% of all melanomas of the uveal tract. They are usually detected early, especially in a blue iris, and have an excellent overall prognosis. For more than 100 years, local excision (iridectomy) has been recommended in these cases to preserve the eye.

Fig. 10.24. Nodular pigmented malignant melanoma of the peripheral iris with involvement of the adjacent ciliary body. M 1167/81: 12-year-old boy with anisocoria for 1 year. A prominent mass of the iris was noticed during examination for anisocoria. Enucleation after biopsy verification of the provisional diagnosis of malignant melanoma.

Intraocular Metastases

Metastases to the eye are usually blood-borne. They most commonly occur in adults and originate from carcinomas of the lung and breast. Intraocular blood-borne metastases usually settle in the uvea. Occasionally, a malignant melanomas and squamous cell carcinomas of the conjunctiva may locally invade the anterior segment of the eye.

Fig. 10.25. Smooth-surfaced choroidal mass with net-like retinal pigment disturbances characteristic of choroidal metastases. M 1093/80: Autopsy eye of a 59-year-old man who had died from metastases from intestinal carcinoma.

Fig. 10.25 A. Metastatic tumor of the choroid. A-scan echograms (**a–c**) and contact B-scan echogram (**d**) of a metastatic choroidal tumor with mainly high reflectivity and rather irregular internal structure (*thick arrows*). R = retina, S = sclera. *Thin white arrows* (**a, d**) = posterior vitreous detachment. Contact B-scan echograms document a more typical flat shape of the metastatic lesions with usually more than one peak and with a more irregular surface appearance (*black arrows*).

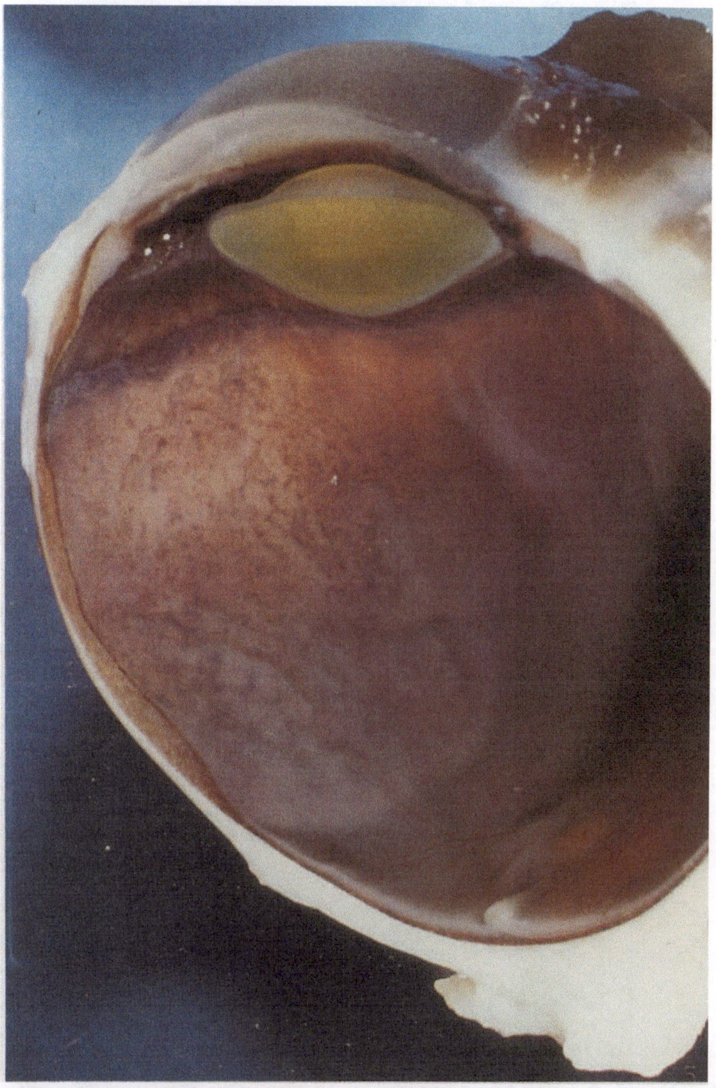

10.25

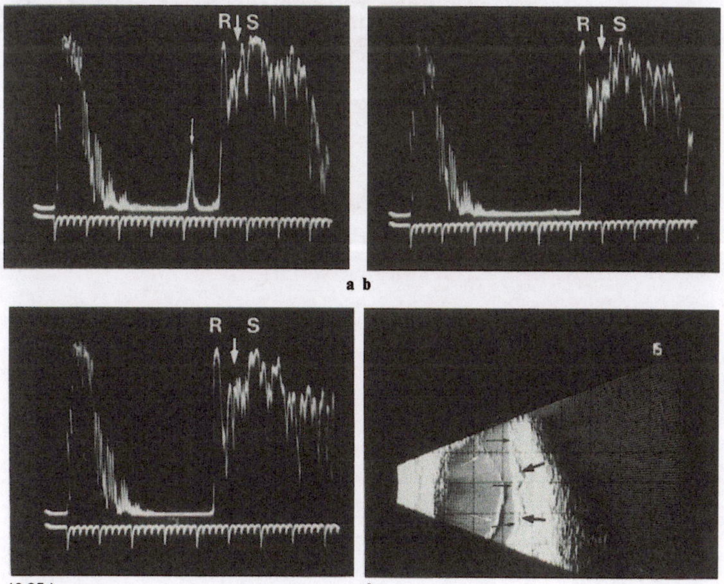

a b

10.25 A c d

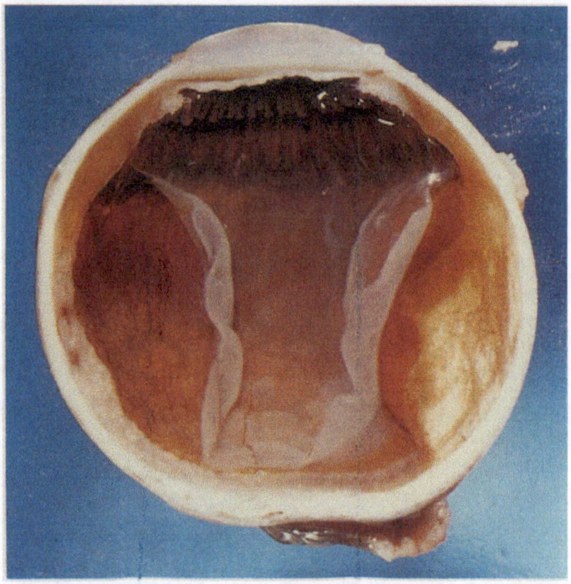

10.26

Fig. 10.26. Diffusely thickened partially detached choroid with total retinal detachment. M 236/79: Autopsy eye of a 64-year-old man who had died from metastatic hypernephroma.

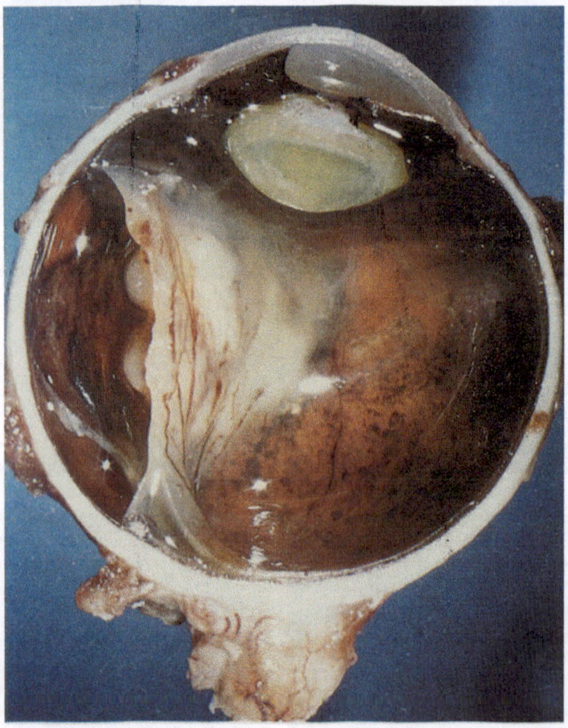

10.27

Pseudotumors

Conditions Simulating Intraocular Malignant Melanoma

There are number of tissue reactions which may clinically simulate a malignant melanoma. Large nevi may be difficult to differentiate even with ultrasonography, transillumination, and fluorescein angiography. The erroneous diagnosis of a malignant intraocular melanoma today is rare (about 3.5%), and is most often associated with conditions which obscure a direct view of the fundus. Hemorrhagic age-related disciform degeneration and intraocular angiomatous tumors with intravitreal hemorrhage, for example, have been mentioned above. Massive gliosis is a reactive proliferation of glial cells (after ocular trauma or inflammation) leading to localized retinal thickening.

Fig. 10.27. Massive gliosis in an area of detached retina following a concussion injury of the eye. The attached retina shows posttraumatic chorioretinal scarring. M 671/76: 41-year-old man who had suffered a severe blunt contusion to the eye 14 months previously.

Fig. 10.28. Higher magnification of the above Fig. 10.27 showing a thickened detached retina with two areas of nodular proliferation.

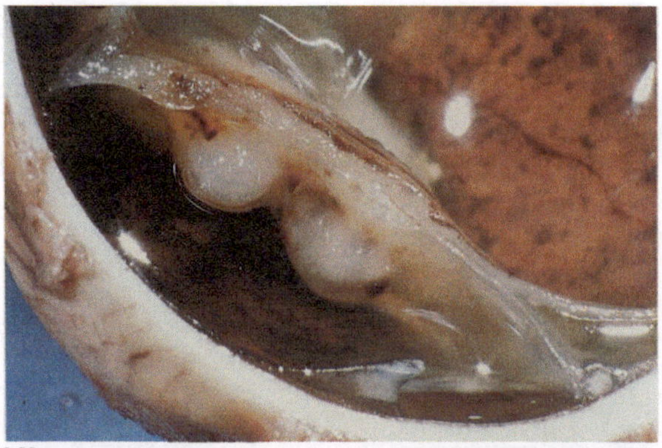

10.28

Retinoblastoma

Retinoblastoma is the most common primary intraocular malignancy in infancy and early childhood arising from the retina. But in Caucasians it is about 10 times rarer than malignant melanoma of the choroid. Signs (strabism, leukocoria) usually occur at the age of 1–2 years. In advanced cases, rubeosis iridis and secondary glaucoma are common findings. After the age of 4 years, this malignant neuroblastic tumor becomes increasingly rare. Over the age of 10 years, it is extremely rare. Ophthalmoscopically, a retinoblastoma may already be present at birth. Some 30% of the patients develop bilateral retinoblastomas with a higher risk in families where one child had already been treated for retinoblastoma. The majority of retinoblastomas, however, occur sporadically possibly due to spontaneous mutation. Besides such sporadic and genetically determined retinoblastomas, occasionally a retinoblastoma occurs with a deletion of chromosome 13/14. If untreated, the slowly growing tumor finally fills the eye and infiltrates the uvea and/or optic nerve within the orbit, leading to a poor prognosis.

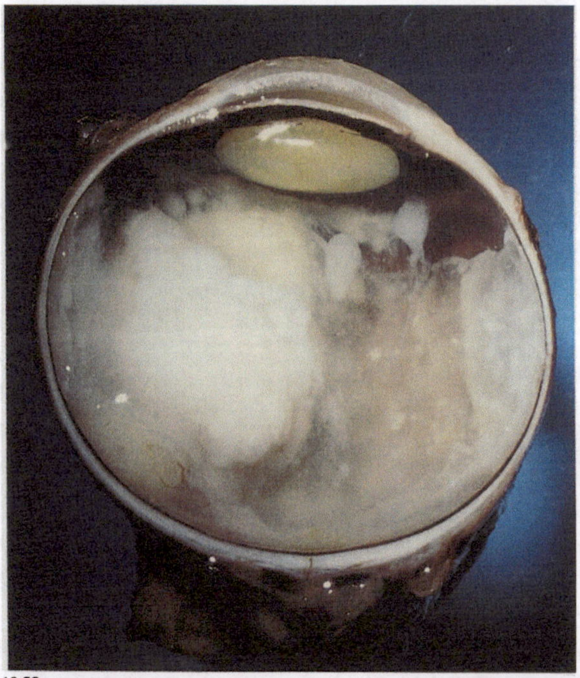

10.29

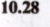

Fig. 10.29. Retinoblastoma with endophytic growth and intravitreal seeding. M 803/77: 3-year-old girl with unilateral sporadic retinoblastoma.

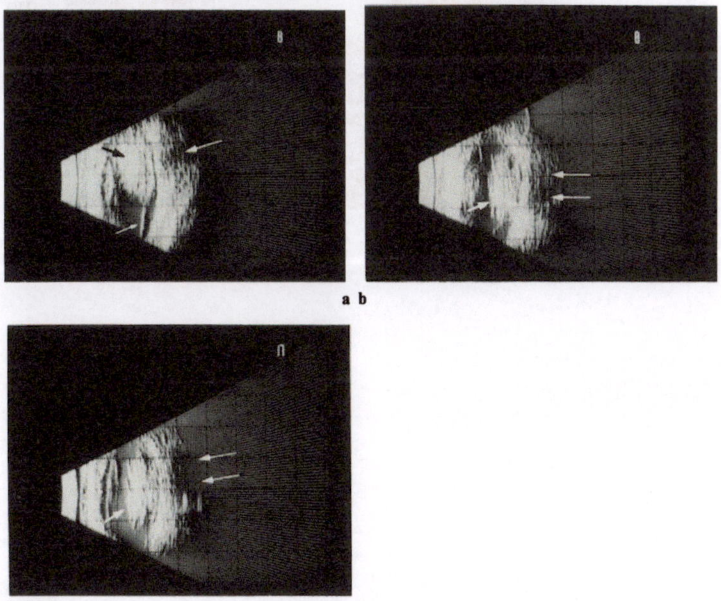

a b

10.29A c

Fig. 10.29A. Retinoblastoma. Contact B-scan echograms of a retinoblastoma with adjacent retinal detachment at three different sections through the lesion, typical acoustic shadowing (caused by calcifications) on the sclera and orbital structures posterior to the tumor (*long white arrows*, **a–c**) and rather bumpy tumor surface (*small white arrows*, **b, c**).

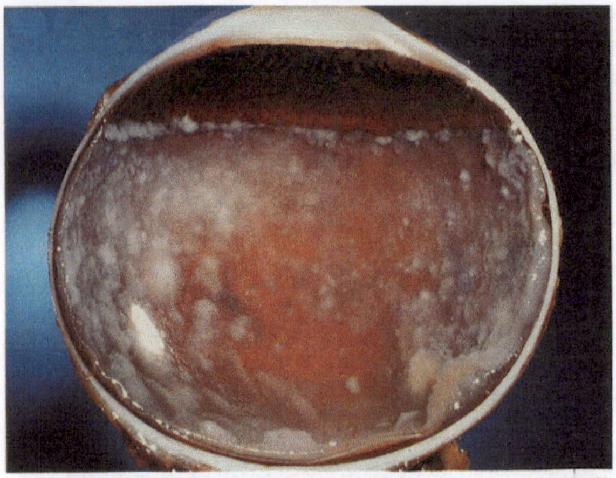

10.30

Fig. 10.30. Multiple foci of retinoblastoma cells in the retina and vitreous of the upper callotte. Same case as Fig. 10.29.

Three major growth patterns are differentiated: diffuse (very rare) within the retina, exophytic from outer layers of the retina into the subretinal space, and endophytic from the inner retinal layers into the vitreous cavity. The latter tend to spread into the vitreous and sometimes cause an appearance similar to uveitis or endophthalmitis. In rare case even a pseudohypopyon may develop. A multicentric origin within the retina is not uncommon. Hematogenous metastases occur in the brain, lungs, and bones. Small retinoblastomas may be treated locally by coagulation or irradiation. Large tumors are enucleated. Necrosis within the tumor is a common histological finding. Sometime scarred remnants of the tumor (spontaneous regression) may be observed during routine examination of relatives of an affected child. The overall prognosis is closely associated with tumor size and the structures invaded. In the developed industrial countries, mortality is about 20%.

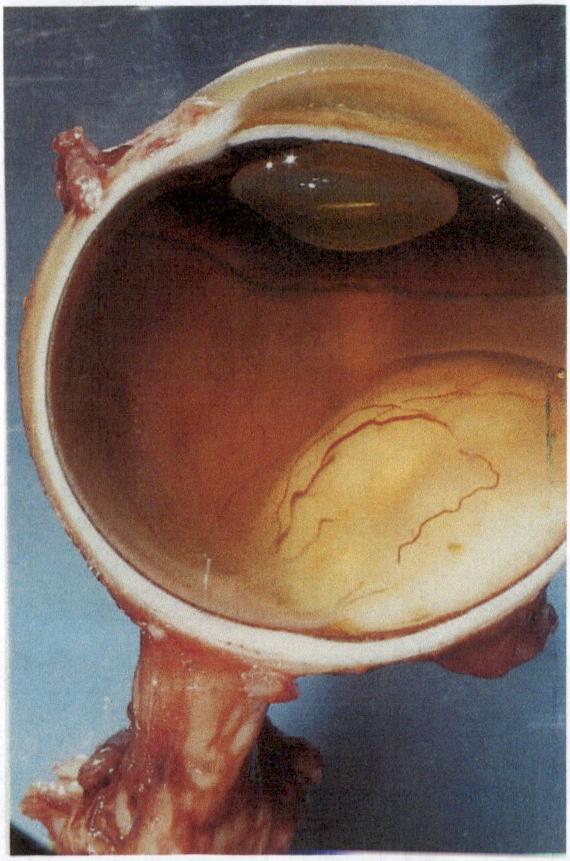

10.31

Fig. 10.31. Retinoblastoma with exophytic growth involving the macula. M 68/83: 2-year-old boy with sporadic unilateral retinoblastoma and strabism.

Fig. 10.31 A. Retinoblastoma. A-scan echograms of a retinoblastoma. Note the high to very high reflectivity (*thick arrows*, **a, b**) with acoustic shadowing (caused by calcifications) on the sclera (*thin arrows*, **a, b**) and the orbital structures posterior to the tumor, whereas the reflectivity of the sclera increases or is normal when the lesion is not centered totally in the sound-beam (**c**).

Fig. 10.32. Retinoblastoma with exophytic growth. M 804/73: 1-year-old male child with sporadic unilateral retinoblastoma and leukocoria.

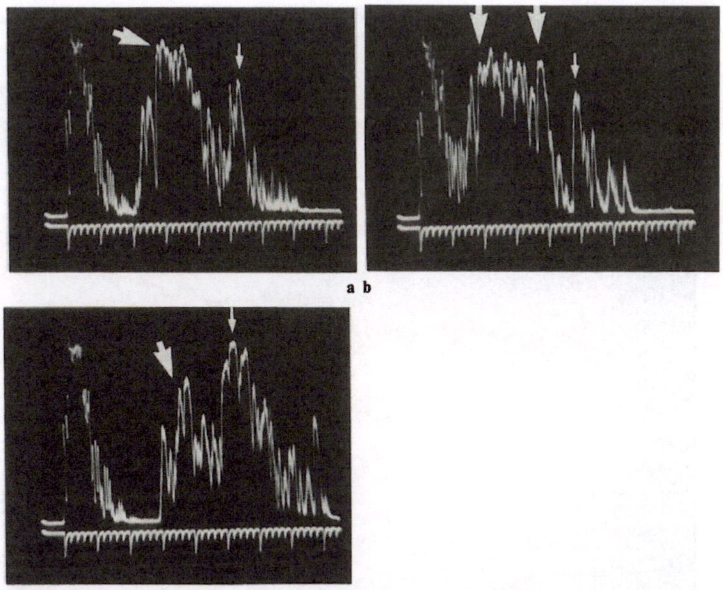

a b

c

10.31 A

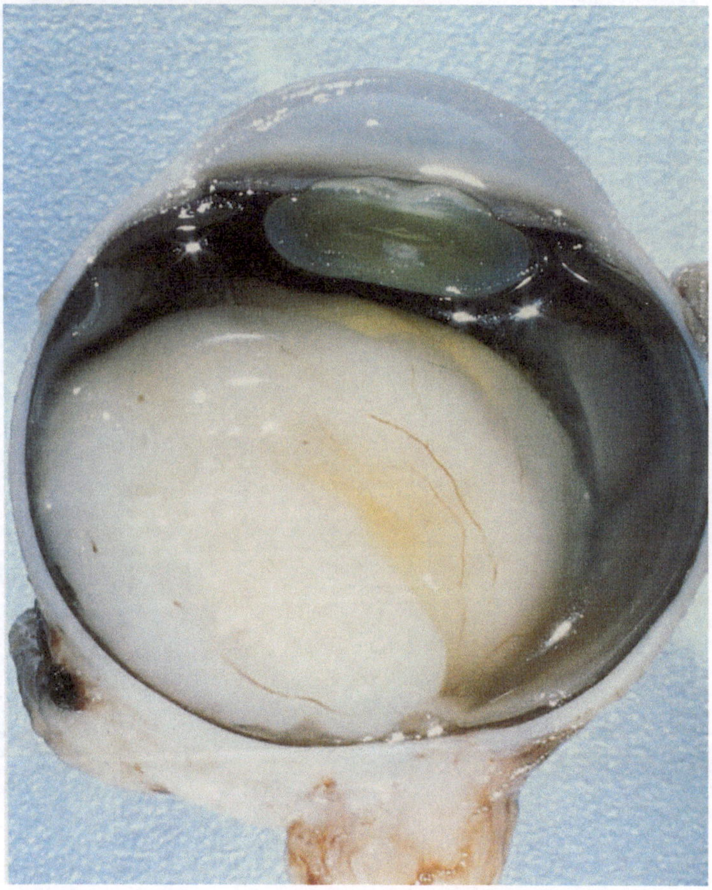

10.32

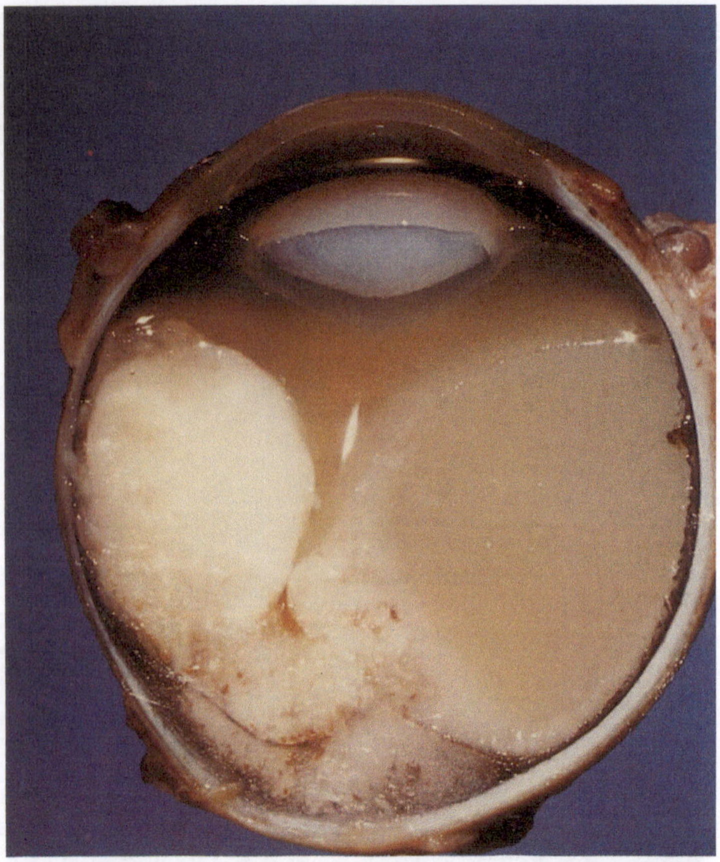

10.33

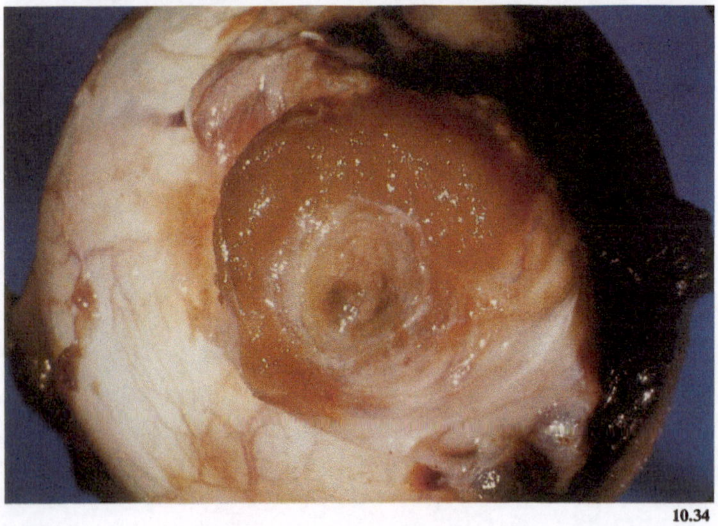

10.34

Fig. 10.33. Retinoblastoma with exophytic growth, total exudative retinal detachment and broad invasion into the posterior choroid. M 763/80: Kenyan boy with familial retinoblastoma and leukocoria.

Fig. 10.34. Posterior aspect of the eye with retinoblastoma infiltrating around the optic nerve. Same Kenyan boy as above.

Fig. 10.35. Retinoblastoma with exophytic and endophytic growth and total retinal detachment. Frontal section of the globe. M 761/73: 16-year-old boy who complained of ocular pain and loss of visual acuity for 1 week. A malignant melanoma or Coats' disease were suspected clinically.

Fig. 10.36. Retinoblastoma with vascular tortuosity and vascular ectasia. Same case as Fig. 10.35.

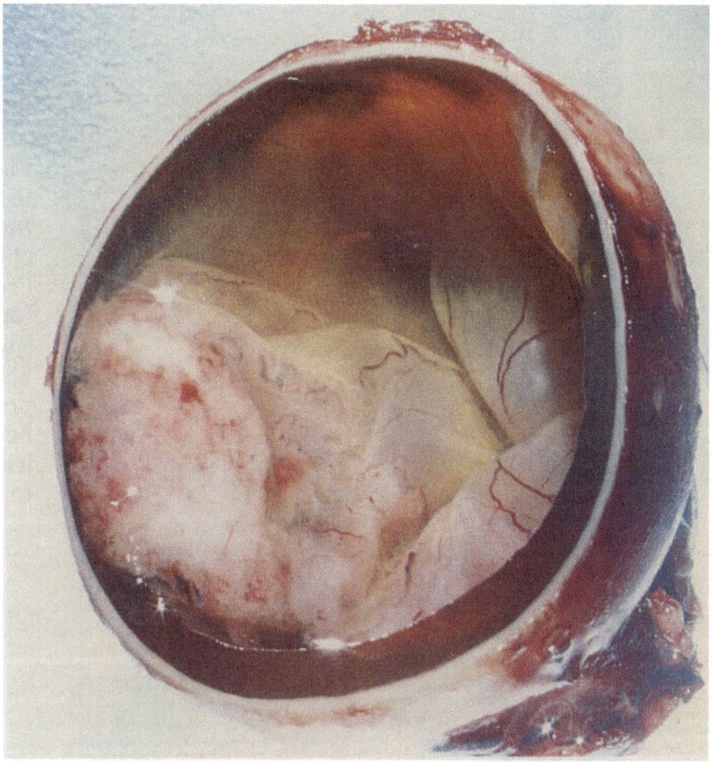

10.35

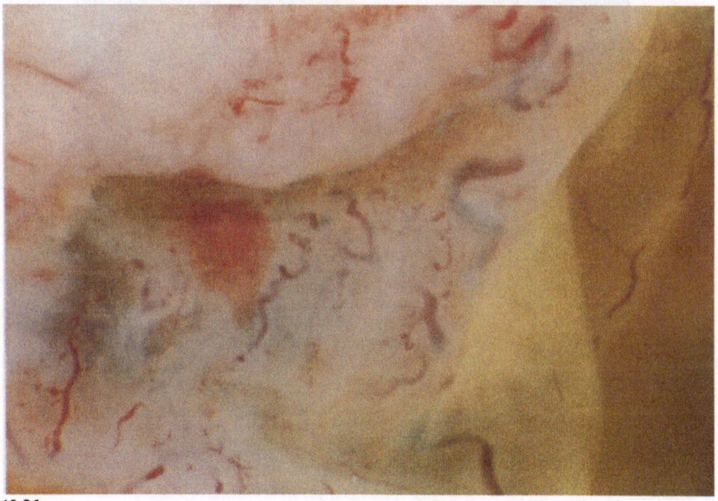

10.36

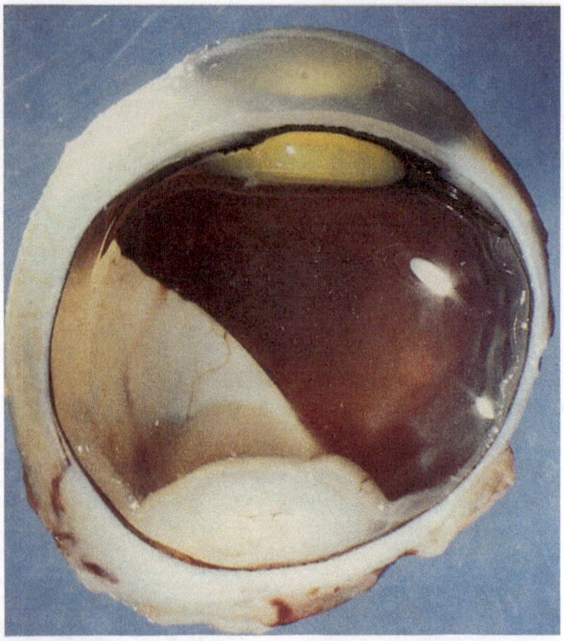

10.37

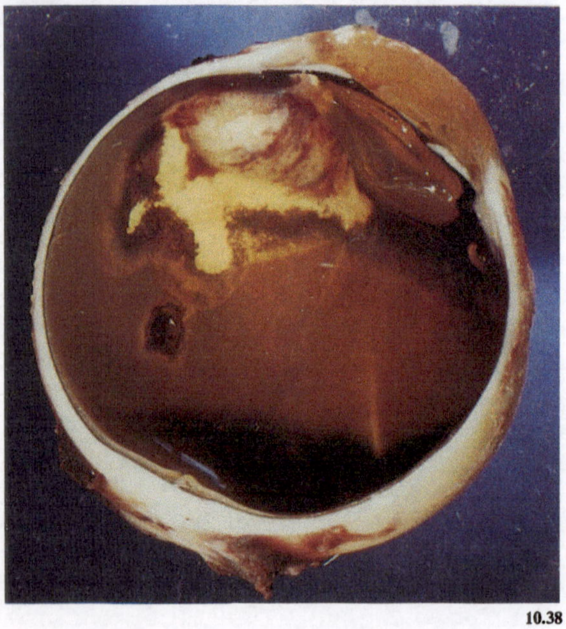

10.38

Fig. 10.37. Retinoblastoma associated with large coloboma of the choroid. M 911/83: 5-month-old female child with 13q-syndrome and bilateral retinoblastoma.

Fig. 10.38. Recurrence of retinoblastoma in scar tissue after local excision of tumor tissue invading the ciliary body and iris root. M 195/85: 4-year-old child with bilateral retinoblastoma. One eye had been enucleated because of advanced retinoblastoma. In this eye, external irradiation of a localized small retinoblastoma was performed (see below) before a grayish iris nodule was observed. The nodule was excised and proved histologically to be a retinoblastoma involving the ciliary body and iris root. A recurrence at the site of surgery led to enucleation of the second eye.

Fig. 10.39. Totally necrotic remnant of an externally irradiated retinoblastoma. Same case as Fig. 10.38.

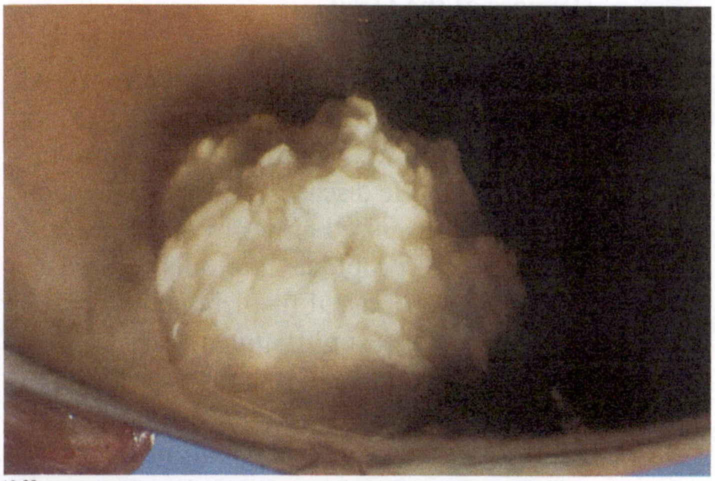

10.39

Conditions Simulating Retinoblastoma

Retinoblastoma may be suspected clinically in a variety of nontumorous conditions (pseudogliomas). One fairly common disease often misinterpreted as retinoblastoma is Coats' disease or a Coats-like lesion. Coats' disease is a retinal vascular disease of unknown etiology, usually uniocular and affecting young boys and men. Rarely it may be present in infants, in girls, or it may be bilateral. Numerous other conditions may simulate retinoblastoma by their secondary intraocular changes. Examples are persistent hyperplastic primary vitreous (see chapter on vitreous), falciform retinal fold with retinal detachment (see chapter on retina), and other malformations. In some of these conditions an associated retinoblastoma has been observed. Even with ultrasonography it may be very difficult to make the correct diagnosis in these cases.

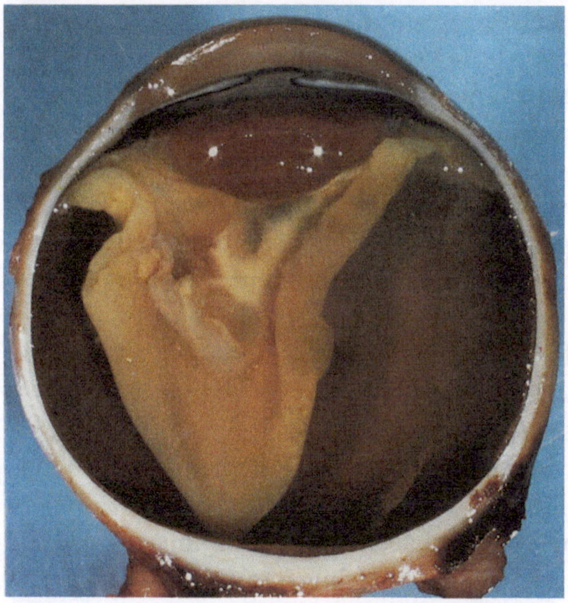

10.40

Fig. 10.40. Total retinal detachment with yellowish remnants of blood in the anterior vitreous behind the lens. M 321/83: 1-year-old boy with unilateral leukocoria.

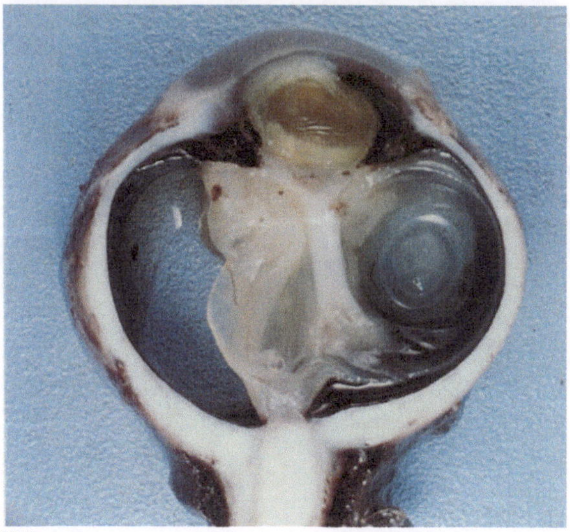

10.41

Fig. 10.41. Retinal detachment with falciform fold of the retina, retrolental fibrous tissue, and cataract.

Tumors of the Orbit

The contents of the orbit may be involved primarily or secondarily by many diseases (malformations, inflammations, immune diseases, muscle diseases, neoplasms) which are often recognized either by displacement of the globe (proptosis, diplopia) or by interference with visual disturbances. Unilateral proptosis (exophthalmos) is a well-recognized clinical sign of larger space occupying lesions. Orbital tumors may develop from any of the structures within the orbit (optic nerve, meninges, peripheral nerves, vessels, connective tissues, muscles, lacrimal gland, bones). The more common primary tumors are hamartomas (hemangiomas), neurofibromas in von Recklinghausen's neurofibromatosis, choristomas (epidermal cyst, dermoid cyst), rhabdomyosarcoma especially in children, benign or malignant lacrimal gland tumors, neural tumors such as schwannomas, tumors of the optic nerve (gliomas, meningiomas). Secondary tumors either reach the orbit as blood-borne metastases (for instance in carcinoma of the lung or breast in adults and neuroblastoma in children) or more commonly by local invasion from adjacent sites (conjunctiva, eye, paranasal sinuses, intracranial structures). Therapy is either nonsurgical (irradiation, cytotoxics) or surgical (local excision or exenteration of the orbit) depending on the type of tumor and its natural course. Taken overall, more tumors are benign and therefore may be locally excised.

Since macroscopy usually adds very little to the understanding of orbital tumors, only a few examples are demonstrated here. For rhabdomyosarcoma, clinically a very important tumor of childhood, exenteration is rarely performed as it responds well to irradiation and supplementary cytotoxic therapy. Therefore rhabdomyosarcoma is not presented here.

Optic Nerve Tumors

Intraorbital tumorous thickening of the optic nerve may be seen mainly in unilateral primary gliomas (juvenile pilocytic astrocytoma) and meningiomas. Other primary optic nerve tumors (for instance, angioblastomas) are very rare. Secondary tumor involvement of the optic nerve occurs in retinoblastoma (see above), intraocular malignant melanoma (see above), intracranial tumors (meningiomas, glioblastomas), and metastases.

Glioma (Juvenile Pilocytic Astrocytoma) of the Optic Nerve

Gliomas of the optic nerve, some of which are possibly hamartomas, occur mainly in children of school age. Clinical signs are proptosis and visual loss. Fairly common is an association with von Recklinghausen's neurofibromatosis. An isolated optic nerve glioma confined to the orbit has an excellent prognosis. Gliomas grow within the optic nerve sheath without a tendency to invade other orbital structures. The signs of intracranial growth (where brain structures may be invaded) are headache and diabetes insipidus. Prognosis then becomes poorer. Often optic nerve glioma is associated with a reactive arachnoid hyperplasia simulating histologically an optic nerve meningioma.

Fig. 10.42. Glioma (juvenile pilocytic astrocytoma) of the intraorbital optic nerve with intact optic nerve sheaths. M 369/75: 7-year-old girl with progressive exophthalmos for 3 years, papilledema, and retinal hemorrhages.

Fig. 10.43. Reactive arachnoid hyperplasia with proliferative thickening of the arachnoid around the proximal optic nerve. M 12/71: 4-year-old girl developing convergent squint with amblyopia for 6 months. Four weeks prior to enucleation, a glioma (juvenile pilocytic astrocytoma) of the optic nerve had been operated by neurosurgeons.

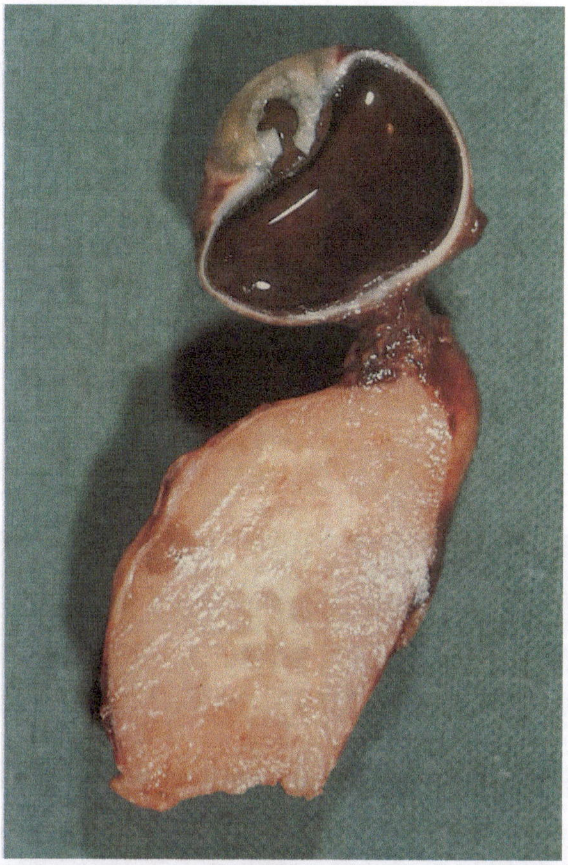

10.42

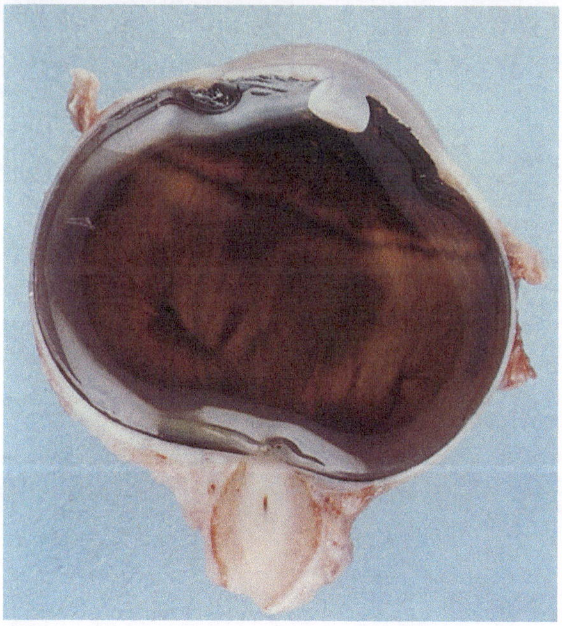

10.43

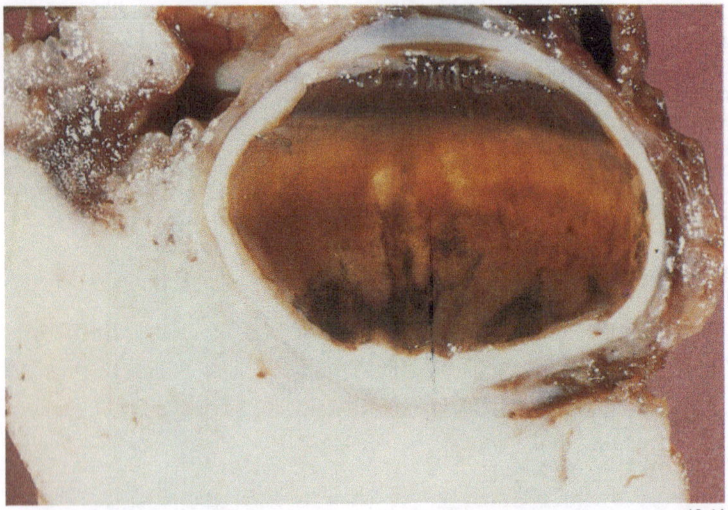

10.44

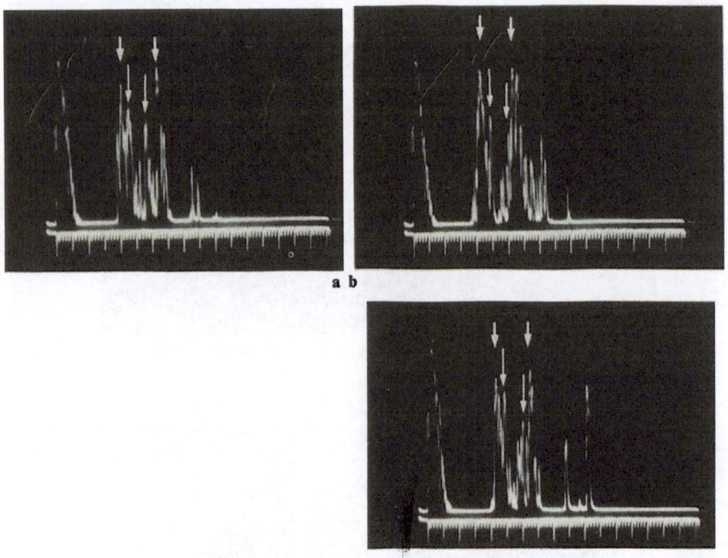

10.44A

Meningioma of the Optic Nerve

Primary meningioma of the intraorbital optic nerve occurs in all age groups and with higher frequency in twins. The clinical signs again are proptosis and visual loss. It may also be associated with von Recklinghausen's neurofibromatosis. Its tendency to invade the orbital tissues and adjacent structure such as bone and the intracranial space result in a poorer prognosis.

Fig. 10.44. Orbital tissue infiltrated by a firm (white) meningioma of the optic nerve. Scleral thickening and folding. Reactive hyperplasia of the retinal pigment epithelium. M 78/76: 65-year-old woman with progressive visual loss over the past decade. Transfrontal orbitotomy with tumor excision had been performed 2 years prior to enucleation for recurrent tumor.

Fig. 10.44A. Meningioma. A-scan echograms (cross sections) of three different parts of a meningioma of the optic nerve. Note the markedly thickened optic nerve sheaths (*short arrows* indicate surface of the tumor; *long arrows* indicate surface of the optic nerve). The solid consistency – in contrast to an enlarged subarachnoid space caused by fluid – can be verified with the 45-degree test (see also Fig. 8.6A).

Hamartomas and Choristomas of the Orbit

Hamartomas are tumors consisting of tissue normally present at the site of tumor growth. Choristomas are composed of tissue not normally present at this site. Common primary tumors of the orbit are hemangiomas (hamartomas) and epidermal and dermoid cysts (choristomas). Less common, except in von Recklinghausen's neurofibromatosis, are neurofibromas (hamartomas).

Hemangioma

Hemangiomas are the most common tumors in the orbit. Cavernous hemangiomas are more common than juvenile hemangioendotheliomas (capillary hemangiomas). They are usually located in the upper nasal quadrant of the orbit. Clinical signs such as proptosis develop with increasing size. Although present from birth, signs may develop at any age, but most frequently appear in adult life.

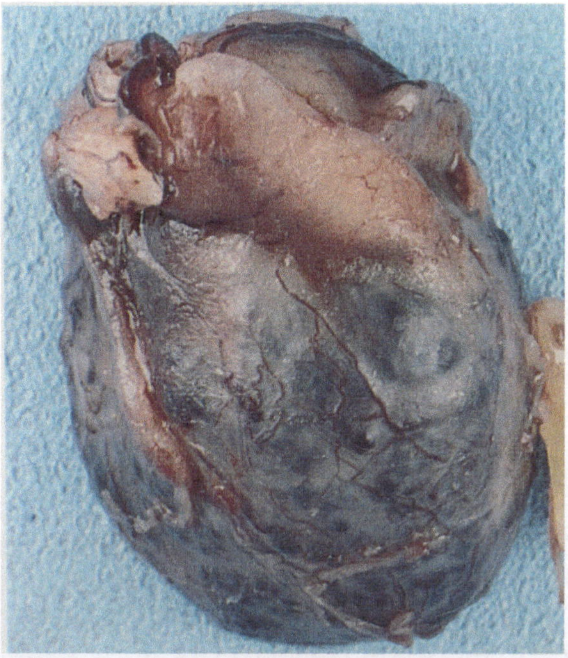

10.45

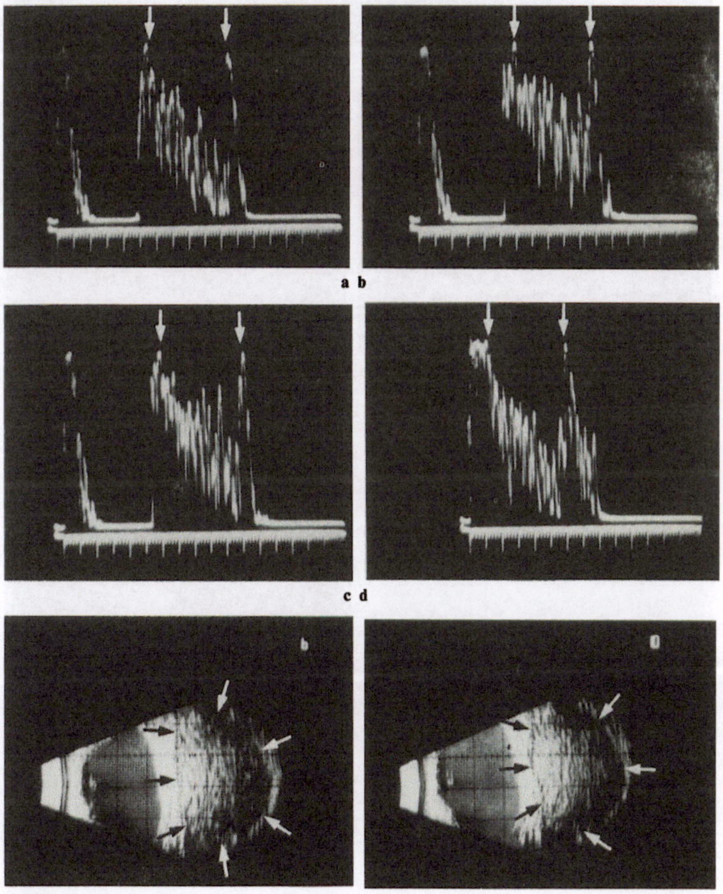

10.45A e f

Fig. 10.45. Encapsulated cavernous hemangioma of the orbit. M 454/71: 60-year-old woman who had noticed an orbital tumor 3 weeks prior to surgery.

Fig. 10.45 A. Cavernous hemangioma of the orbit. A-scan echograms (**a–c** transocular, **d** paraocular examination technique) and contact B-scan echograms (**e, f**) of an orbital cavernous hemangioma (*arrows* = very distinct tumor surface = capsule of the hemangioma). Note, in the A-scan, the high reflectivity and homogeneous structure of the tumor. The progressive decrease from left to right of the height of the homogeneous internal echo signals, indicates sound attenuation of the tumor. B-scan sections show the typical rounded shape and the sometimes scalloped surface of the cavernous hemangioma.

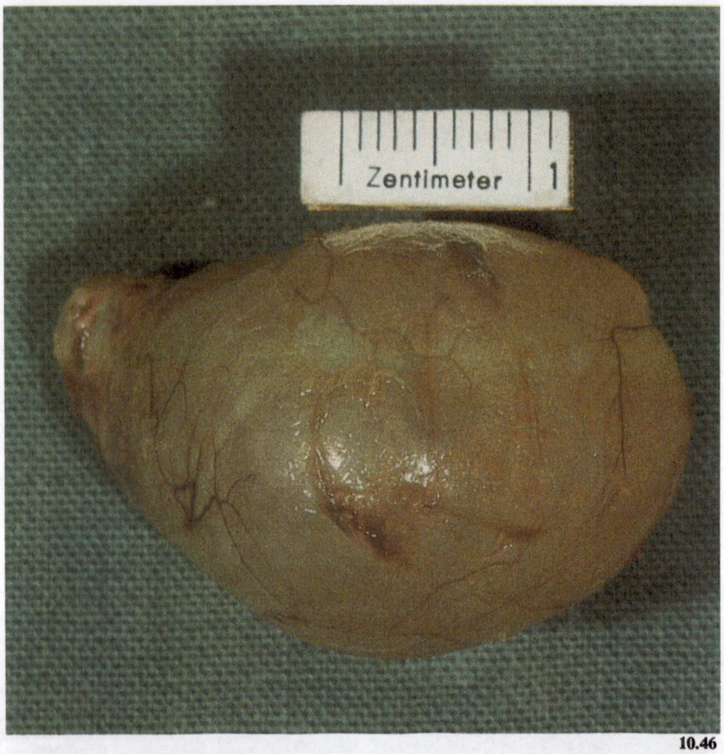

10.46

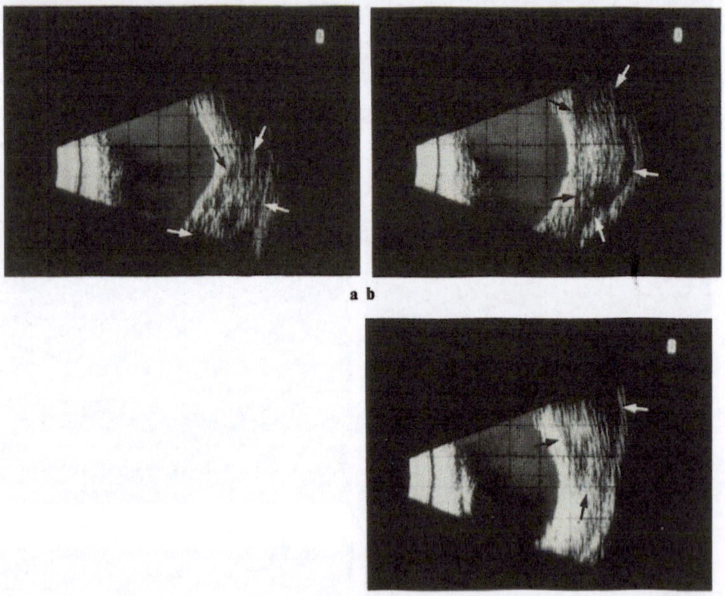

a b

c 10.46A

Epidermal/Dermoid Cysts

Congenital epidermal cysts (consisting of epidermal tissue without epidermal appendages and thus containing only keratin) and dermoid cysts (consisting of additional epidermal appendages such as hair follicles and sebaceous glands) are usually found at the upper temporal quadrant of the orbit.

Fig. 10.46. Epidermal cysts of the orbit. M 816/74: 36-year-old man who developed an increasing lid swelling.

Fig. 10.46A. Dermoid cyst of the orbit. Contact B-scan echograms of a dermoid cyst (*OS*). Transverse sections at 12:00 (**a** nasal side = top of the echogram), at 1:30 (**b** 12:00 = top, 3:00 = bottom of the echogram), and at 3:00 (**c** 1:30 = top, 4:30 = bottom of the echogram).

Fig. 10.46 B. Dermoid cyst of the orbit. A-scan echograms (transocular examination technique) of a dermoid cyst. Note the very pronounced heterogeneity of the internal structure in three different sections representing the tissue variation normally encountered in dermoid cysts (= *long arrows; short arrows* = surface of the dermoid).

Fig. 10.46 C. Dermoid cyst of the orbit. A-scan echograms (paraocular examination technique) of a dermoid cyst. *Arrows* indicate the very distinct borders of the dermoid, the cyst surface is usually double or triple peaked (**c**). Also note the heterogeneity of the internal echo signals seen in three different sections of the lesion (**a–c**).

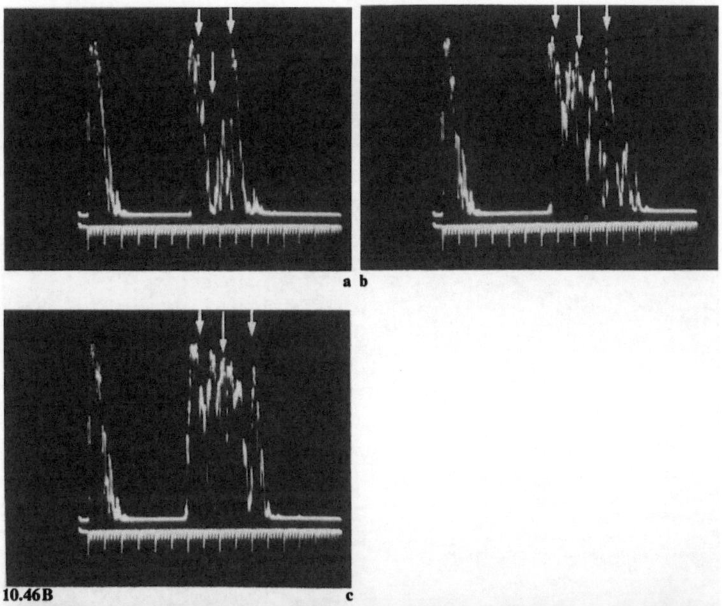

10.46 B a b c

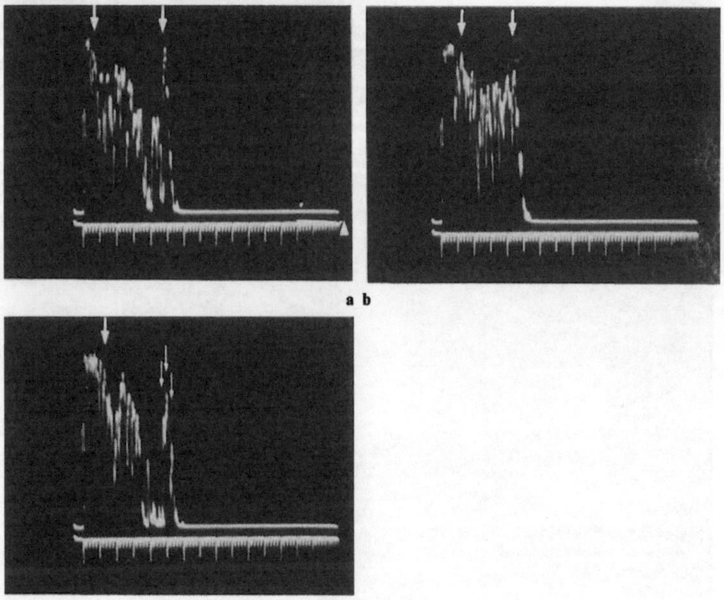

10.46 C a b c

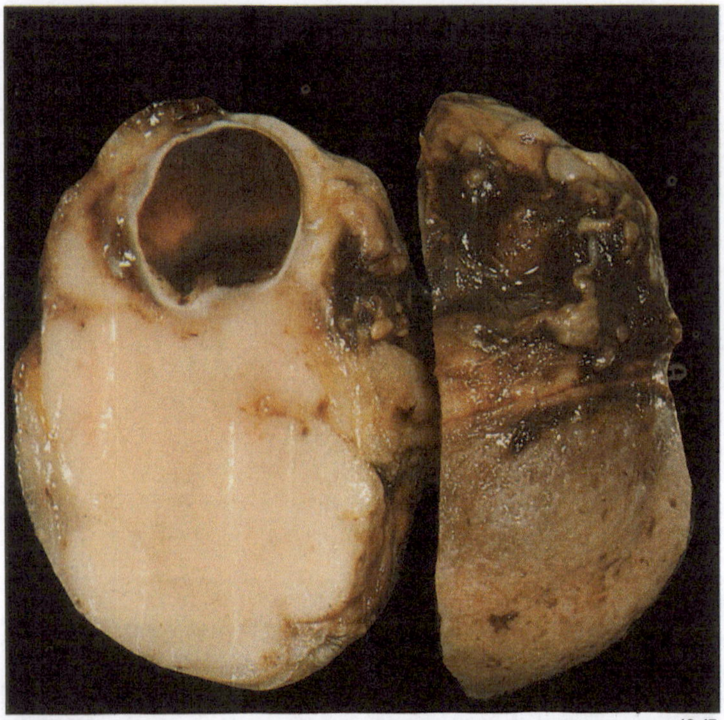

10.47

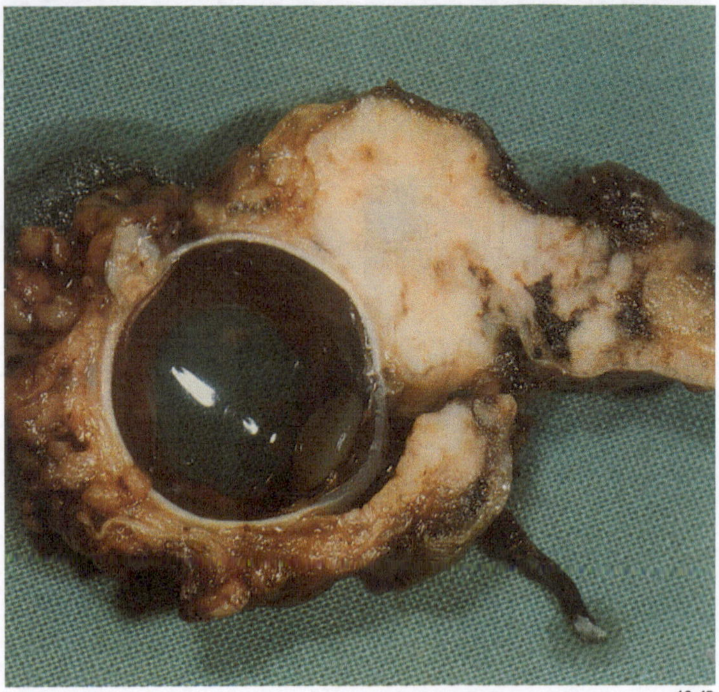

10.48

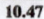

Lymphoid Tumors of the Orbit

Malignant lymphomas may occasionally have their primary site in the orbit causing signs long before the systemic character of the disease can be demonstrated.

Fig. 10.47. Diffuse infiltration of the orbital tissues by a reticulum cell sarcoma (histiocytic malignant lymphoma). 65-year-old man with severe exophthalmos, loss of vision, and loss of motility.

Secondary Tumors of the Orbit

Secondary tumor growth within the orbit results either from local invasion of tumors from adjacent sites (eyelids, conjunctiva, intraocular structures, paranasal sinuses, brain) or from bloodborne metastases.

Fig. 10.48. Large recurrent basal cell carcinoma of the lower lid invading the anterior orbital tissues; 67-year-old man.

Fig. 10.49. Large recurrent malignant melanoma of the conjunctiva invading the anterior orbital tissues. 46-year-old woman with a long history of recurrent malignant melanoma. She died from a second unrelated malignancy. There were no melanoma metastases.

Fig. 10.50. Large orbital tumor invasion of a diffuse malignant melanoma of the choroid. M 389/74: 56-year-old woman with progressive exophthalmos following the diagnosis of central retinal vein thrombosis and uniocular glaucoma.

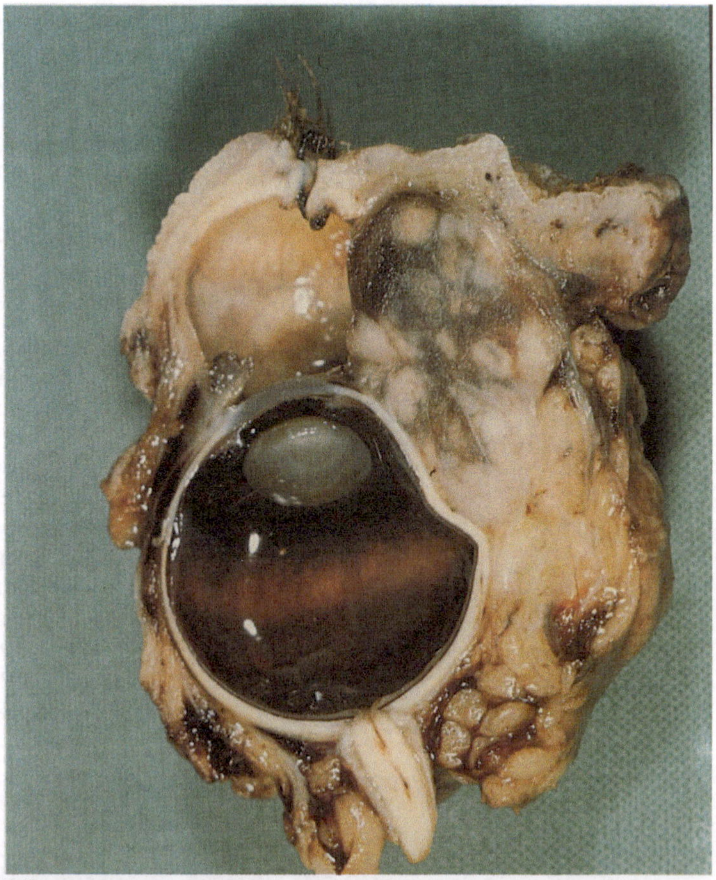

10.49

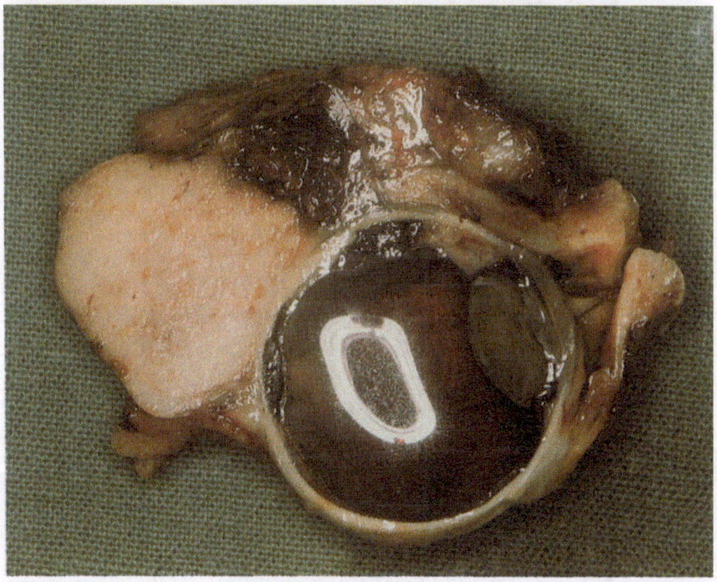

10.50

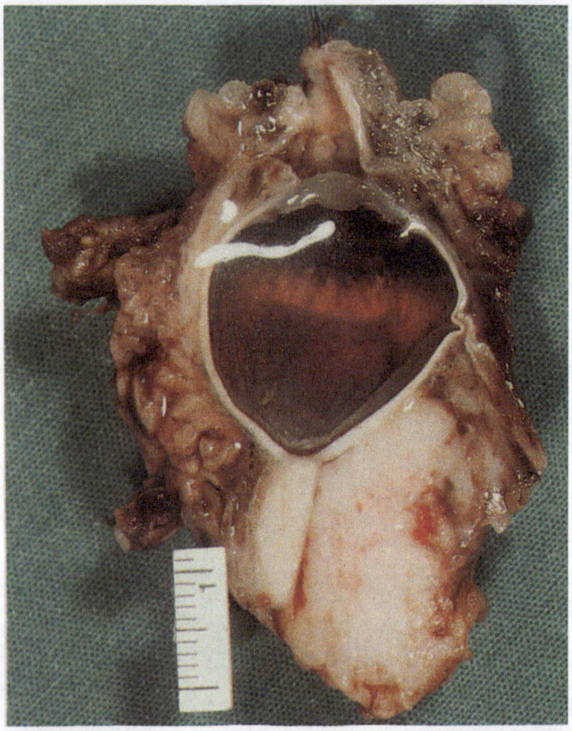

10.51

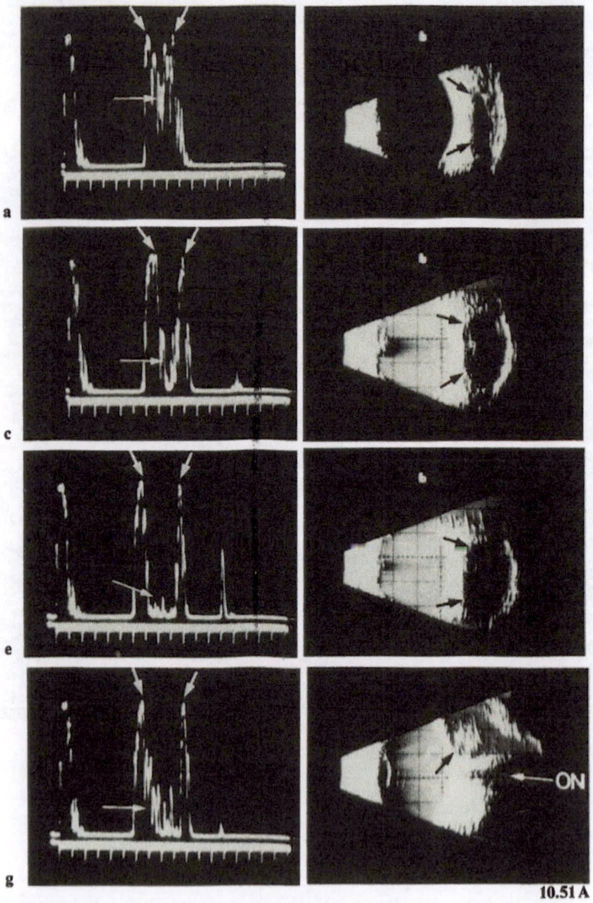

10.51 A

Fig. 10.51. Large metastasis of the orbit from a bronchial carcinoma compressing the temporal posterior segment of the eye. The retina is folded. M 63/72: 63-year-old man with progressive exophthalmos and previously unknown bronchial carcinoma.

Fig. 10.51 A. Orbital metastasis (medial rectus muscle). A-scan echograms and contact B-scan echograms of a metastatic lesion in the medial rectus muscle. **a, c, e, g** Cross sections through the thickened medial rectus muscle obtained by angling the sound probe from the anterior muscle insertion (**a**) to the posterior parts of the muscle (**g**). Note the decreased internal reflectivity of the muscle due to its infiltration by metastatic tumor cells (*short arrows* = muscle surface; *long arrows* = low reflectivity and homogeneous internal echo signals from muscle tissue apart from the most anterior part of the muscle near its insertion). **b, d, f** Cross sections obtained with B-scan. Note the topographic relationship of the thickened muscle to the optic nerve (**h** longitudinal section/*ON* = optic nerve).

Inflammatory Pseudotumor of the Orbit

Frequently, unilateral progressive exophthalmos is caused by inflammatory reactions. In children, a secondary inflammatory reaction is usually due to paranasal sinusitis; in adults, primary idiopathic inflammatory pseudotumor is an additional important cause. The clinical diagnosis is one of exclusion. Biopsy shows chronic inflammation and connective tissue scarring. No specific cause of the entity is known. Treatment consists of high-dose corticosteroids and low-dose irradiation.

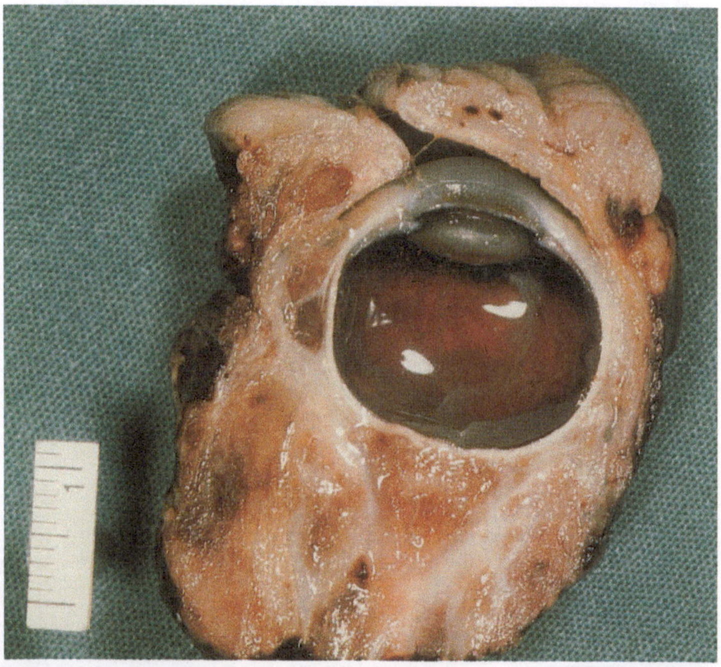

10.52

Fig. 10.52. Inflammatory pseudotumor of the orbit with white scar tissue and brownish discoloration of orbital fat due to chronic inflammatory infiltration. M 627/71: 55-year-old woman with progressive exophthalmos and loss of motility. Exenteration for suspected recurrence of a reticulum cell sarcoma of the maxillary sinus, which had been treated 9 years previously.

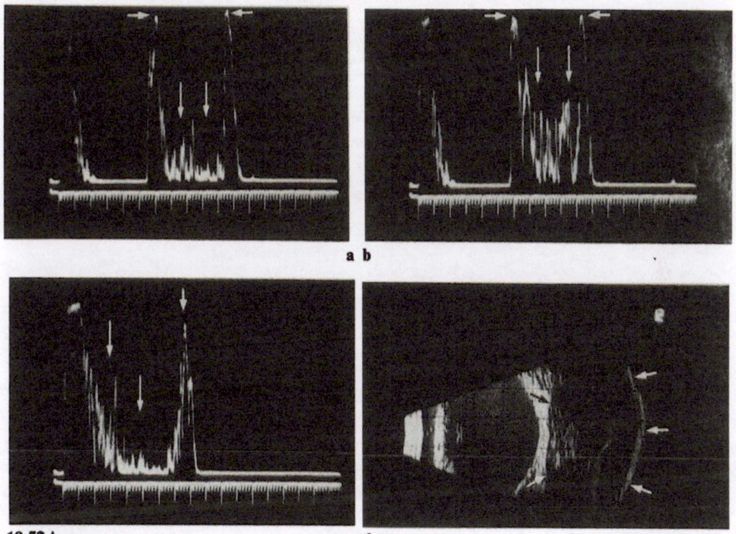

a b

10.52A c d

Fig. 10.52A. Inflammatory pseudotumor of the orbit. A-scan echograms (**a, b** transocular and **c** paraocular examination technique) and contact B-scan echogram of an orbital inflammatory pseudotumor. Note the low reflectivity and the rather homogeneous internal structure of this lesion (**a–c** *long arrows*). The borders of orbital pseudotumors may appear well-outlined (as presented here; *short arrows*), poorly outlined, or diffuse. Measurements of maximum size are important for follow-up examination during therapy.

11. Trauma

Surgical trauma: *Cataract extraction · Retinal detachment surgery · Vitrectomy · Glaucoma surgery · Retinal photocoagulation · Keratoprosthesis*

Accidental (nonsurgical) injuries: *Traumatic retinopathy · Iris tears · Retinal dialysis · Avulsion of the optic nerve · Luxation of the globe · Laceration · Burns · Foreign body · Infection · Surgical repair*

Phthisis bulbi

Any kind of trauma carries some risk of complications which may lead to blindness. Ocular structures are very thin and distortion of the globe may readily cause breaks in the various tissues. Surgical trauma has a defined risk while accidental trauma is often preventable. Sudden lowering of intraocular pressure by surgery, penetrating injury, or rupture of the globe (in nonpenetrating injury or in corneoscleral inflammation) may cause leakage of uveal veins or breaks in uveal blood vessels. Acute severe complications such as uveal effusion, intraocular hemorrhage, intraocular infection, tissue prolapse, and loss of intraocular contents may occur from both surgical and accidental trauma. In the long run, these complications may lead to intraocular scarring with shrinkage of the eye (phthisis bulbi). Major long-term complications of surgical and accidental trauma are chronic corneal edema, glaucoma, and retinal detachment. Injury of the vitreous is often associated with the formation of bands or strands; the combination of vitreous injury with hemorrhage and lens injury may be especially harmful. Preoperative ultrasonography and intraocular microsurgery (vitrectomy and irrigation/aspiration devices) nowadays are important procedures in the management of such complications and thus in the prevention of blindness.

After primary surgery and surgical repair of accidental ocular trauma, it is generally the more severe cases which ultimately require enucleation. Therefore, this chapter is devoted to complications following surgical and accidental trauma.

Surgical Trauma

Surgical trauma of the eye is a controlled injury with a low incidence of severe complications. These surgical procedures (cataract extraction, retinal detachment surgery, vitrectomy) have a defined goal attained using standard techniques which vary only slightly. Thus the success rate is high in uncomplicated situations. Surgical techniques utilized in treatment of glaucoma vary to suit the differing pathogeneses. Complications may occur at the time of surgery or arise later.

Cataract Extraction

Cataract extraction (intracapsular, extracapsular) is a highly standardized operation with a very low complication rate. Intraocular lens implantation is experiencing a renaissance today. The most serious but fortunately rare complications of cataract extraction are expulsive (arterial) hemorrhage with massive prolapse of intraocular tissues (expulsive hemorrhage) and postoperative endophthalmitis (see vitreous). Both lead usually to blindness and often enucleation of the operated eye. If intraoperative hemorrhage is less severe, vitreous loss and incarceration into the wound may occur. Small anterior chamber hemorrhages resolve quickly but hemorrhage into the vitreous causes long-standing blurring of vision. Venous (nonexpulsive) hemorrhage into the suprachoroidal space may organize forming a spongy thickening of the peripheral uvea and fixed ciliochoroidal detachment. Uveal effusion from uveal veins with ciliochoroidal detachment is not so rare and is less serious with waterlight wound closure. If interciliary (cyclitic) membranes develop, the ciliochoroidal detachment may persist. Delayed complications of cataract extraction are multiple. Examples include retinal detachment, infection, glaucoma, uveitis, corneal edema, chronic cystoid macular edema, and wound rupture.

Intraocular Hemorrhage

Fig. 11.1. Posterior vitreous detachment with incarceration of vitreous into a limbal incision. Vitreous traction on the peripheral retina. Marked hemolytic (yellow) subretinal hemorrhages. Some preretinal hemorrhages. M 878/78: 62-year-old man who developed secondary glaucoma and retinal detachment after complicated cataract extraction with vitreous loss.

Fig. 11.2. Higher magnification of the upper callotte of the same eye as Fig. 11.1. Incarceration of hemorrhagic vitreous in the cataract wound and traction on the peripheral retina. Old hemolytic hemorrhage underneath the retina.

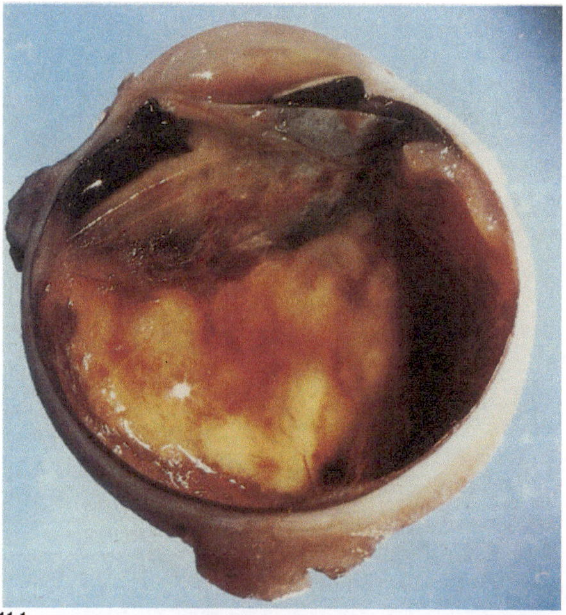

11.1

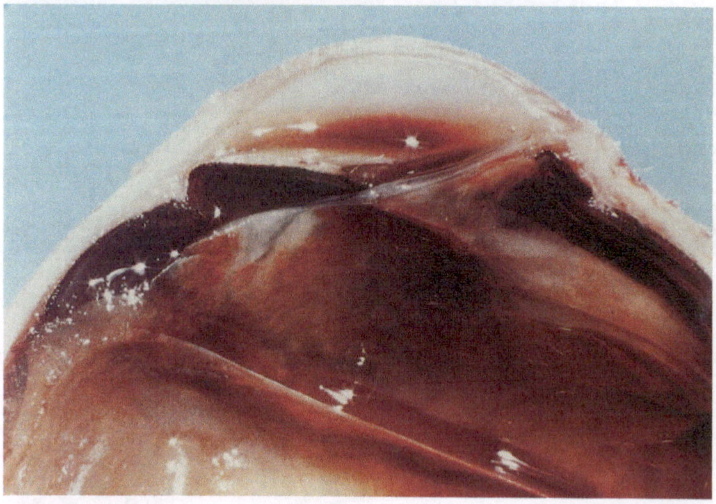

11.2

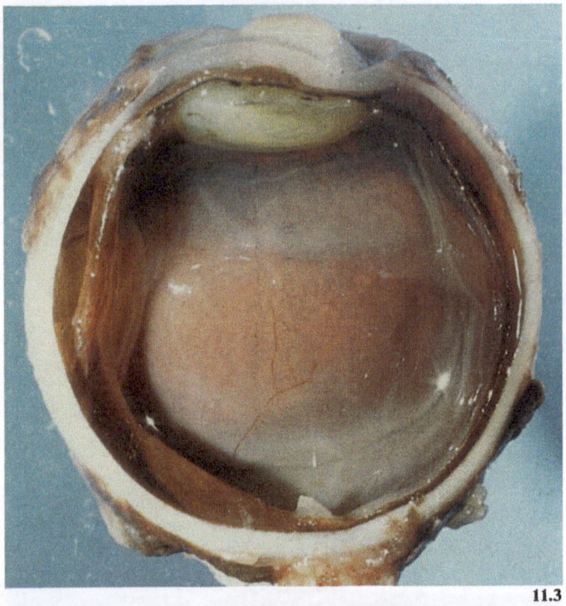

11.3

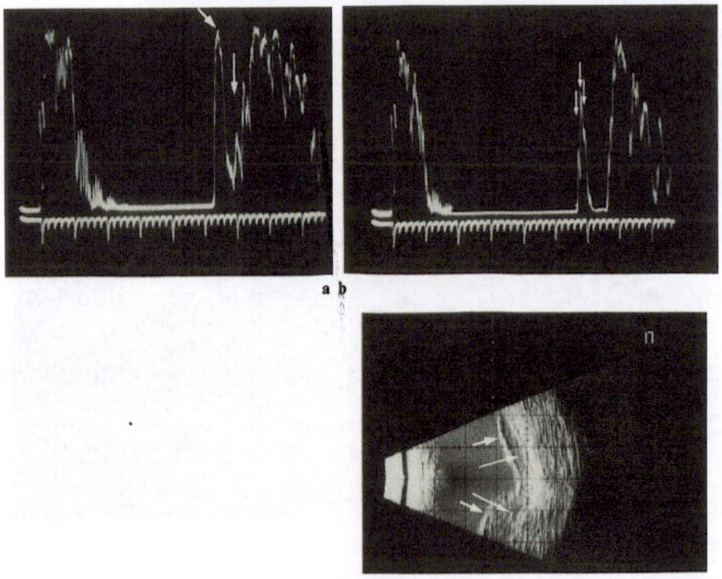

a b

c 11.3A

Ciliochoroidal Detachment

Ciliochoroidal detachment is not a rare complication in penetrating injuries of the eye. It also occurs after external ocular surgery such as retinal detachment surgery. It develops from increased leakage of the uveal veins following surgical or accidental opening of the eye or obstruction of vortex veins and leads to ocular hypotony. At the end of cataract extraction, some degree of ciliochoroidal detachment is often present. Characteristically, the surface of the detachment is smooth. Watertight wound closure and reestablishment of the intraocular pressure quickly leads to reattachment of the ciliary body. Persisting ciliochoroidal detachment is either due to a fistulizing wound with flattened anterior chamber or due to interciliary membrane formation with traction on the ciliary body.

Fig. 11.3. Ciliochoroidal detachment showing the smooth surface of the elevated choroid. M 31/78: 63-year-old man with a history of long-standing glaucoma. Acute keratitis had led to corneal perforation.

Fig. 11.3A. Choroidal detachment. A-scan echograms (**a, b**) and contact B-scan echogram (**c**) of a hemorrhagic choroidal detachment. Note the high surface signal that has an increased width (*short arrows*) as compared to a retinal detachment which can be tested at "measuring sensitivity" of the standardized A-scan instrument (see Table 1/Preface) and thus appears double or triple-peaked (**b**). The echo signals in the subchoroidal space represent fresh hemorrhage (*long arrows,* **a, c**).

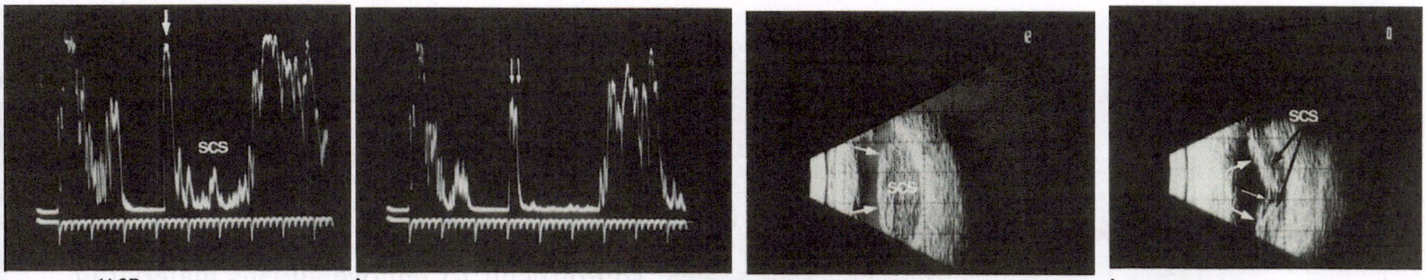

11.3B a b c d

Fig. 11.3B. Fresh hemorrhagic choroidal detachment. A-scan echograms (**a, b**) and contact B-scan echograms (**c, d**) of hemorrhagic choroidal detachments in the nasal (**c**) and temporal (**d**) periphery (*arrows* = surface of the choroidal detachment; *thin arrows* (**b**) = at low "measuring-sensitivity" setting of the standardized A-scan instrument (see Table 1/Preface), the double peaked surface spike representing retina and choroid is shown; *thin arrow* (**d**) = retinal detachment between two bullae of choroidal detachment; *SCS* = opacities in the subchoroidal space).

Fig. 11.4. Large long-standing ciliochoroidal detachment with interciliary membrane formation and retinal detachment. M 542/75: 79-year-old man with history of recurrent iritis and secondary glaucoma. Glaucoma surgery had been successful, but ocular hypotony developed after intracapsular cataract extraction with vitreous loss.

Fig. 11.4A. Thickened choroid after hemorrhagic choroidal detachment. A-scan echogram (**a**) and contact B-scan echogram (**b**) of flat, diffusely thickened choroid in an area of previous hemorrhagic choroidal detachment.

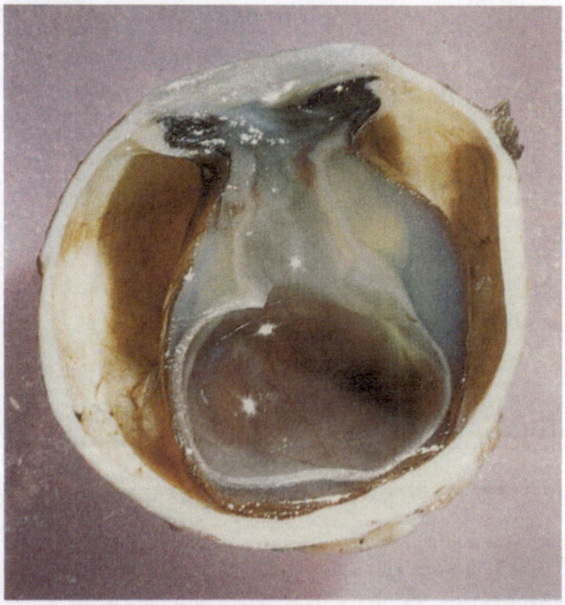

11.4

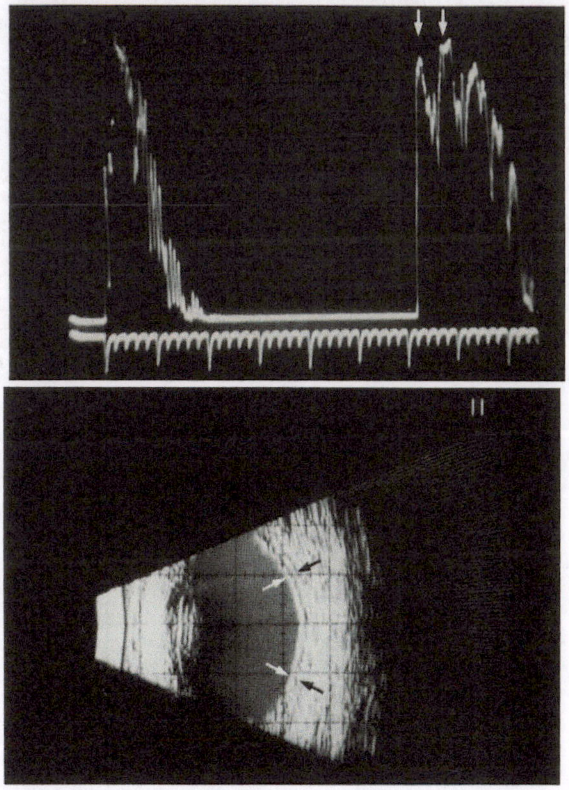

a b

11.4A

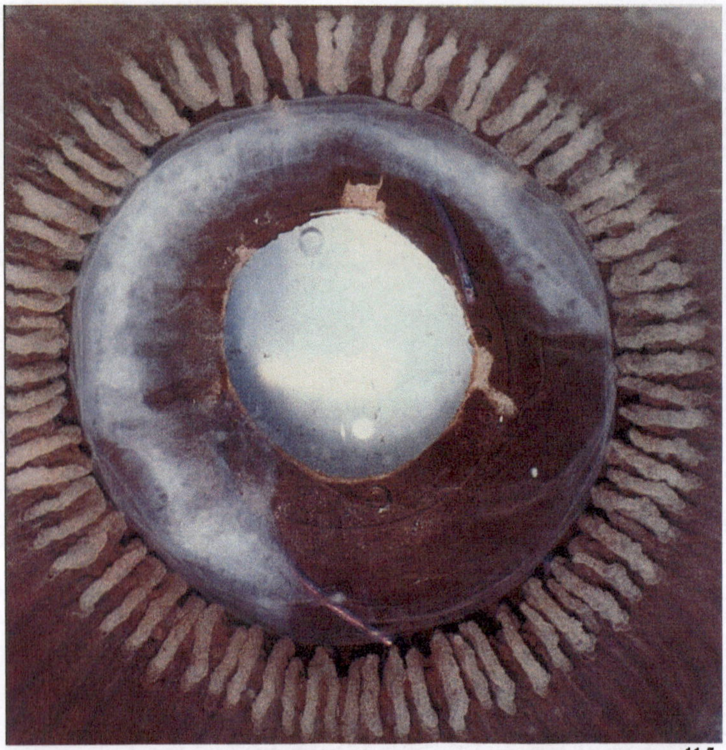

11.5

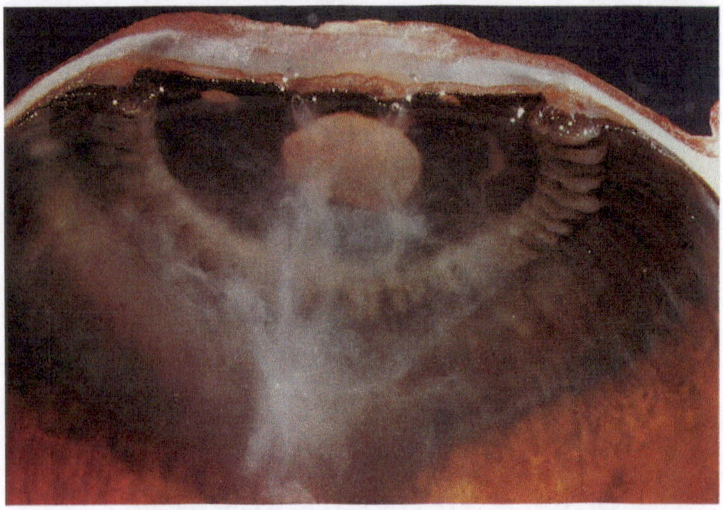

11.6

Intraocular Lens Implantation

The revival of intraocular lens implantation today is attributable to technical progress in surgery and lens manufacturing. Irrigation-aspiration systems have dramatically influenced operation techniques. Yet it is still difficult to remove all lens material (a strong antigen) from behind the iris. The reintroduction of lens implants began with iris-fixed intraocular lenses after intracapsular cataract extraction. But today, most surgeons have turned to posterior chamber lens implants with fixation of the lens haptic either in the ciliary sulcus or in the lens bag after performing an extracapsular cataract extraction.

Fig. 11.5. Clinically successful implantation of a posterior chamber lens (Sinsky type) with the haptics in the ciliary sulcus. Remnants of lens cortex in the remaining lens capsule after extracapsular cataract extraction. Some defects of iris pigment epithelium. M 599/84: Autopsy eye of an 83-year-old man with age-related cataract operated a few days prior to his death.

Fig. 11.6. Postoperative infection with iris-fixed four-loop intraocular lens (Binkhorst type) after intracapsular cataract extraction. Severe intraocular infection with hypopyon, yellow-whitish infiltrates over the ciliary body and within the anterior vitreous. M 143/85: 78-year-old man who developed signs of endophthalmitis 3 days after intracapsular cataract extraction and intraocular lens implantation for age-related cataract.

Retinal Detachment Surgery

Retinal detachment surgery with modern techniques of external scleral buckling has a high success rate in sealing retinal holes and relieving vitreous traction. At the beginning of modern retinal surgery, Custodis used polyviol (polyvinylalcohol plus gummi arabicum plus Congo red) for buckling. But this caused severe toxic intraocular inflammation in many cases. Today, solid silicone and silicone sponge are the materials of choice. Scleral infolding is sometimes performed as an alternative to placing a silicone exoplant. Complications of retinal detachment surgery are intraocular hemorrhage, ciliochoroidal detachment, postoperative inflammation, glaucoma, anterior segment ischemic syndrome (string syndrome), and massive vitreoretinal reaction.

Fig. 11.7. Two brownish Custodis' polyviol rods with discoloration of the adjacent sclera. The attached retina shows chorioretinal scarring. M 377/82: Autopsy eye of a 54-year-old man who had retinal detachment surgery more than a decade before death.

Fig. 11.7 A. Globe with 360-degrees encircling band after retinal detachment. A-scan echograms (**a, c, e**) and contact B-scan echograms (**b, d, f**) of a globe after retinal detachment surgery with a 360-degree encircling band. Sections central to the buckle (**a, b**) show free vitreous and attached retina with a slight enlarged globe diameter (**a**). When angling the sound probe towards the buckle (**c, d**) and then centering the buckle (**e, f**), it is represented in the echogram by a high surface spike (sclera/anterior surface of the band) and a somewhat lower posterior spike (posterior surface of the band) with acoustic shadowing on the orbital pattern behind the buckle.

Fig. 11.7 B. Vitreous opacities/Posterior vitreous detachment/Scleral buckle. Contact B-scan echograms after retinal detachment surgery (buckling procedure). *Thick arrow* = buckle/superotemporal equatorial periphery; *long thin arrows* = acoustic shadowing on the orbital patterns caused by the silicone material; *small white arrows* = posterior vitreous surface; *small black arrow* = point of adhesion of the vitreous at the buckle. **a** before, **b** immediately after the beginning, **c** during and **d** after eye movement on command.

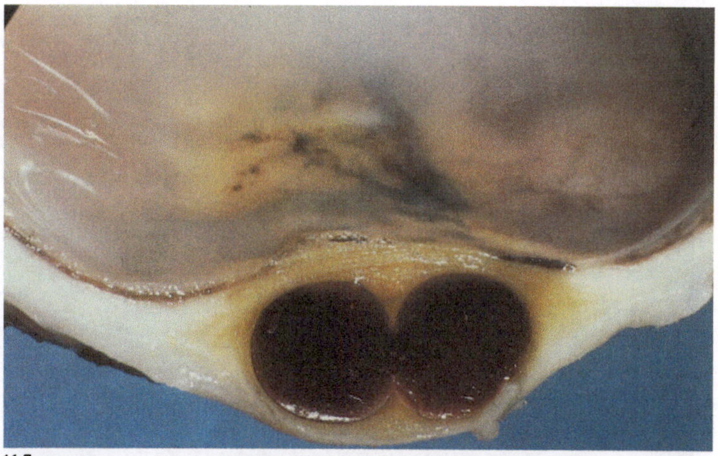

11.7

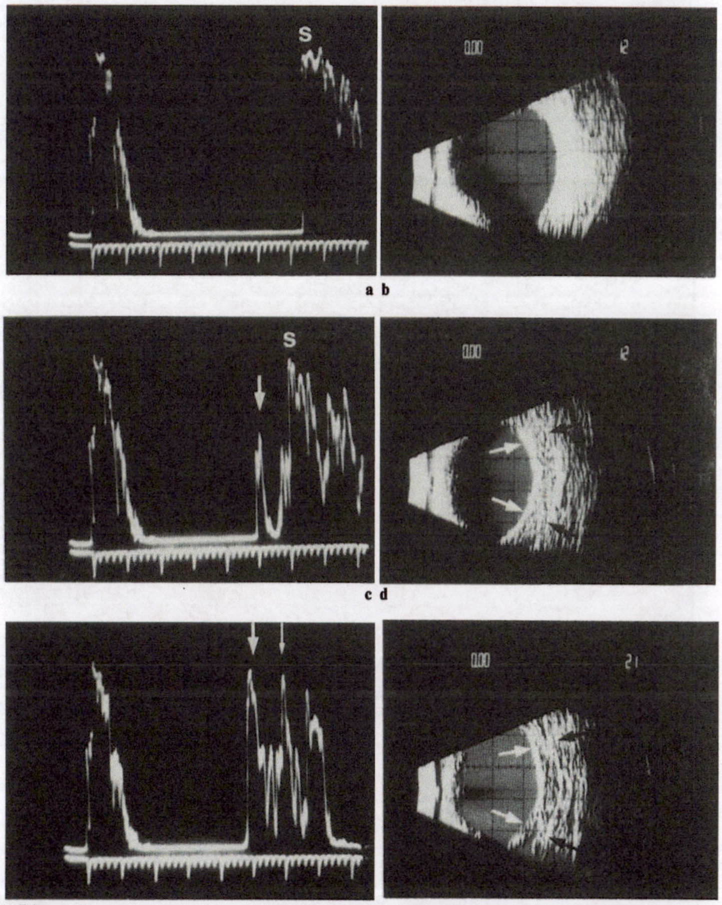

a b
c d
11.7A e f

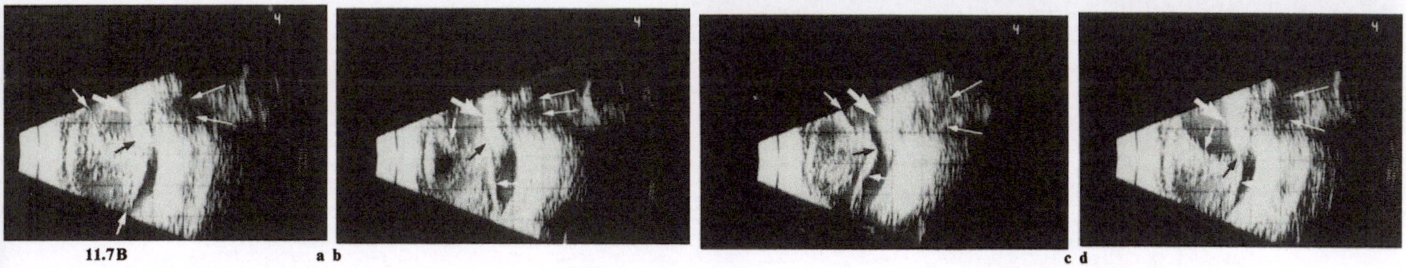

11.7B a b c d

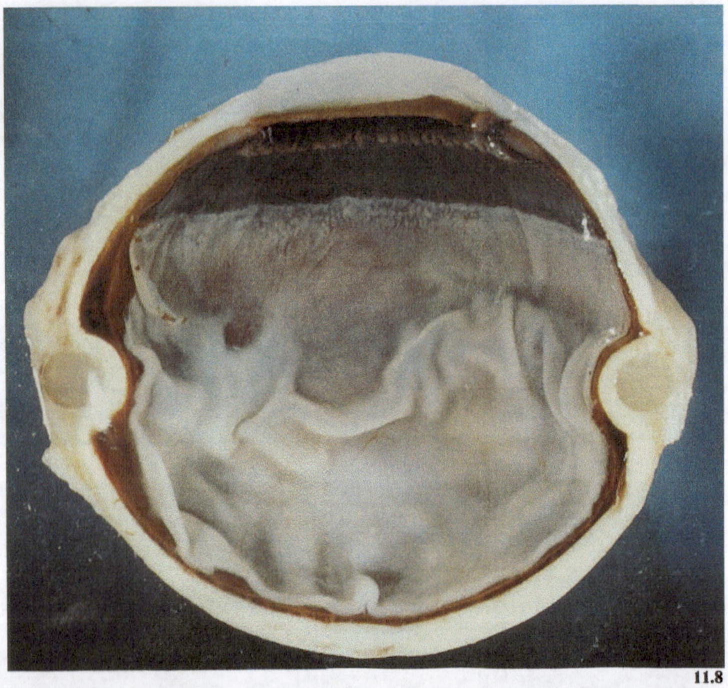

11.8

Fig. 11.8. Silicone band encircling the eye. Detached folded retina and ciliochoroidal detachment. M 919/81 73-year-old man who had unsuccesful retinal detachment surgery.

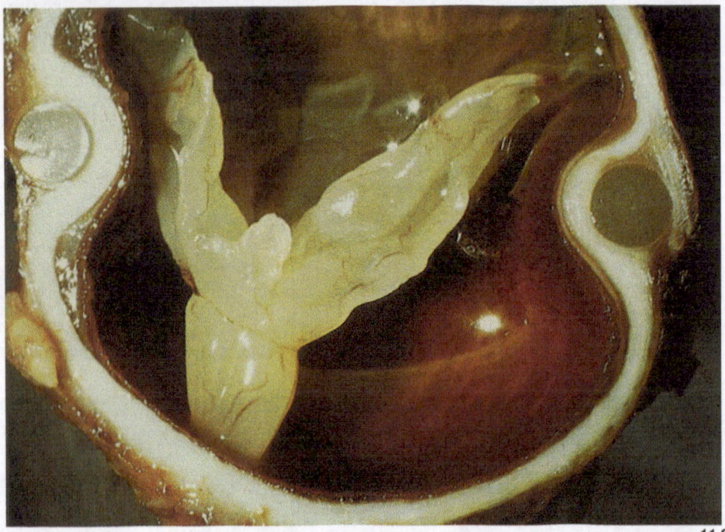

11.9

Fig. 11.9. Silicone band encircling the eye. Total retinal detachment with subretinal membrane formation (constriction of the retinal stalk). M 464/77: 56-year-old man who had had retinal detachment surgery and subsequent massive vitreoretinal reaction with redetachment of the retina.

Fig. 11.10. Scleral buckle with chorioretinal scar due to intraoperative cryotherapy. Fibrous reaction of the overlying cloudy vitreous. M 645/74: 59-year-old man who had had retinal detachment surgery following intracapsular cataract extraction.

Fig. 11.11. Scleral buckle after scleral infolding surgery with marked proliferative reaction of the retinal pigment epithelium. Some fine glistening cholesterol crystals are present as a sign of previous hemorrhage. M 635/79: 53-year-old woman who had had complicated cataract surgery with large subretinal hemorrhage and scleral infolding for subsequent retinal detachment.

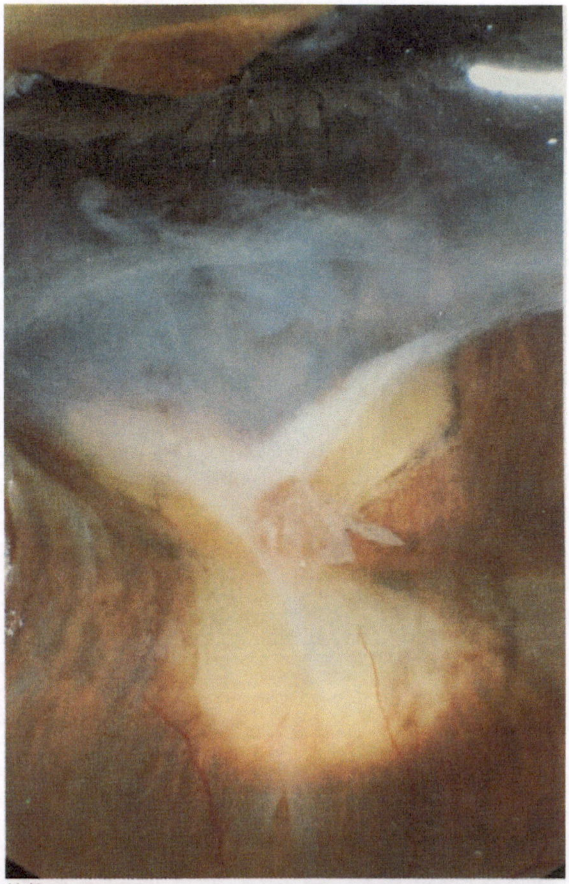

11.10

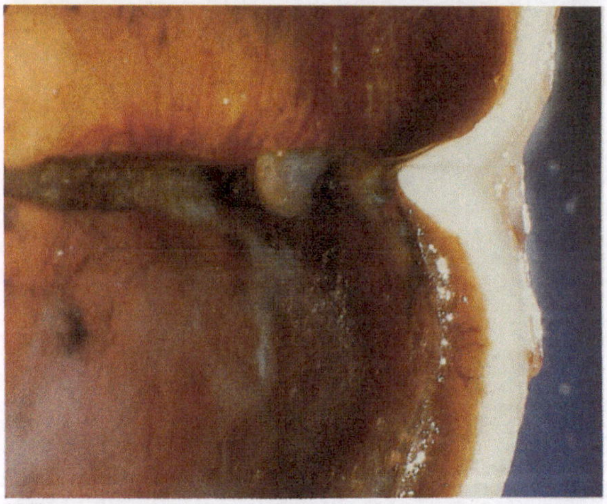

11.11

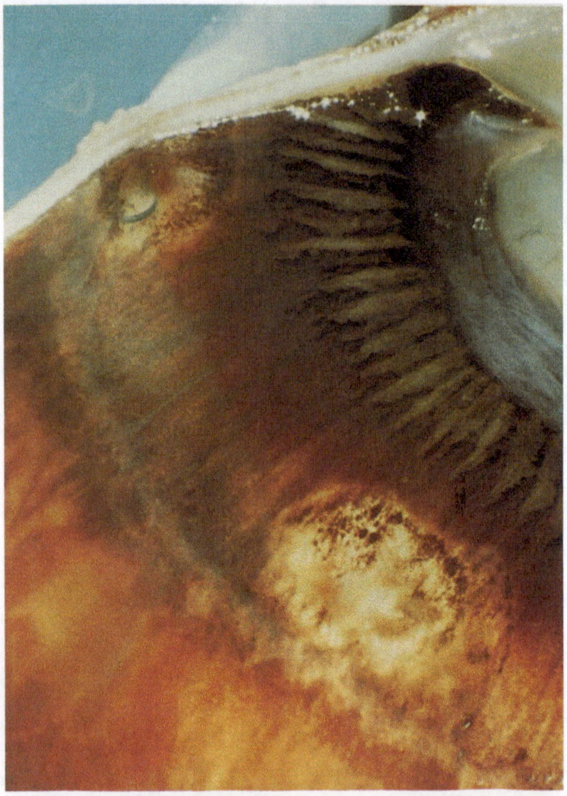

11.12

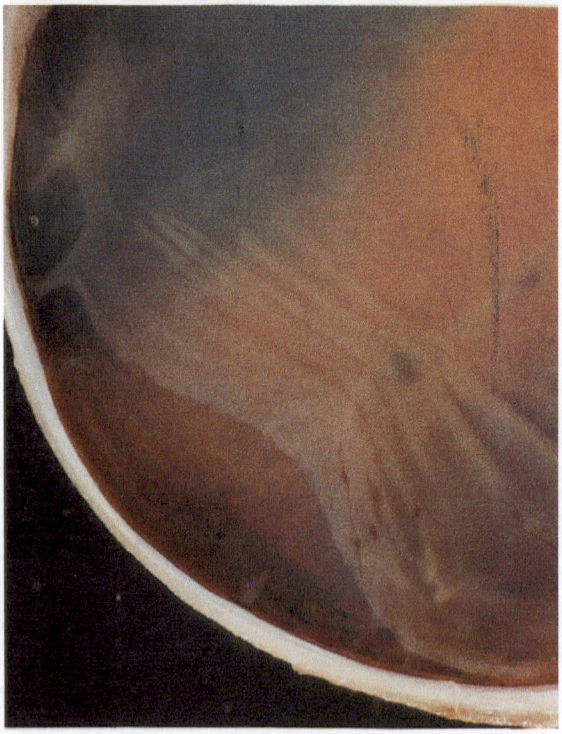

11.13

Vitrectomy

Intraocular microsurgical vitrectomy with endodiathermy and endocryotherapy is an increasingly important procedure in the management of the complications of trauma, intravitreal hemorrhage of various origin, vasoproliferative disease, complicated retinal detachment, and idiopathic periretinal membranes. The common introduction site of the light source, the infusion device, the vitreous cutter, scissors, hooks and other intraocular instruments is the pars plana, thus avoiding damage to nearby lens and sensory retina at the ora serrata. Moreover, if cataract abscures the view, the lens may be removed at the same procedure. Secondary scar formation from the pars plana wound is a fairly rare cause of tractional retinal detachment.

Fig. 11.12. Two uncomplicated scars of the pars plana of the ciliary body after vitrectomy. Remnants of the lens behind the iris. M 543/77: 56-year-old man with a history of penetrating injury and pars plana vitrectomy with lensectomy for secondary complications. Enucleation because of postthrombotic neovascular glaucoma.

Fig. 11.13. Scar of the pars plana of the ciliary body with fibrous plaque. Detachment of the nonpigmented ciliary epithelium and the peripheral retina. M 840/83: 56-year-old diabetic man who had been treated with laser photocoagulation for diabetic retinopathy and by pars plana vitrectomy for vitreous hemorrhage. Enucleation for untreatable secondary glaucoma.

Glaucoma Surgery

The general aim of glaucoma surgery is to reduce intraocular pressure and thus to prevent visual field loss and optic nerve damage. The mechanisms leading to glaucoma vary widely (see chapter on glaucoma) as do the surgical procedures. A number of fistulizing operations have been developed mainly for primary open-angle glaucoma. Trabeculectomy with scleral flap is a standard filtering procedure today. Goniotomy is widely used for infantile glaucoma. Iridectomy is the method of choice after an acute attack of angle-closure glaucoma or in prophylaxis. Controlling glaucoma due to trauma (accidental or surgical) or to neovascularization may be especially difficult. For the latter, many different surgical procedures have been tried with little success. One type of surgery aims to reduce the filtration area of the ciliary body.

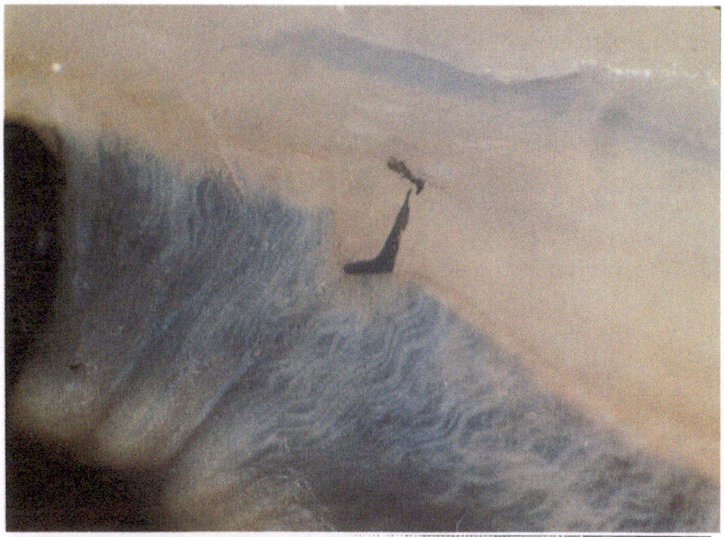

11.14

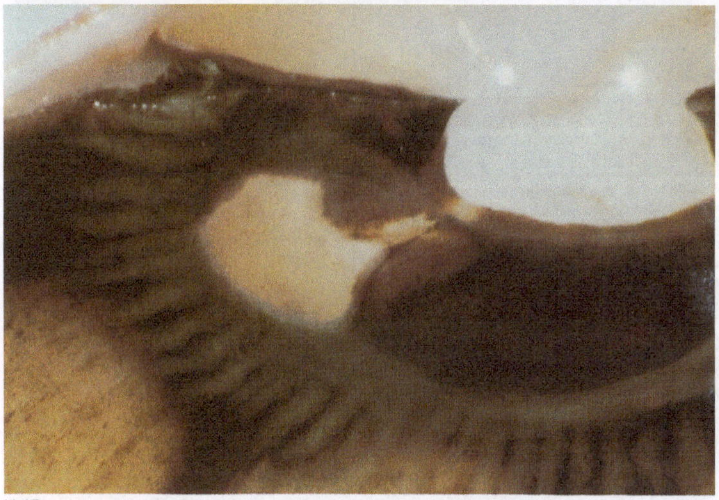

11.15

Iridectomy

Peripheral iridectomy is used prophylactically for angle-closure glaucoma due to a multiplicity of causes. As an isolated operation, it has few risks or side effects. In cataract extraction this procedure has been performed for more than 100 years as a preventative measure. In patients with a history of iritis it may be more difficult to fashion a patent iridectomy because of posterior fibrovascular proliferation at the iris base in the ciliary sulcus.

Fig. 11.14. Iris pigment epithelium layer between small peripheral iridectomy and zone of limbal corneal incision. Surgical aphakia in an autopsy eye without clinical history.

Fig. 11.15. Large peripheral iridectomy performed during intracapsular cataract extraction. The central portion of the iris in front of the iridectomy shows atrophy. Depigmented scars of the ciliary body from cryotherapy. M 448/82: 66-year-old woman enucleated because of secondary glaucoma due to diffuse epithelial invasion of the anterior chamber after cataract extraction.

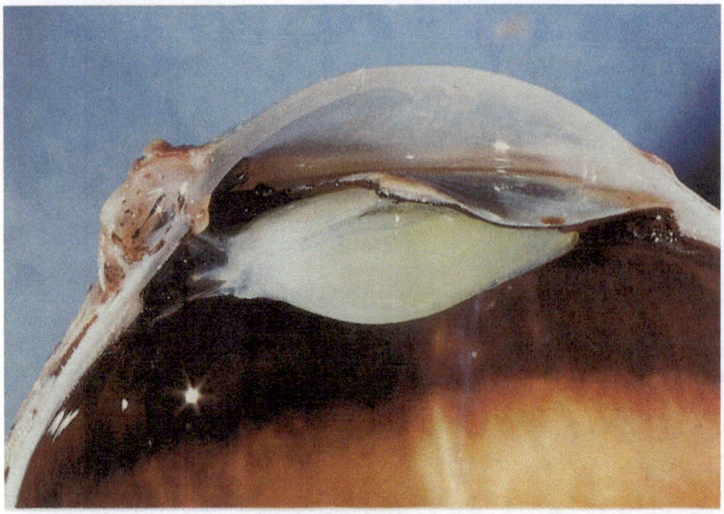

11.16

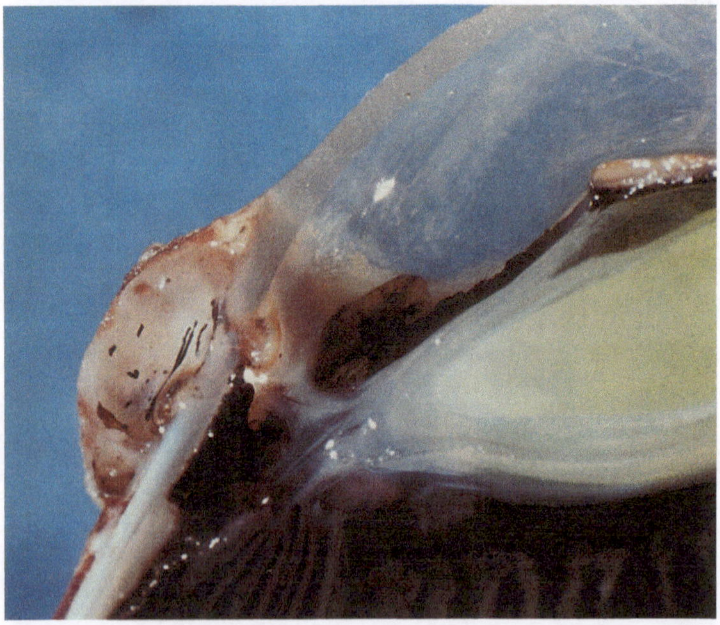

11.17

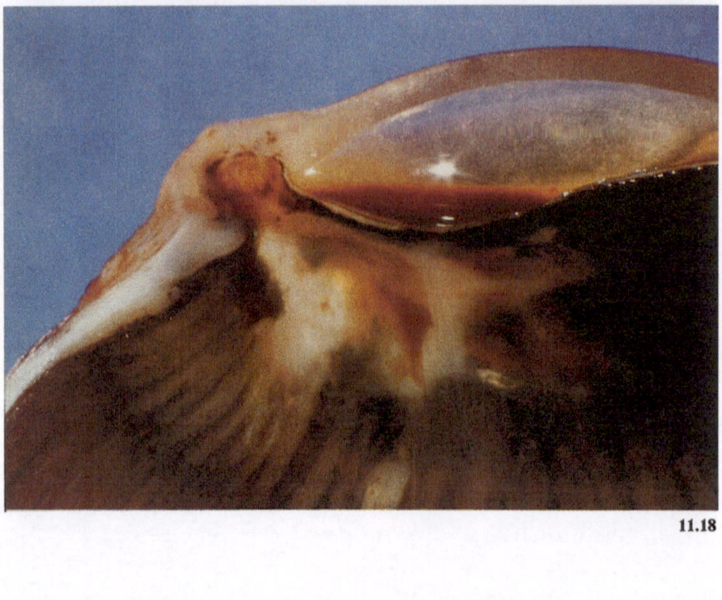

11.18

Filtering Procedure

Fig. 11.16. Conjunctival filtering bleb after Elliot's filtering procedure without scleral flap with total iridectomy. The lens equator is attached to connective tissue from the site of surgery. M 510/85: 16-year-old boy who had been operated several times for infantile glaucoma with buphthalmos (hydrophthalmos) before Elliot's filtering procedure was performed 10 years previously.

Fig. 11.17. Higher magnification of Elliot's filter with conjunctival filtering bleb.

Fig. 11.18. Trabeculectomy with peripheral anterior synechia, scar formation, and hemorrhage into the anterior and posterior chamber. Surgical aphakia. M 836/79: 72-year-old woman who had had primary chronic simple glaucoma, trabeculectomy, cataract extraction, and central retinal vein occlusion.

Reduction of Aqueous Filtration

The aim of several procedures for otherwise untreatable glaucoma is to reduce ciliary body filtration. Cyclectomy, diathermy of the ciliary body, and cryotherapy have been used. One of the risks is progressive loss of intraocular pressure (hypotony) and subsequent phthisis bulbi.

Cyclectomy

Cyclectomy generally is performed for local excision of small tumors of the ciliary body. It has also been used to control glaucoma.

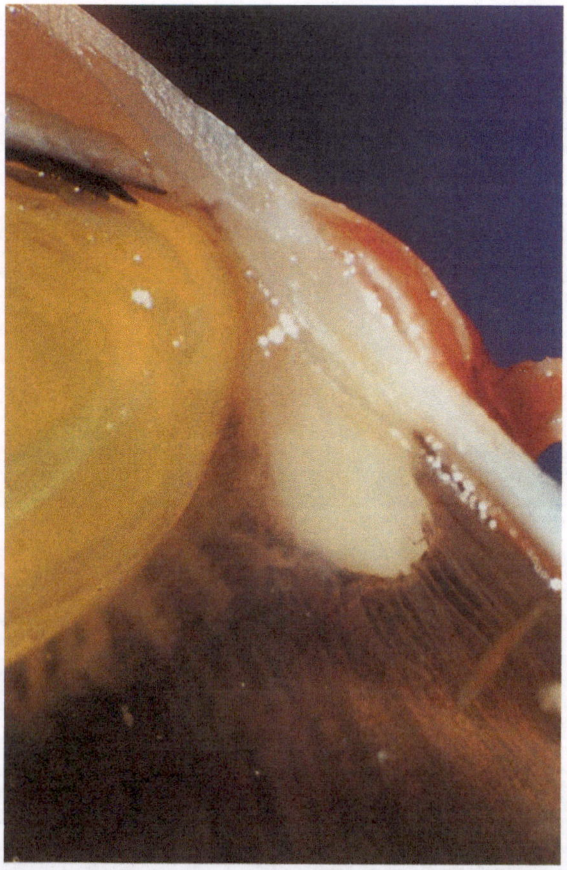

11.19

Fig. 11.19. Defect of the anterior ciliary body and adjacent iris after cyclectomy. The lens is located close to the cyclectomy area and there is some hemorrhage in the anterior vitreous. M 77/85: 67-year-old woman with malignant melanoma located in the anterior ciliary body and invading the iris root.

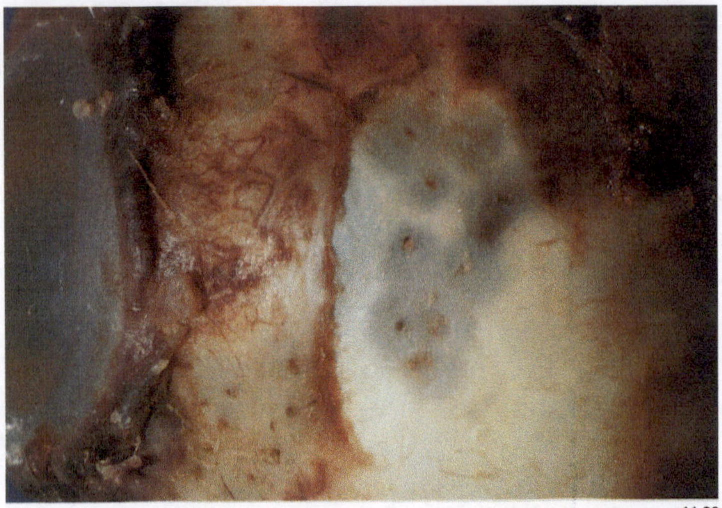

11.20

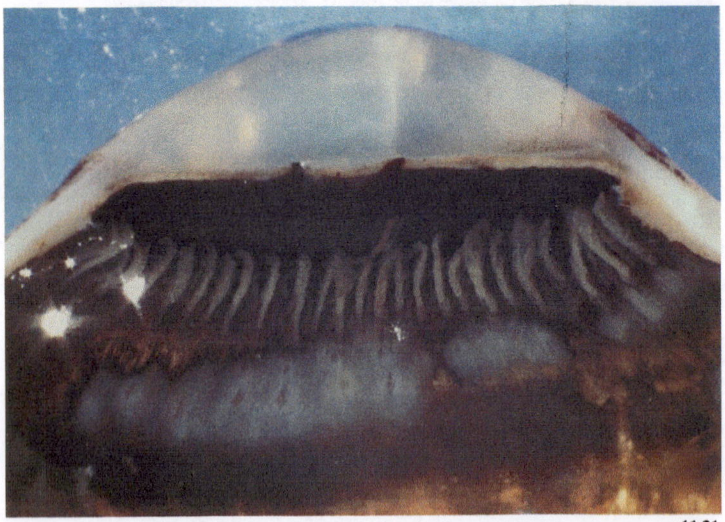

11.21

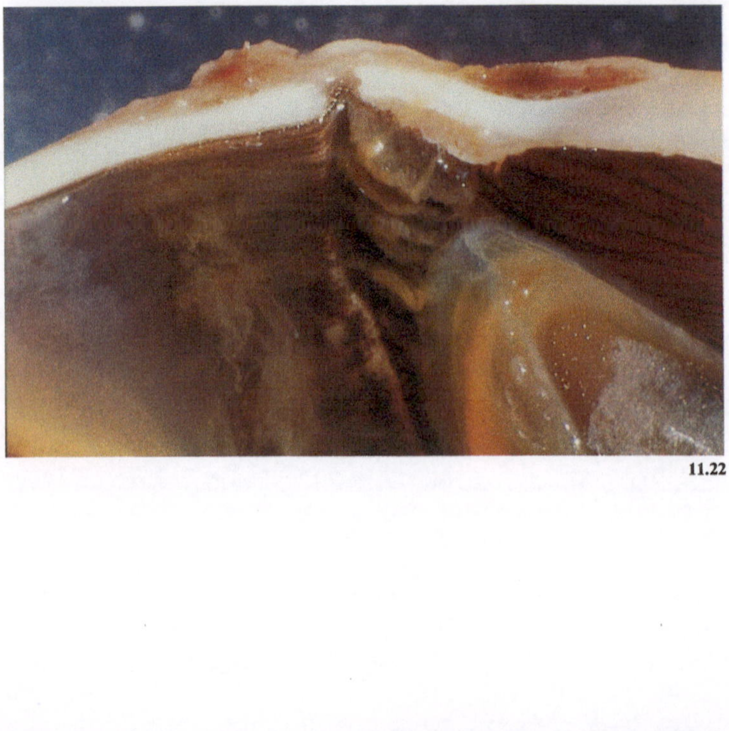

11.22

Diathermy of the Ciliary Body

Transscleral diathermy of the ciliary body results in coagulation of both sclera and the underlying structures of the ciliary body. In using a long diathermy needle, one must avoid the nearby lens.

Fig. 11.20. Grey diathermy coagulation marks in the sclera around a central needling defect. M 198/80: 67-year-old man with secondary glaucoma due to untreated total retinal detachment with chronic iridocyclitis, rubeosis iridis, and peripheral anterior synechias.

Fig. 11.21. Scarring ciliary coagulations from diathermy. Anterior peripheral synechias (goniosynechias). M 680/84: 39-year-old man who had developed neovascular glaucoma following ocular contusion.

Direct Diathermy of the Ciliary Body

After reflecting a scleral flap, direct diathermy is applied to the exposed ciliary body. Some surgeons combine this procedure with excision of the coagulated ciliary body.

Fig. 11.22. Dehiscent (staphylomatous) scar of the sclera following direct diathermy of the ciliary body. The adjacent ciliary processes show some atrophy. M 321/79: 73-year-old woman who had central retinal vein occlusion 14 years ago. Postthrombotic neovascular glaucoma was diagnosed 2 years previously. Direct diathermy of the ciliary body was unsuccessful.

Cryotherapy of the Ciliary Body

Cryotherapy is widely used today for reducing ciliary secretion of aqueous. It has proven less complicated than diathermy of the ciliary body, can easily be repeated, and is effective in a number of patients.

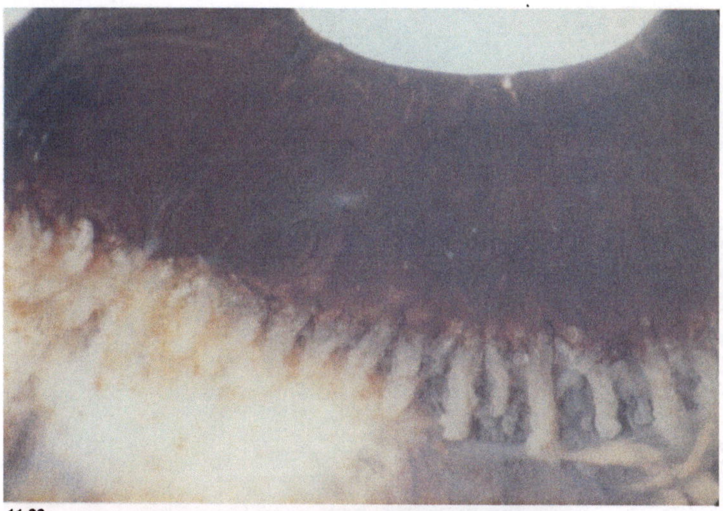

11.23

Fig. 11.23. White scar of the ciliary body after cryotherapy. M 568/82: 62-year-old aphakic man with postthrombotic untreatable neovascular glaucoma.

Retinal Photocoagulation

Retinal photocoagulation is widely used in the prophylaxis of a variety of proliferative and degenerative retinal diseases. In diabetic retinopathy, central retinal vein occlusion and retinal breaks, it is a sight saving procedure. The xenon arc light or laser light focused on the retinal pigment epithelium results in a thermal burn of the sensory retina which subsequently heals by scarring. Laser photocoagulation has mainly replaced xenon-photocoagulation during the past 10 years.

Xenon Arc Photocoagulation

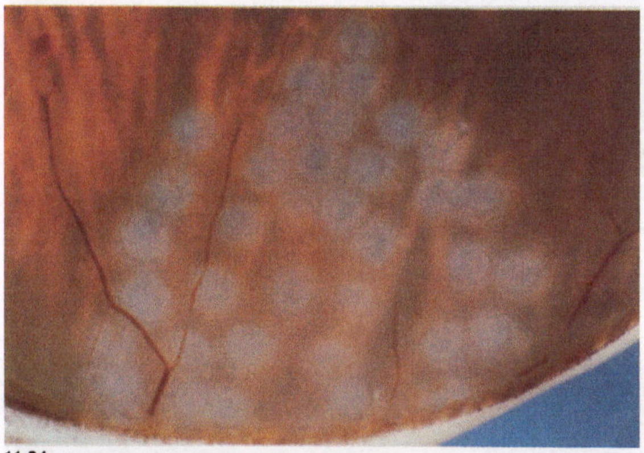

11.24

Fig. 11.24. Initial xenon arc photocoagulation burns of the retina. M 943/78: 48-year-old diabetic man enucleated for malignant melanoma of the choroid. Photocoagulation was performed 30 min before enucleation.

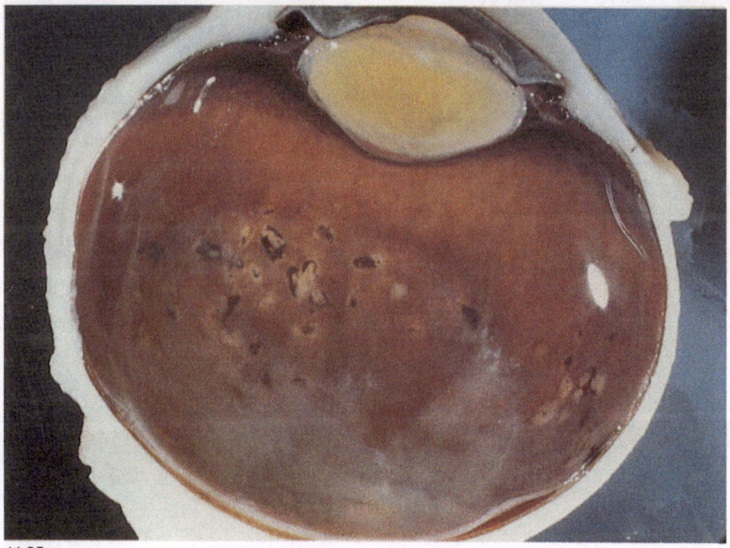

11.25

Fig. 11.25. Old chorioretinal scars from xenon arc photocoagulation in proliferative diabetic retinopathy. M 1088/82: Autopsy eye of a 73-year-old woman with diabetic retinopathy. Photocoagulation had been performed some years previously.

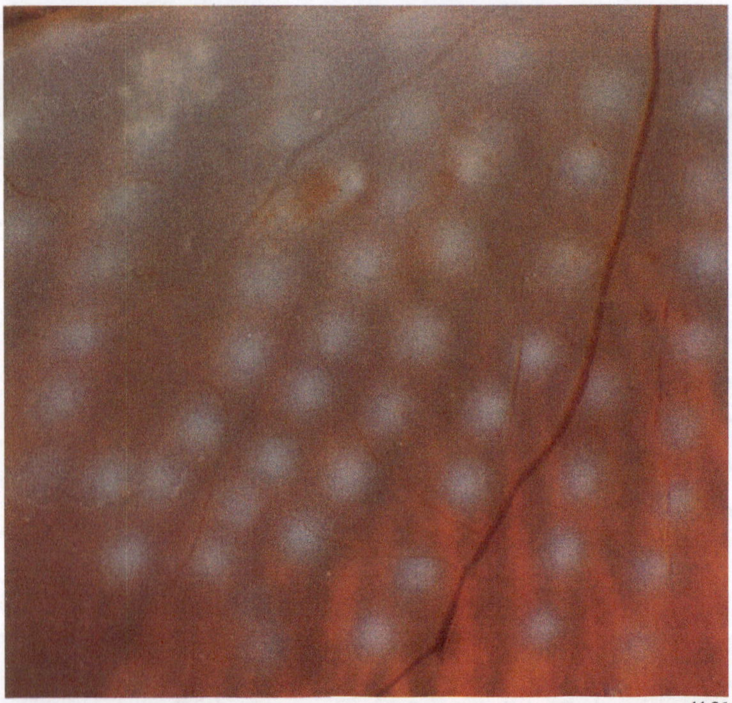

11.26

Laser Photocoagulation

Fig. 11.26. Initial laser burn of the retina. M 943/78: 48-year-old diabetic man enucleated for malignant melanoma of the choroid. Photocoagulation was performed 30 min before enucleation.

Fig. 11.27. Old scars of retinal laser burns. M 37/85: Autopsy eye of a 74-year-old diabetic man treated in the past for diabetic retinopathy by laser photocoagulation.

Fig. 11.28. Elevation of the retina showing clumps of pigment of the outer surface of the retina and small proliferations of retinal pigment epithelium. Same patients as in Fig. 11.27.

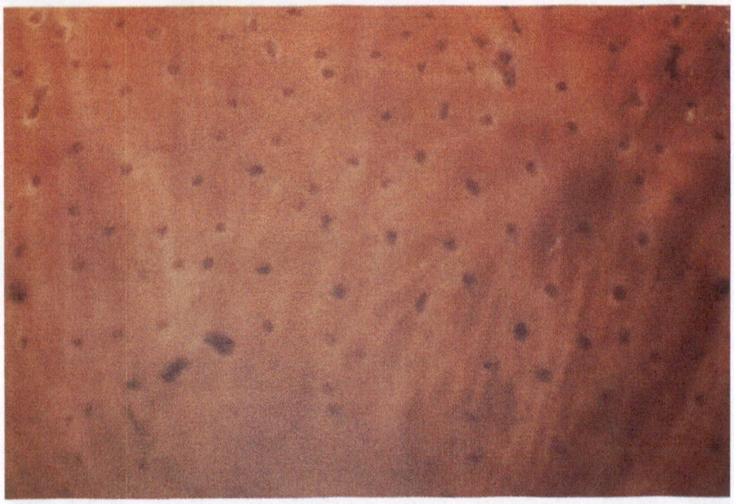

11.27

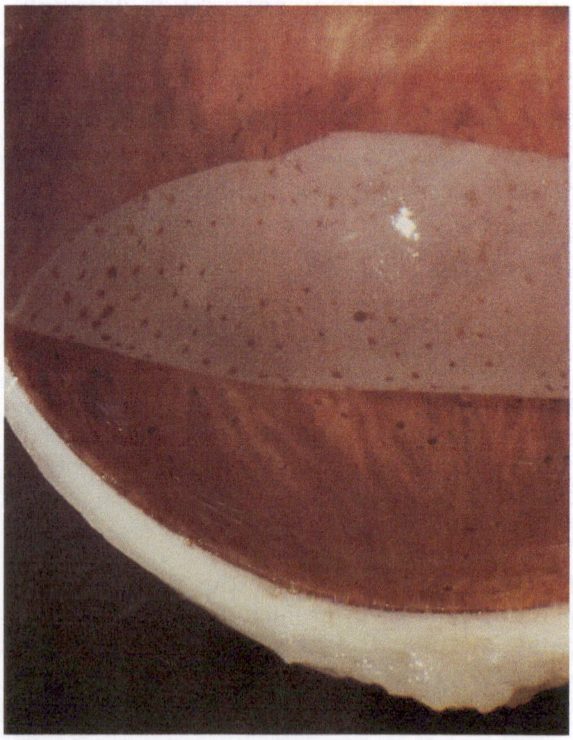

11.28

Keratoprosthesis

The implantation of an artificial optical cylinder (keratoprosthesis) has been used by several surgeons to treat severe scarring of the cornea and after failed corneal grafting. Strampelli was fairly successful with an osteo-odonto-keratoprosthesis, which uses tooth and bone for fixation of the implant. Choyce used an all plastic haptic and others have used ceramics for fixation. Some patients have a navigation visual acuity. A number have even achieved a 20/20 (6/6) visual acuity. The postoperative complications are unrecognized elevation of intraocular pressure, extrusion of the optic cylinder, and retinal detachment.

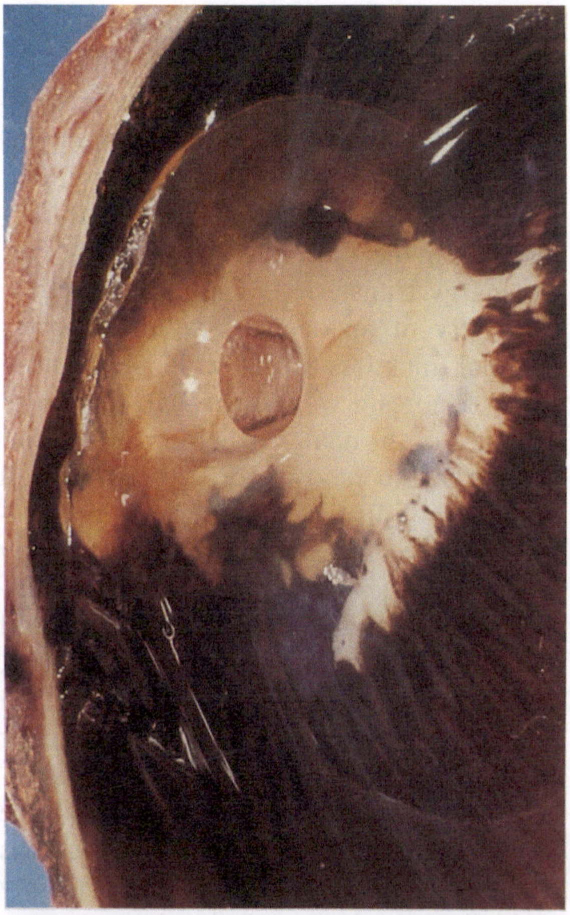
11.29

Fig. 11.29. Osteo-odonto-keratoprosthesis in place viewed from the back of the iris. The optic cylinder is seen passing through remnants of the lens. There is marked loss of iris pigment epithelium. The corneal surface is thickened by tooth, bone, and mucosal graft. M 795/78: 33-year-old man with a history of bilateral corneal scarring after severe lime burn. Several earlier keratoplasties had been unsuccessful.

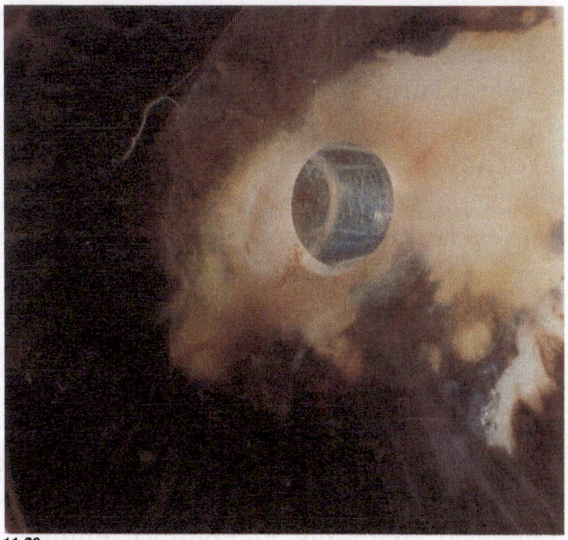
11.30

Fig. 11.30. Higher magnification of Fig. 11.29 showing the optical cylinder in the lens remnants.

Accidental (Nonsurgical) Ocular Injuries

Although the eye represents only a small percentage of the body surface, it is involved in at least 10% of accidental trauma. The resulting eye injuries vary greatly according to the mechanism of trauma and the energy transferred. The term penetrating injury of an ocular structure denotes a partial thickness wound while perforating injury denotes a wound through the entire thickness of the ocular structure. Superficial injuries of the eye with or without a small foreign body usually have a good prognosis. Contusion and penetrating foreign body injuries may cause tissue breaks with intraocular disorganization, hemorrhage, and tissue loss. Besides mechanical damage, other damage such as thermal burns and chemical burns may occur. A great number of eyes are lost every year by traumatic intraocular lesions although many could have been prevented by simple measures such as protective goggles or seat belts. Highly sophisticated microsurgical techniques save many of these eyes, but few that are severely damaged, are left functionally normal. General surgical principles are, immediate surgical repair of ocular lesions and removal of any intraocular foreign body. Enucleation as a primary procedure is performed only very rarely even when the prognosis appears extremely poor from the clinical appearance at surgery. This clinical impression may later prove wrong with the eye in time regaining useful vision. Severe injuries of the eye have a poor prognosis because of frequently developing traumatic cataract, secondary glaucoma, retinal detachment, hypotony, and phthisis bulbi.

Contusion

Blunt trauma to the eye may lead to traumatic edema, pressure increase, pupillary disturbances, breaks in various intraocular tissue and even rupture of sclera or cornea. Tissue repair processes may lead to further complications. Typical sites for tissue breaks are, the trabecular meshwork, the zonules, the pupillary zone of the iris, the choroid, and the retina. Dialysis of the iris (disinsertion at the iris base), dialysis of the ciliary body (disinsertion of the ciliary muscle from the scleral spur), dialysis of the anterior vitreous (disinsertion of the vitreous base), and retinal dialysis (retinal disinsertion at the ora serrata) are also common intraocular injuries. Dialysis of the iris may have cosmetic and optical implications and dialysis of the ciliary body may cause globe hypotony. Both are treated by surgical refixation of the disinserted iris or ciliary body. Rupture is common at the corneal limbus and posterior to the scleral insertion of the rectus muscles. The loss of intraocular tissue in global rupture contributes to the poor prognosis. Avulsion of the optic nerve at the optic disc or rupture of the nerve within its sheaths, or rupture of external muscles of the eye are rare events in blunt trauma. With this range of potential tissue damage, ocular contusion is regarded as a serious injury.

Traumatic Retinopathy

Berlin's retinal edema in commotio retinae may develop at the site of contrecoup. It resolves spontaneously and may then cause retinal ischemia with hole formation or retinal scarring (traumatic retinopathy) with atrophy of the retina, hyperplasia, and atrophy of retinal pigment epithelium and gliosis.

Fig. 11.31. Partial posttraumatic retinal detachment. Traumatic retinopathy in the area of attached retina and giant drusen of the pigment epithelium beneath the detached retina. Cataractous small lens. M 1057/77: 54-year-old man who had suffered a penetrating injury caused by a knife at the age of 5 years. Enucleation for untretable secondary glaucoma.

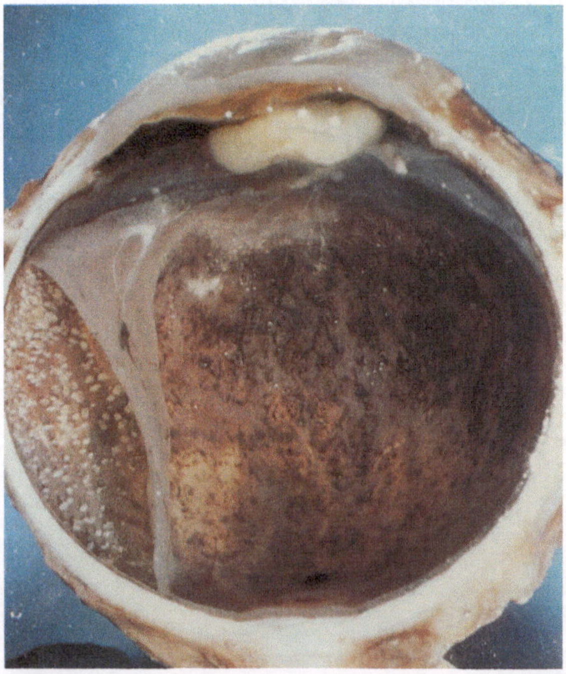

11.31

Iris Tears

In concussional injuries, the iris may tear in the pupillary zone or at its base (dialysis of the iris). The latter often is associated with tears in the trabecular meshwork and secondary glaucoma. For cosmetic and optical reasons, a dialysis of the iris may be repaired surgically.

Fig. 11.32. Large dialysis of the iris with atrophy of the adjacent ciliary body. M 41/84: 71-year-old woman who had suffered severe ocular concussion. Later she developed secondary glaucoma.

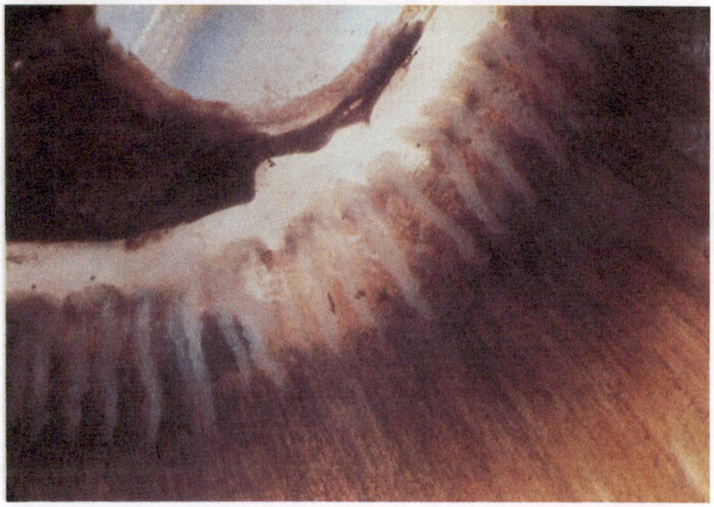

11.32

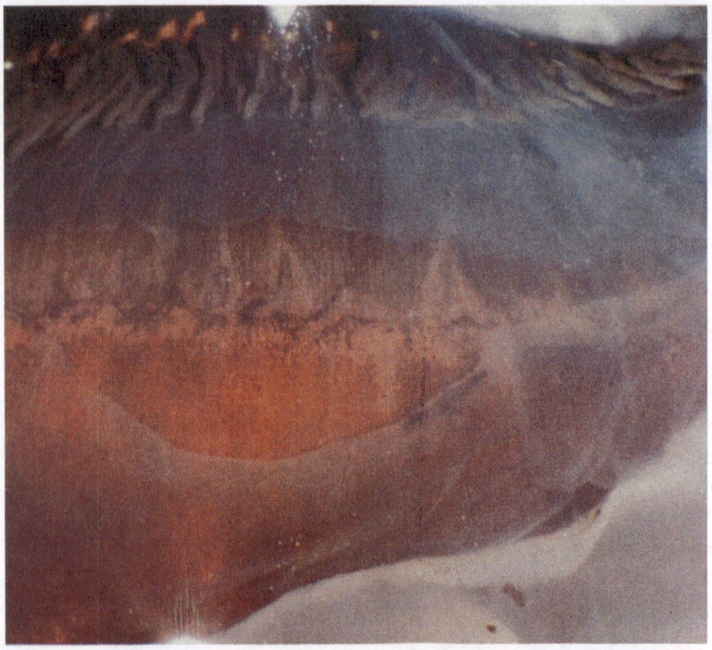

11.33

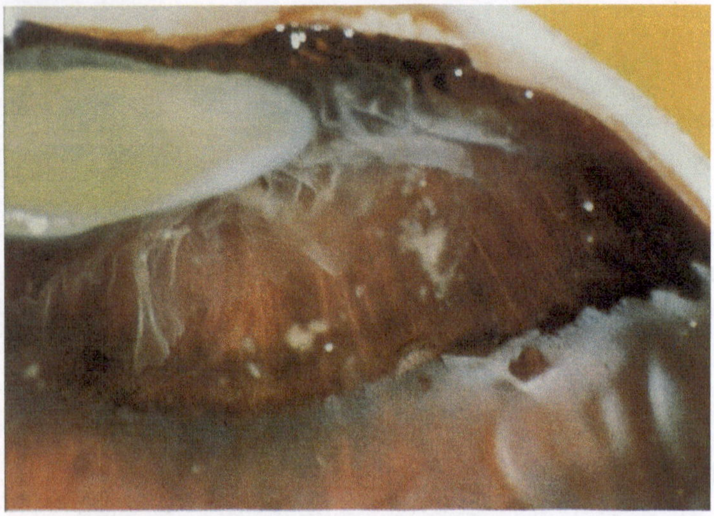

11.34

Retinal Dialysis

Tearing of the pars plana epithelium or of the sensory retina is often associated with disinsertion of the vitreous base. In rare instances, retinal dialysis may extend more than 180 degrees. It may even be total. Clinically, retinal detachment in smaller retinal dialyses may develop a long time (a year or more) after the initial trauma. The prognosis depends on the size of the dialysis and of the duration of the detachment prior to treatment.

Fig. 11.33. Large traumatic tear of the pars plana epithelium. M 767/78: Autopsy eye of a young man who suffered a severe accidental head injury.

Fig. 11.34. Large tear at the ora serrata with anterior detachment of the vitreous base and pars plana epithelium. There is also a small retinal tear close to the ora serrata. M 162/75: 17-year-old man who developed traumatic luxation of the globe with rupture of the optic nerve and horizontal eye muscles in a motorcycle accident. Enucleation as a primary procedure 3 hours after injury (see also Fig. 11.37).

Avulsion of the Optic Nerve

Avulsion of the optic nerve with total disinsertion of the retina at the optic disc is a rare complication of blunt trauma. Vision is lost immediately. Usually the tear is not visible ophthalmoscopically because of hemorrhage in the vitreous.

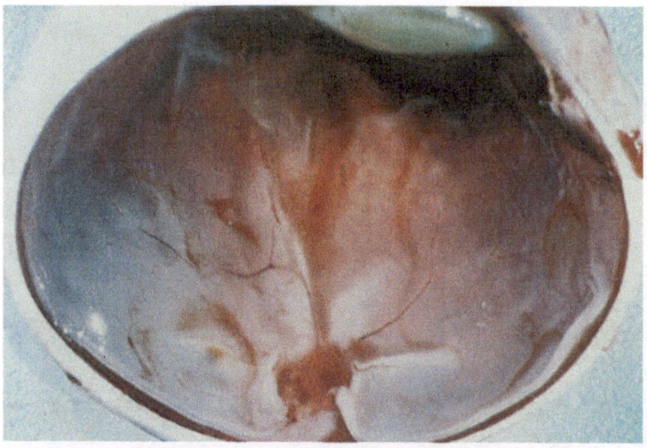

11.35

Fig. 11.35. Total disinsertion of the retina from the optic disc and some intraocular hemorrhage. Histology also showed tears of the trabecular meshwork and at the ora serrata. There was a large hematoma within the ciliary body. M 114/74: 24-year-old man with traumatic luxation of the globe and rupture of the extraocular muscles and the optic nerve 1 cm behind the globe. Enucleation as a primary procedure 2 hours after injury.

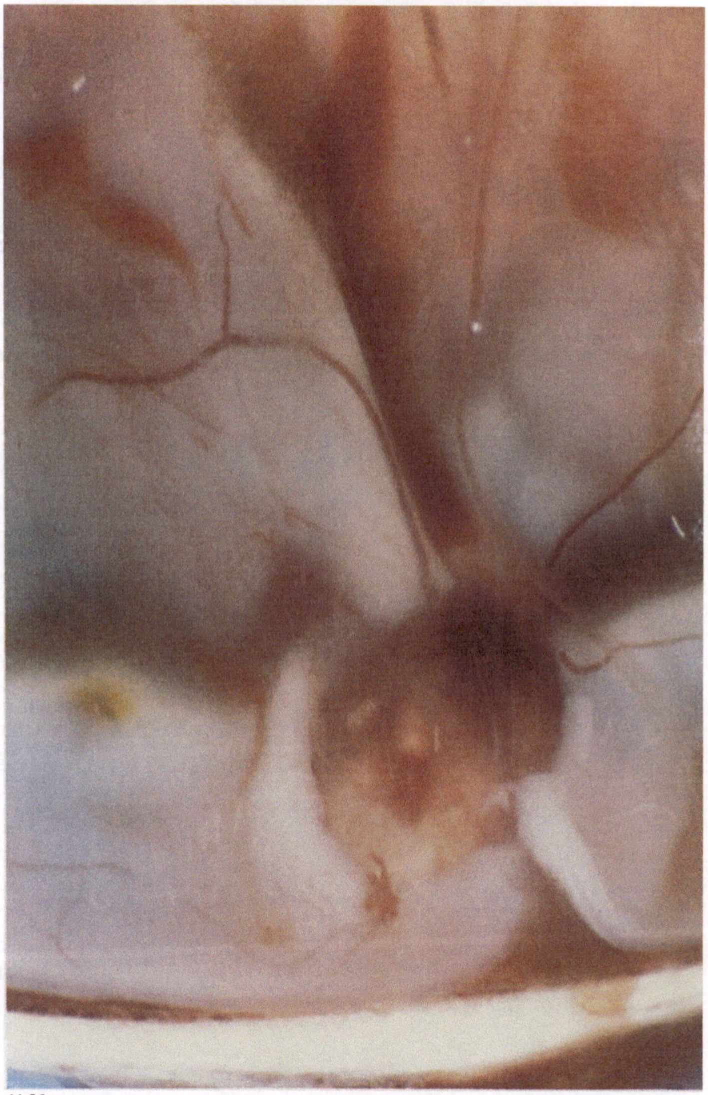

11.36

Fig. 11.36. Higher magnification of Fig. 11.35 showing the elevated edges of the torn retina at the site of the optic disc and some hemorrhages.

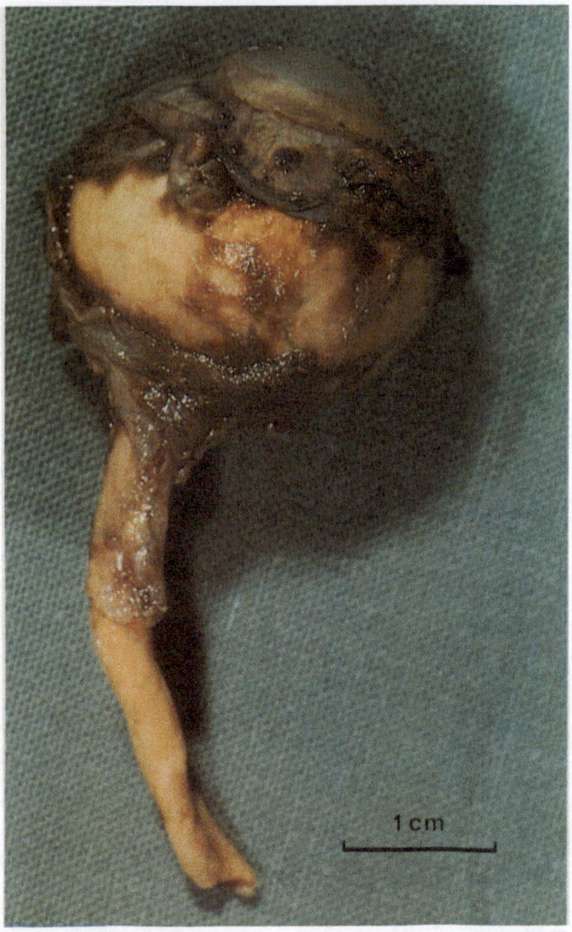

11.37

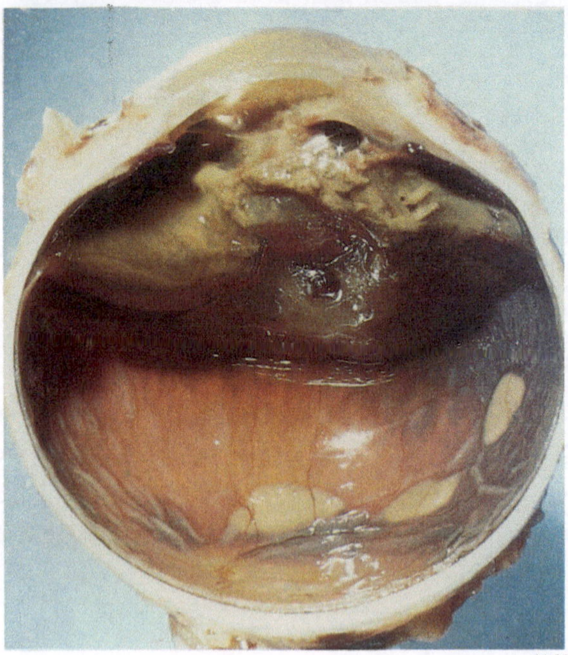

11.38

Traumatic Luxation of the Globe

Traumatic luxation of the globe is usually associated with rupture of the optic nerve with its sheaths and of the horizontal extraocular muscles. The eye is immediately blinded. Sometimes a rupture of the optic chiasm may also occur.

Fig. 11.37. Traumatic rupture of the optic nerve. The optic fascicle is ruptured more than 3 cm behind the globe and the optic nerve sheaths are ruptured about 1.5 cm behind the eye. M 162/75: Same patient as Fig. 11.34. Visual field in the remaining eye was normal.

Laceration

Severe blunt ocular trauma may cause rupture of intact sclera or cornea. Commonly the eye ruptures at the limbus of the cornea and underneath the rectus muscles. Pressure on an eye with previous surgical incisions may cause wound rupture, which, in principle is comparable to laceration. Usually there is loss of intraocular tissues and marked intraocular hemorrhage, which obscures the view of the internal eye structures. The intraocular hemorrhage may be massive with loss of ocular contents, then termed expulsive hemorrhage. Wound rupture or laceration following intraocular surgery is always a very severe injury.

Fig. 11.38. Laceration wound at the temporal limbus of the cornea. Aphakia. Hemorrhagic imbibition of the vitreous with secondary posterior vitreous detachment. Subretinal hemorrhages from choroidal tears. M 1212/80: Concussional injury in a 39-year-old man with laceration wound at the limbus of the cornea, loss of the lens, and intraocular hemorrhage 1 month previously.

Fig. 11.39. Massive clotted hemorrhage in the anterior segment of the eye. Aphakia and aniridia. Hemorrhagic retinal detachment nasally. M 820/74: 33-year-old man whose blind eye had ruptured along an old traumatic corneal scar after a first blow. The lens, the iris, and part of the vitreous were lost. Enucleation was performed because of hemophthalmos.

Fig. 11.40. Laceration of the sclera underneath a horizontal rectus muscle with extraocular luxation of the lens and fibrous ingrowth from the wound into the eye. Distorted intraocular contents. Large dialysis of the ciliary body. The dislocated iris is adherent to the ingrowing fibrous tissue. Total retinal detachment. Marked hyperemia of the choroid. M 965/76: 37-year-old man who had blunt trauma to the eye from a metallic rod 3 months before seeing an ophthalmologist for blurred vision in his other eye (sympathetic ophthalmitis).

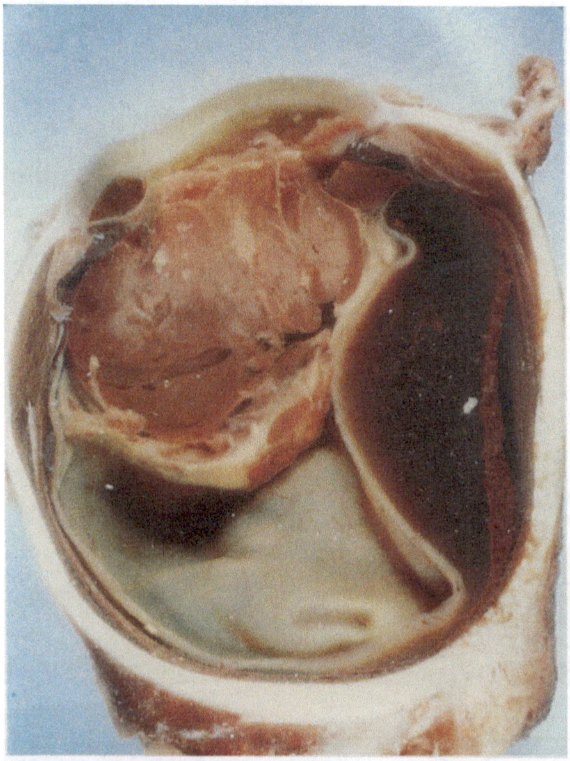
11.39

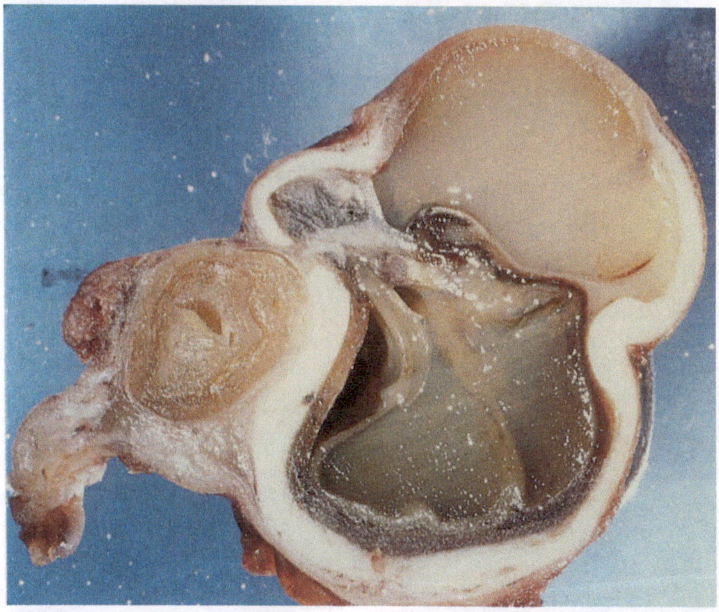
11.40

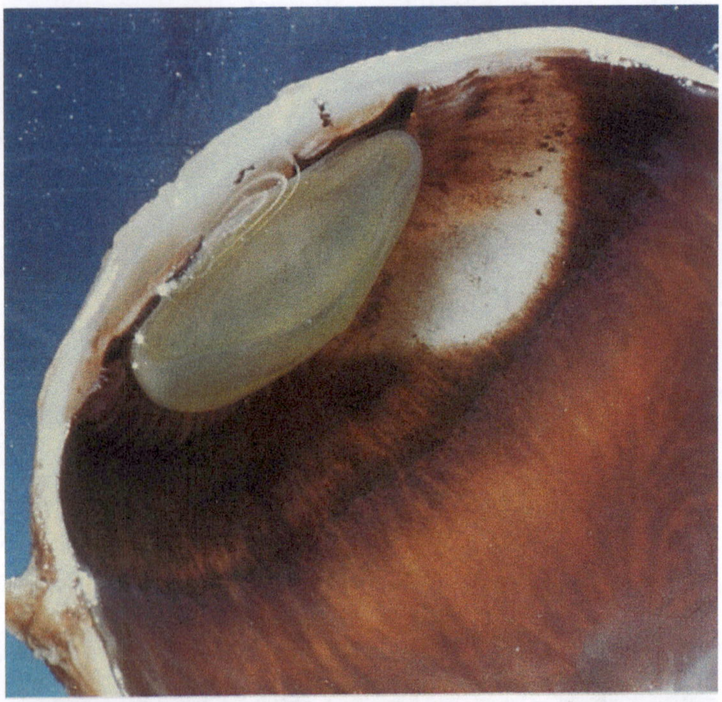

11.41

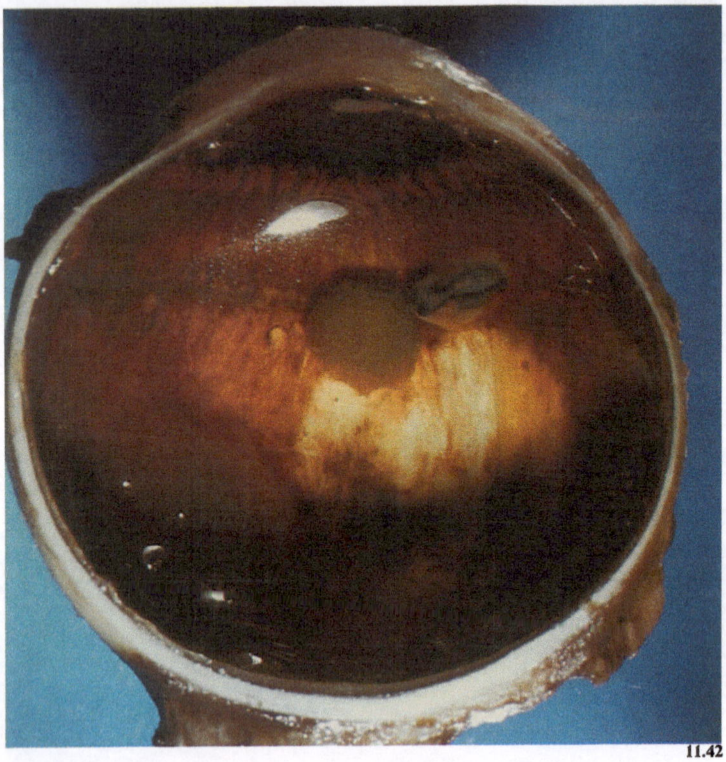

11.42

Burns

Chemical burns such as alkali, which severely damage the anterior eye have been mentioned previously. They may also cause peripheral anterior synechias.

Thermal burns as they occur in metal factories from fluid metals coagulate the outer eye tissues. If heat exposure is long enough intraocular tissues may also coagulate.

Fig. 11.41. Large coagulation scar of the ciliary body. M 953/78: 34-year-old man who suffered from a severe thermal burn of one eye from fluid aluminum. Enucleation because of complete loss of the lids and marked corneal scarring.

Penetrating Foreign Body Injuries

In foreign body injuries, the structures of the anterior segment of the eye are usually involved. The depth of ocular penetration depends on the velocity, speed, and sharpness of the foreign body, while the degree of tissue damage is related to foreign body size. Foreign bodies such as metal splinters or glass or stone fragments may be retained. Others, such as knives or tree twigs cause large cuts with a certain degree of tissue deformation at the time of perforation. Small foreign bodies at high velocity may perforate the globe and reach the orbital tissues including the optic nerve. Many penetrating metallic foreign body injuries occur from hammering metal on metal. The risk

Fig. 11.42. Large iron splinter at the equator of the lower half of the eye surrounded by chorioretinal scarring. Brownish pigmentation of the intraocular tissues, which is most prominent at the ciliary processes. Aphakia. M 712/78: 56-year-old man who had an untreated foreign body injury of one eye 35 years previously. Later cataract extraction from the blind glaucomatous eye was performed for cosmetic reasons.

of bacterial infection from an intraocular foreign body is to some extent related to the size and composition of a foreign body. Small foreign bodies in general are less infectious than larger ones. The clinical history may provide a clue to the risk of ocular infection. Organic materials such as wood are practically always infectious. Large foreign body perforations of the outer coats of the eye cause the same complications as lacerations. These include hemorrhages, tissue tearing, and loss of tissue. Immediate wound repair with foreign body removal and watertight suturing is essential. Any chemically or mechanically active intraocular foreign body (e.g., iron, copper) must be removed. Untreated or undiagnosed chemically active intraocular foreign bodies may destroy an eye functionally as well as morphologically. Iron leads to intraocular siderosis with loss of retinal ganglion cells,

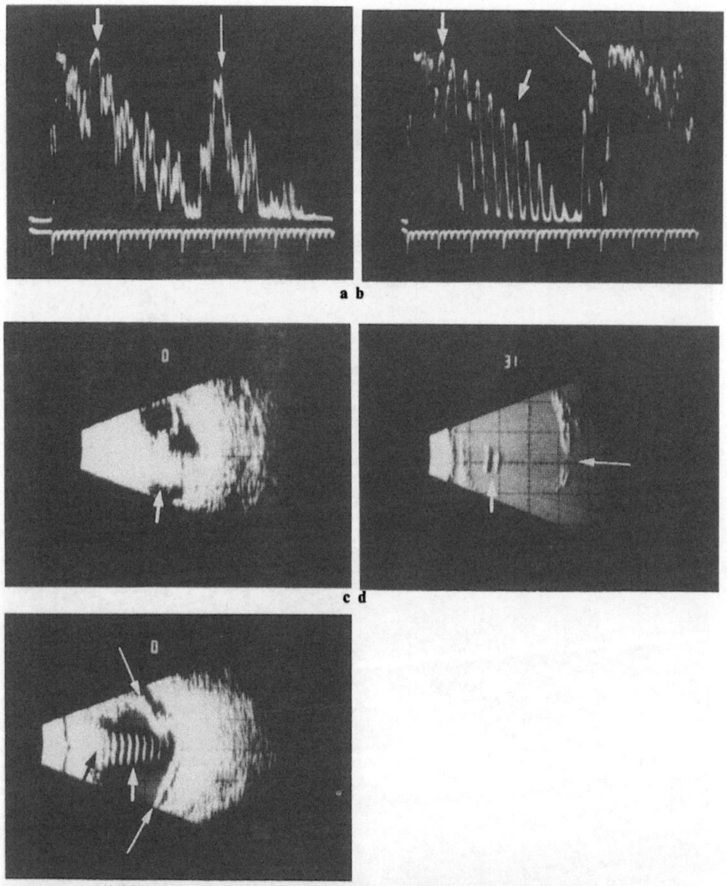

11.42A

Fig. 11.42A. Common and spherical intraocular foreign bodies. A-scan echograms (**a, b**) and contact B-scan echograms (**c–e**) of a common (**a, c, d**) and a spherical (BB-shot) (**b, e**) intraocular foreign body, both located in the most anterior vitreous. The common foreign body lies within the opacified vitreous but clearly shows a very high reflectivity (*short arrows*) and causes acoustic shadowing on more posterior structures (*long arrows*). When a spherical foreign body is centered in the soundbeam it produces typical multiple reverberation signals (*small arrows*). (*Long arrows* = adjacent retinal detachment.)

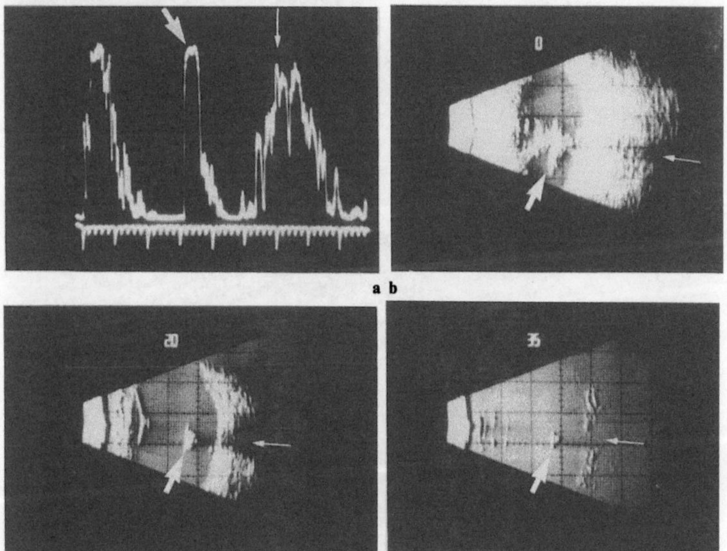

11.42B

Fig. 11.42B. Intraocular foreign body (common). A-scan echogram (**a**) and contact B-scan echograms (**b–d**) of a common intraocular foreign body. Note the very high reflectivity and the rather wide signal of the foreign body at "tissue-sensitivity" setting of the standardized A-scan (**a**). When centered in the sound beam, the foreign body typically causes an acoustic shadow with decreased reflectivity of more posterior structures, e.g., sclera, orbital patterns (*long arrows*). Even at the lowest sensitivity of the instrument (documented here in the B-scan **c, d**) the foreign body is well displayed.

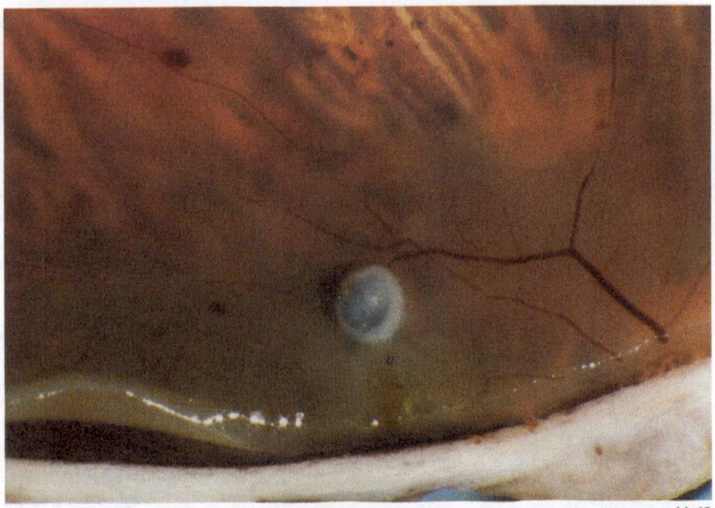

11.43

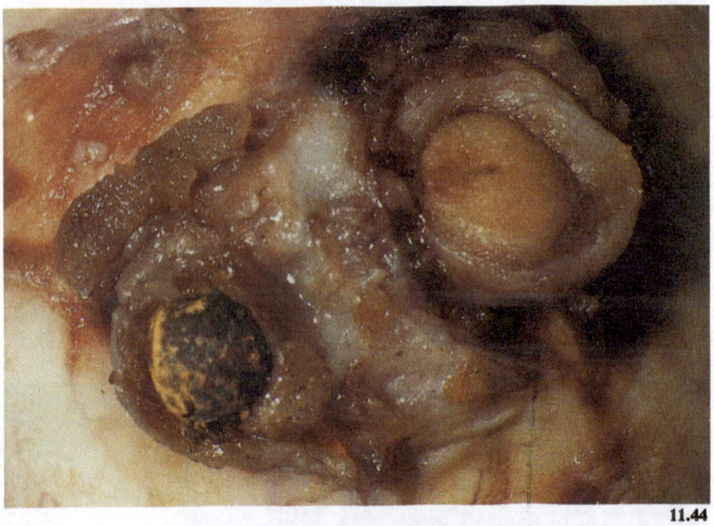

11.44

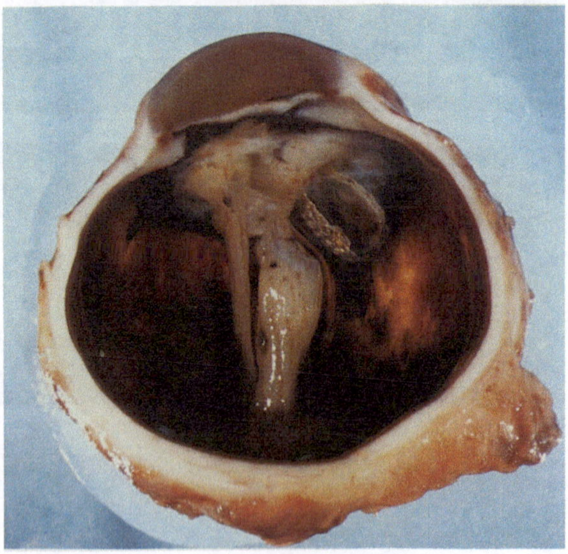

11.45

marked gliosis of the remaining retina, cataract, and glaucoma. Copper containing foreign bodies may cause a severe sterile endophthalmitis or chalcosis of intraocular structures. Therefore X-ray examination is most important in any type of ocular injury. A chemically inert intraocular foreign body such as glass may be left in situ if there is a high risk of the removal causing further intraocular damage. Most small foreign bodies outside the eye carry little risk of damaging important ocular structures. Further preventative surgical measures such as vitrectomy, retinal coagulation, scleral buckling, lens extraction, or corneal grafting may become necessary during primary surgical repair or during a second operation. Prognosis after foreign body injuries to the eye depends on the amount of tissue damage and on secondary intraocular tissue reactions. In general, the visual prognosis with small foreign bodies is fairly good while it is poor with large particles.

Fig. 11.43. Small encapsulated iron containing 1 mm foreign body on the surface of the retina with yellow-brownish discoloration of the adjacent retina. M 406/72: 66-year-old man who had an untreated foreign body injury to one eye at age 39. At age 42 he developed glaucoma which led to blindness in this eye.

Fig. 11.44. Extrascleral iron foreign body adjacent to the optic nerve after perforating injury of the eye. M 479/82: 22-year-old man, who had suffered a foreign body injury of one eye while hammering on a piece of metal. Enucleation after second stage vitrectomy for suspected (not verified) sympathetic ophthalmitis.

Fig. 11.45. Total retinal detachment with retained air gun pellet in the subretinal space. Aphakia. The retina is fixed to a fibrous membrane which is continuous with fibrous ingrowth at the site of the limbus and ciliary body scar. M 40/81: 12-year-old boy who had been injured by an air gun pellet 3 months previously.

Fig. 11.46. Radial scar involving the cornea, iris, ciliary body, and peripheral retina. Aphakia. Tractional retinal detachment with strong adhesion of the retina to a choroidal scar. M 128/76: 29-year-old man who had suffered a penetrating injury due to a piece of glass.

Fig. 11.47. Traumatic aniridia and vitreous hemorrhage. Remnants of the lens with central defect. M 720/75: 38-year-old man who had a transcorneal penetrating injury of his eye by an iron nail with loss of the entire iris and damage of the lens. Enucleation for untreatable secondary glaucoma.

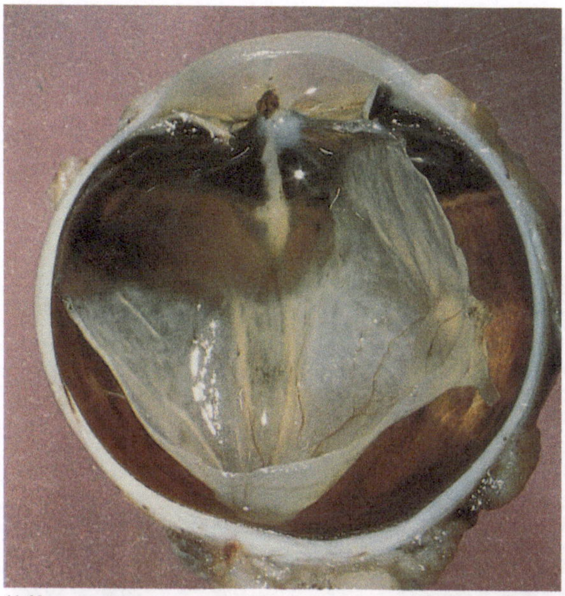

11.46

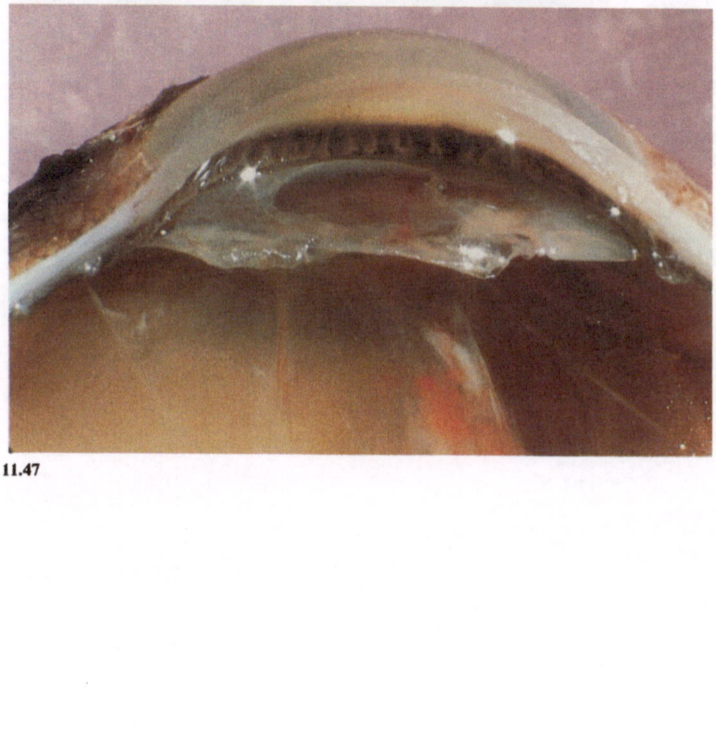

11.47

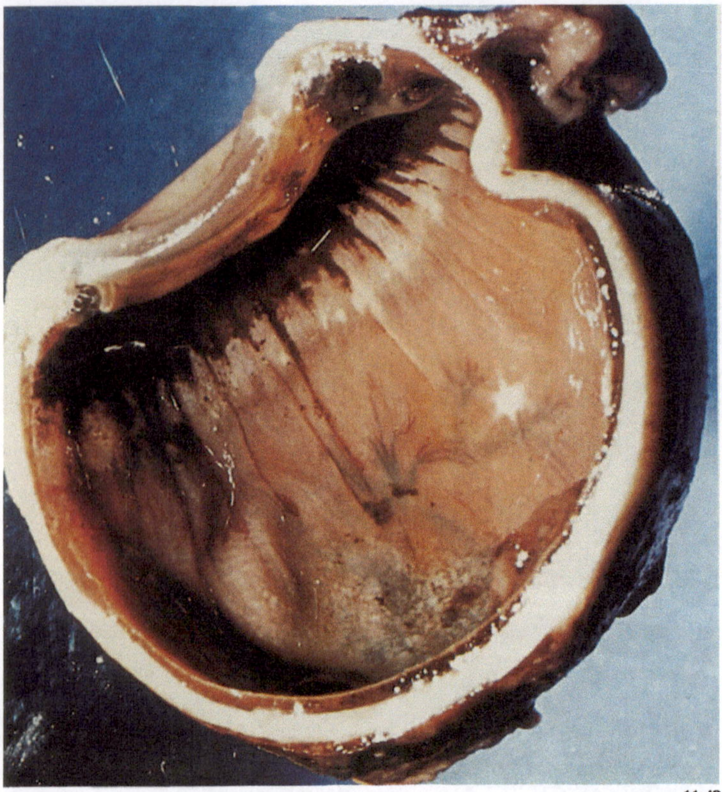

11.48

Infection

Usually it takes bacteria some days to multiply to the extent that the clinical signs of endophthalmitis manifest themselves. Clostridium perfringens is an organism which causes complete tissue destruction and lysis within a few hours after infection. Infections most commonly result from infected penetrating foreign bodies during work in an infected environment (garden, stables, septic tanks). Clinically, the conjunctiva and anterior chamber contents show a characteristic chocolate-brown discoloration from hemolysis even before a gas bubble appears in the anterior chamber (gas gangrene). The infection rapidly leads to blindness. The lens may luxate early into the liquefied vitreous because of zonular lysis. In gas gangrene endophthalmitis, enucleation is mandatory.

Fig. 11.48. Intraocular lysis with marked loss of pigment from a Clostridium perfringens infection a few hours after penetrating intraocular foreign body injury. M 715/79: 67-year-old man who sustained a foreign body injury while hammering in a septic tank. Eight hours after the trauma, the eye was completely blind and painful showing the characteristic chocolate-brown appearance and a gas bubble in the anterior chamber.

Surgical Repair

In penetrating injuries of the eye, surgical repair should be performed as soon as possible by a highly experienced ocular surgeon using microsurgical techniques and fine suture material. The aim is not only the removal of any foreign body and watertight wound closure, but the repair and prophylaxis of intraocular damage. After the initial surgical repair, a second or third operation on the injured eye may be required to prevent blindness or alert enucleation.

Fig. 11.49. Corneal and scleral perforation after surgical repair. Traumatic aniridia and aphakia. Hemorrhage in the anterior vitreous. M 1086/83: In a traffic accident a 27-year-old man suffered a severe penetrating ocular injury from windshield glass. He had not used a seat belt.

Fig. 11.50. Limbal perforation after surgical repair. Traumatic aniridia and aphakia. Hemorrhage in the anterior vitreous. M 1178/79: 38-year-old man who had suffered from perforating injury 2 months prior to enucleation.

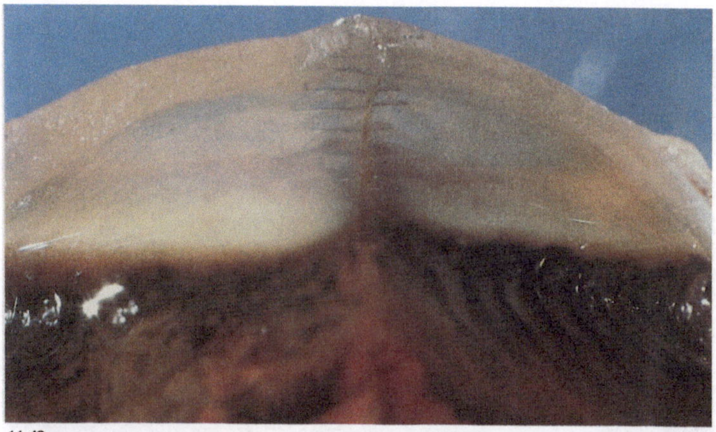

11.49

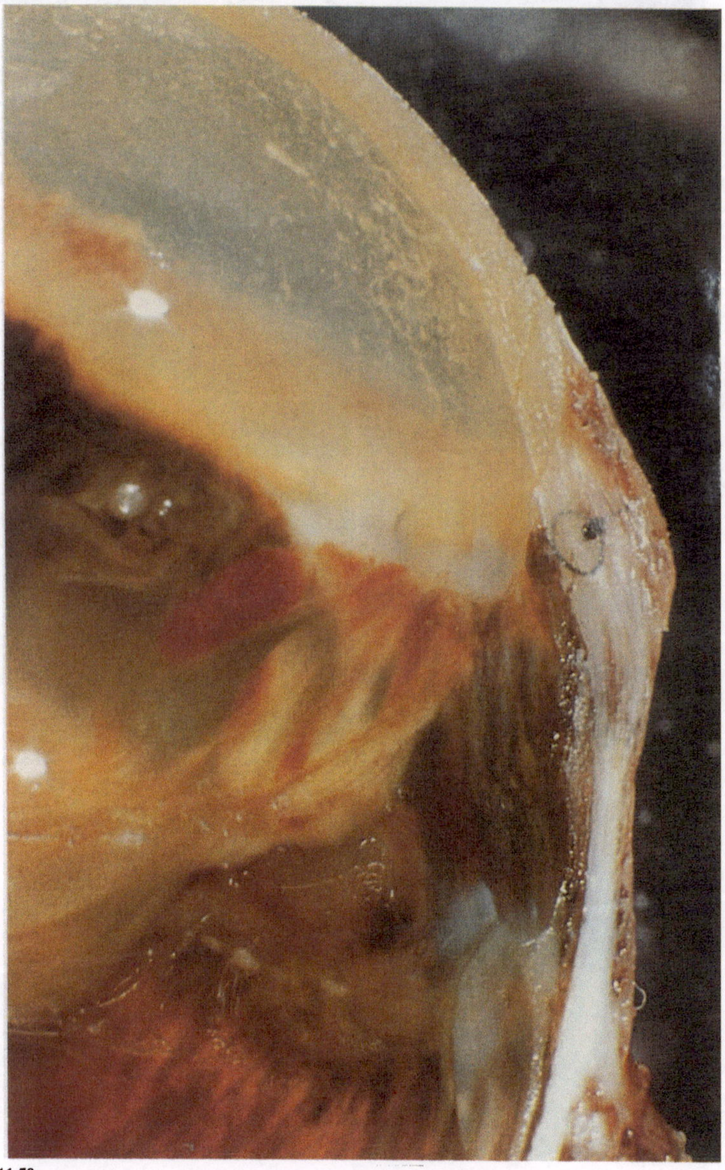

11.50

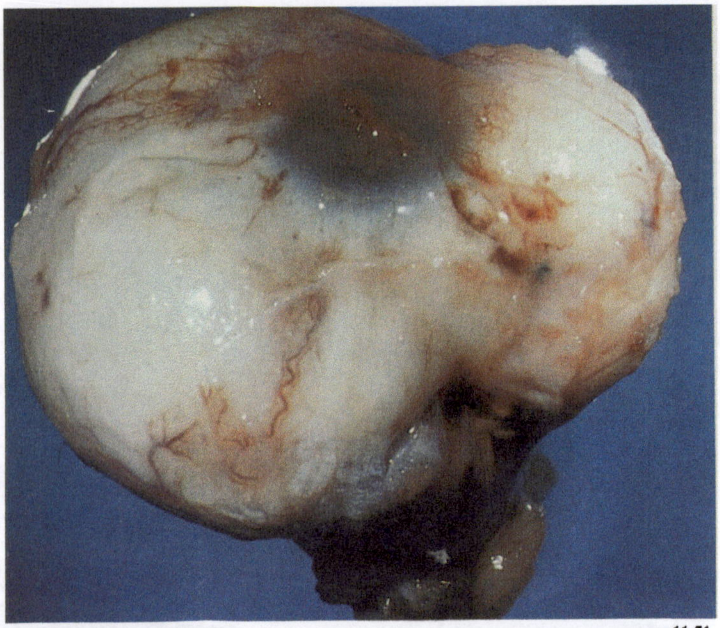

11.51

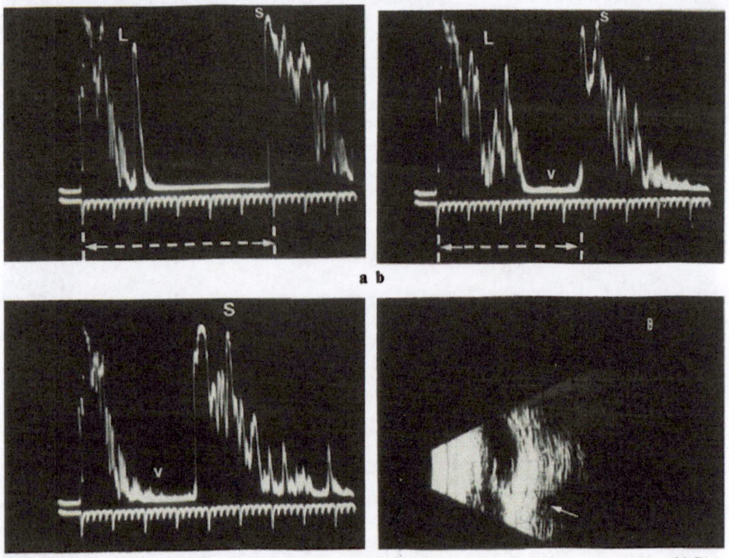

11.51A

Phthisis Bulbi

Phthisis bulbi results from a florid proliferative intraocular reaction in a variety of severe intraocular lesions such as accidental or surgical trauma, intraocular inflammation, vascular disease, long-standing retinal detachment, or necrotizing tumors. If the florid proliferative reaction persists, a hypotonic shrunken globe with disorganized intraocular contents results. It is largely the hypotony which may cause severe ocular pain leading to enucleation. Macroscopically, these eyes often show radial scleral folding and scleral thickening, small corneal diameters, and marked intraocular scarring with ciliochoroidal detachment, usually from an interciliary (cyclitic) membrane. Intraocular calcification and ossification are not rare findings.

Fig. 11.51. 13.5 × 15.5 × 15.5 mm measuring shrunken globe with extreme shrinkage of the corneal diameter. There was marked intraocular ossification. M 923/83: 27-year-old man with phthisical eye 5 years after penetration by an iron foreign body which had been extracted using a magnet.

Fig. 11.51 A. Phthisis bulbi. A-scan echograms of a normal eye (**a**) and A-scan (**b, c**) and contact B-scan (**d**) of a phthisical eye. Note the decreased axial diameter (**b** compared to **a**; *L* = lens; *S* = sclera; *V* = vitreous opacities in the phthisical eye) and the thickening of the retinochoroidal layer with secondary changes (e.g., calcification) in this layer causing acoustic shadowing manifested by decreased scleral spike and orbital patterns (**c, d**).

Fig. 11.52. Shrunken globe with marked spongy detachment of the ciliary body and choroid (organized ciliochoroidal hemorrhage). Total retinal detachment. Mature cataract. M 128/75: 40-year-old woman with shrunken globe 4 years after scleral laceration caused by a bull's horn.

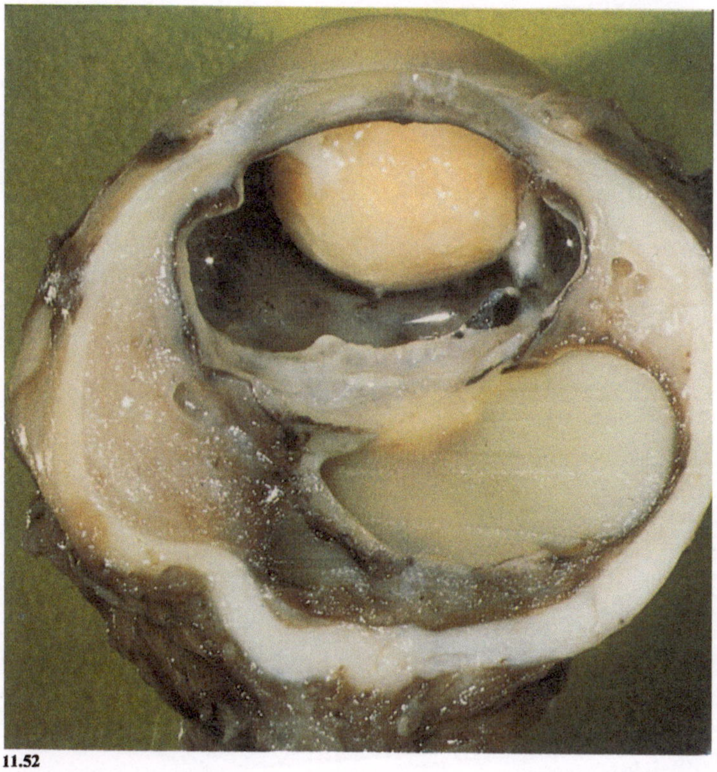

11.52

Subject Index